"No patient should be in pain. Those health care providers who allow pain are guilty of sins far worse than malpractice. This book is every patient's Bill of Rights when it comes to pain control."

—Bob Arnot, M.D.
Medical Correspondent, *CBS News*

"Pain can kill."

—John Liebeskind, Ph.D., UCLA
Former President, American Pain Society

"Inappropriate or inadequate assessment of patients is the single biggest cause of poor pain management."

—Charles Cleeland, Ph.D.
University of Wisconsin Medical School

"So long as one person remains in pain and we cannot help, our knowledge of pain remains inadequate."

—Patrick D. Wall, M.A., D.M.
University College, London

"It is impossible to predict or guess how much drug a patient will need for relief. The right dose is the right dose."

—Peter Koo, Pharm. D.
University of California, San Francisco

"It is a disservice to the patient not to appreciate the complexities of pain."

—Wayne O. Evans, Ph.D.

"Suffering is a personal, private, internal event whose existence can only be inferred."

—Gerald Losser, M.D.
iversity of Washington

"Parents must act as advocates for their children when there is pain."

—Nancy Hester, Ph.D., R.N.
University of Colorado

"Pain is not a passive symptom. It is an aggressive symptom in the central nervous system."

—Ronald Dubner, D.D.S., Ph.D.
National Institutes of Health

Pain Relief!

JANE COWLES, Ph.D.

PAIN RELIEF!

How to Say "No" to Acute, Chronic, and Cancer Pain

MASTERMEDIA LIMITED *New York*

MASTERMEDIA and colophon are registered trademarks
of MasterMedia Limited.

Library in Congress Cataloging-in-Publication Data
Cowles, Jane.
    Pain Relief! How to Say "No" to Acute, Chronic, and Cancer Pain/
Jane Cowles, Ph.D.
        p.   cm.
    Includes bibliographical references and index.
    ISBN 0-942361-77-6: $20.95
    1. Pain—Popular works.   2. Intractable pain.   3. Cancer pain.
I. Title.
RB127.C74 1993
616'.0472—dc20   93–4106
                                                           CIP

Designed by Jacqueline Schuman
Manufactured in the United States of America
Production services by Martin Cook Associates, Ltd., New York
10 9 8 7 6 5 4 3 2 1

In memory of my sister Susan.
Her insight and bravery guide me at all times.

To Peter, David, and Charles.

With thanks and love to my husband, Hanford.

Contents

Acknowledgments ix

Preface xiii

Introduction 1

1 PLANNING PAIN MANAGEMENT
WITH YOUR DOCTOR *19*

2 CHRONIC NONMALIGNANT PAIN *60*

3 INFANTS AND CHILDREN *140*

4 ADOLESCENTS *186*

5 CANCER PAIN *199*

6 HIV AND AIDS-RELATED PAIN *284*

7 HOME CARE *292*

8 ELDER PAIN CARE *302*

9 NURSING HOMES *310*

10 NEAR THE END OF LIFE *321*

11 PAIN CENTERS *342*

12 ALTERNATIVE HEALTH CARE   *357*

Postscript   361
Guide for the Consumer   363
General Pain Resources   383
Glossary   387
Index   395

Acknowledgments

In 1973 my sister Susan was diagnosed with breast cancer. She suffered the pain of biopsy, surgery, radiation therapy, and disease-related fractures, as well as emotional pain. Through it all, her pain was never adequately managed. I remember one day when she was dying she asked the nurse for more pain medication. The nurse began to lecture her on the necessity of "bearing the pain." Susan was my introduction to the horrors of undertreated acute, chronic, cancer, and end-of-life pain.

In 1977 I fractured my femur and experienced excruciatingly acute pain as well as an aftermath of chronic pain that often still bothers me today.

In 1990 a dear friend had his spleen removed. He was in agony. When his family asked for more medication, not only was his request denied, his dose was cut.

In 1992 my secretary fell and sustained a serious wrist fracture that required surgery; her pain was never adequately managed.

For the last twenty years I have been concerned about the under-treatment of pain. I have written about pain as a medical journalist, authoring the Pain Patient's Bill of Rights. I have tried to help patients learn how to ask their doctors for adequate pain control. Patients usually have met resistance from the medical and health care community. The message has been "This is not open to discussion or debate." The result has been poor pain control and needless suffering. I decided that nothing will change until the consumer becomes involved.

This book is to acknowledge all those patients who have endured needless pain. It is also the voice of the researchers and clinicians who have dedicated their lives to end the suffering caused by pain. My hope is that others learn from this book.

I would like to thank:

Susan Stautberg, of MasterMedia Limited, who received my proposal at five o'clock one afternoon and bought *Pain Relief!* at eight the next morning!

Mr. Richard Gelb, Chairman of Bristol-Myers Squibb, for his support, and George Blewitt, M.D.

And special thanks to those who have been so generous with their knowledge and time:

John Liebeskind, Ph.D., of the Department of Psychology at UCLA, who guided me early on.

Antonio Gotto, M.D., Chairman of Medicine at Baylor College of Medicine.

With special thanks to my critical reviewers:

Russell Portenoy, M.D., Director of Analgesic Studies of the Pain Service at Memorial Sloan-Kettering Cancer Center, who has always been generous with his time in interviews we have had over the last four years.

Cancer Pain: Kathleen Foley, M.D.; C. Richard Chapman, Ph.D.; Betty Ferrell, Ph.D., F.A.A.N.; Russell Portenoy, M.D.

Infants, Children, and Adolescents: Nancy Hester, Ph.D.; Myron Yaster, M.D.; Marilyn Savedra, D.N.S., R.N.; Philip Pizzo, M.D.

How to Talk to Your Doctor: Peter Koo, Pharm.D.

Chronic Pain: John Reeves, Ph.D.

HIV and AIDS-Related Pain: Richard Payne, M.D.

Those who were so generous with their time and material: Margo McCaffery, R.N.; C. Stratton Hill, Jr., M.D.; David Joranson, Ph.D.; Diana Wilkie, Ph.D., R.N.; Jo Anne Dalton, Ed.D., R.N., F.A.A.N.; Stuart Grossman, M.D.; Ronald Melzack, Ph.D.; John Loeser, M.D.; Dennis Turk, Ph.D.; the Rev. Robert Smith, Ph.L.; Gayle Page, Ph.D.; Jamie Von Roenn, M.D.; Jeffrey Ngeow, M.D.; Charles Cleeland, Ph.D.; Gary Bennett, Ph.D.; Robert Kerns, Ph.D.; Brian Ready, M.D.; Christine Miaskowski, R.N., Ph.D., F.A.A.N.; Steven B. Graff-Radford, D.D.S.; Lloyd Saberski, M.D.

Thanks to Lawanda Katzman, Ph.D., a friend and associate, and Bob Arnot, M.D., for his early support of the book.

Thank you to my "readers" Dorothy Mitchell, Paul Goldenheim, M.D., and Ellen Ingler.

To Matthew C. Dugan, who foraged in the medical libraries with my endless lists, for resources and general assistance, and Elizabeth

Mersey, whose good old-fashioned medical editing made the difference.

The American-Italian Foundation for Cancer Research, especially our Executive Director, Gilda Zane.

Not to be forgotten, Ben and Barney of Future Computers of New York, who not only brought me a computer but had the patience to teach me computer literacy.

Most importantly, to my husband and our extended "lively" family of eleven!

—Jane Cowles

Preface

Excellence in managing patients' acute and chronic pain has not been achieved.

National studies show that up to 50% of acute pain due to injury, surgery, childbirth, or disease is undertreated. Up to 50% of all cancer pain is undermanaged. Chronic pain from backaches, headaches, arthritis, old injuries, and progressive disease often go unrelieved because of inadequate therapy.

Treatment of a patient's pain often takes a back seat to treatment of the medical problem. Studies show that unrelieved acute pain can slow the healing process, pose life-threatening complications, and add to the number of inpatient days. Undertreated cancer pain can compromise patients physically and can affect their emotional, family, and work life.

Doctors and nurses often undermedicate and undertreat acute and cancer pain, due to a lack of education about pain and unfounded fears of addiction, depression of respiration, and side effects. Poor assessment of patients' pain, underutilization of multidisciplinary nondrug techniques, and state or federal regulations restricting access to pain-relieving drugs add to inadequate pain control. In addition, doctors infrequently assess the complex emotional and psychosocial aspects of chronic pain.

Patients share many of the same misconceptions about pain and pain treatments as doctors and nurses. Furthermore, patients rarely participate in how their pain is managed. The process that allows patients to make informed decisions about all of their other medical and surgical choices is generally absent when it comes to pain control decisions. This is one of the few areas of medicine in which patients often lack "informed consent".

Pain management is not a national priority. This results in untold human misery costing patients physically and emotionally, and also adds billions of dollars to the health care system.

Pain is a dehumanizing and isolating experience, which health care providers have a moral, ethical, and legal duty to alleviate.

The information in this book will teach you how to assess pain by using a simple Pain Assessment Scale. "The Pain Patient's Bill of Rights" will instruct you about your rights as a patient. You no longer have to be a bystander. You can make informed choices about your pain care, just as you currently make informed decisions about your medical and surgical care. Making good choices can lead to faster healing, better quality of life, and less expense.

Adults are not the only ones at risk for undertreatment of pain. Infants, children, the elderly, and those who do not speak English must have their pain care needs diligently monitored by family as well as doctors and nurses.

The information in this book has been researched from medical journals, pain conferences, government and corporate studies, and interviews with top pain researchers, doctors, nurses, and other specialists.

You must ask your doctor to include you in pain control decisions. It may not be easy. Old habits die hard. You have an opportunity to help accomplish what no one, not even federal guidelines, has been able to do: make pain management a national health care priority for you and your family.

This book is for all who have suffered needless pain, and was made possible by the researchers, doctors, nurses, and others in health care who specialize in pain management and have labored tirelessly and compassionately to make pain control a reality for every patient.

You don't have to suffer pain needlessly while you are trying to cope with your medical problem.

You have an opportunity to exercise your basic human right to adequate pain control.

Pain Relief!

Introduction

Generally, when you sustain an injury, fracture a bone, have a diagnostic procedure, opt for surgery, or are treated for disease, you don't think about what kind of pain you may experience, how long the pain may last, what kind of medication you will get, how often it will be administered, or what to do if the medication does not work.

Pain medications and treatments usually "just happen" to you. You are rarely involved in the process. You routinely make responsible medical or surgical choices, but when it comes to how your pain will be managed, you seldom know your options, nor do you benefit from state-of-the-art pain management. Pain management is the one area left in medicine in which informed patient involvement and informed consent[5] are often absent. And, as studies show, pain control is often absent.

National studies show that 50% of acute pain due to trauma, surgery, and labor is undertreated. Poorly treated acute pain can lead to life-threatening physical complications such as pneumonia and blood clots, resulting in increased days spent in the hospital.[1] More than 50% of chronic cancer pain is also undermanaged. Chronic pain resulting from arthritis, old injuries, headache, and backache is also undermanaged.[2] Chronic pain impairs the quality of a patient's family relationships, work, and social life.[3] This failure of adequate pain management results in millions of adults and children suffering physically and emotionally, adding billions of dollars to health care costs. Poor pain management is the norm, despite irrefutable medical evidence that *patients who are adequately treated for pain have fewer medical complications, reduced number of inpatient days, better quality of life, and therefore lower health care costs.*[4]

THE ETHICAL, MORAL, AND LEGAL
IMPERATIVE TO RELIEVE PAIN

"Treatment of pain is a moral imperative. Health care providers have a clear moral duty to alleviate pain. It's not just enough to treat pain. There must be a clearly developed strategy of how to treat the pain," says the Reverend Robert Smith of the Institute for Medicine in Contemporary Society at Stony Brook.[6]

Wayne O. Evans, Ph.D., states, "To allow a patient to suffer unnecessary pain does harm to the patient—a violation of the first ethical principle of medicine."[7]

In 1990 a North Carolina jury ruled that an elderly man suffering from cancer that had spread to the bones was denied pain medication that was prescribed for him; the nurse substituted a placebo for the pain medication. After his death, his family brought legal action. The court awarded $7.5 million in punitive damages and $7.5 million in compensatory damages to the plaintiff. The nursing home was found in violation of both state and federal regulations for withholding the prescribed dose of morphine that was to be given every three to four hours. It was the first case in which a health care provider was held liable for failing to provide adequate pain relief.[8]

If there is an ethical, moral, and legal obligation to relieve pain, then why are patients still suffering?

DOCTORS AND NURSES UNDERTREAT PAIN

Lack of Knowledge

Doctors and nurses have traditionally treated injury or disease as the top priority in patient care. Pain has never been considered a health care problem in its own right. John Bonica, M.D., the noted authority on pain management, states, "Doctors don't know how to treat physical suffering because they are never taught to think of pain as anything but a symptom of something else. Pain has never been part of the standard medical school curriculum." In his textbook, *The Management of Pain,* Dr. Bonica writes that pain education in the medical school curricula is deficient. He reviewed ten textbooks on medicine and surgery and eleven on cancer. The texts "are used as standard texts for medical students, house officers, and practitioners. *Out of 27,000 pages, only 0.6% are devoted to the description of symptomatic therapy of acute and chronic pain.*"[9]

Russell Portenoy, M.D., the Director of Analgesic Studies of the Pain Service at Memorial Sloan-Kettering, says, "Physicians are not trained in school and have little access to state-of-the-art pain treatments. As a result, the physician can have a simplistic view. Either the patient has pain or does not have pain. Period. The patient does not get asked about the intensity, quality or flux of pain. The preoccupation is how is the disease or illness doing, not how is the patient doing."[10]

Betty Ferrell, Ph.D., F.A.A.N., a specialist in pain management at City of Hope Hospital, says, "We must stop the practice of letting humans suffer. The vast majority of nurses do not believe in pain relief and how it affects the quality of life. For the record, pain management is pathetic. We do a poor job."[11]

Deborah McGuire, Ph.D., R.N., Director of Nursing Research at the Johns Hopkins School of Nursing, cites a recent survey of pain education in the curriculum of Illinois nursing schools. The survey covered general, pediatric, and cancer pain management. Of the forty-eight schools that responded to the questionnaire, "4.9 hours were spent on general pain management, 1.5 hours on pediatric pain, and 1.9 hours on cancer pain."[12]

Joyce Zerwekh, Ed.D., R.N., an assistant professor at the University of Washington, comments, "Patients are having pain and nurses are missing it. We need to change the system of care. We need to reduce the pain experience. Nurses need to regain beginners' eyes and ears when it comes to pain management."[13]

Hospitals Have No Pain Policy

To compound doctors' and nurses' lack of knowledge, hospitals remain steadfast in making medical treatment the priority and generally allowing pain to be undertreated. Administrators fail to acknowledge that treating patients adequately for pain will result in fewer medical complications and a lower number of inpatient days. There is no hospital policy to offset the staff's lack of pain education by making a commitment to state-of-the-art pain management. Patients continue to suffer in the dark ages of pain care.

Misconceptions about how pain evolves, lack of knowledge about the pharmacology of drugs, fear of patient addiction, overconcern about side effects, disbelief of patients' reporting of pain, failure to aggressively assess patients' pain, not treating each patient's pain individually, and not making a commitment to the prevention of pain result in unnecessary suffering. Little emphasis is given to alternative pain control measures, such as heat/cold therapy, massage, meditation, distraction, and other nondrug treatments.[14]

State Laws, Regulations, and Agencies Restrict Pain Control

The war on drugs unfortunately penalizes pain patients and their doctors who wish to prescribe opioids (morphine-like drugs) to manage pain.

Some of the problem rests with state medical boards and some pharmacy boards. Although federal law clearly recognizes the use of drugs for intractable pain, that message does not get through to the individual states.[15]

The problem also rests with state programs to monitor physicians' prescribing practices. The boards have created and enforced anti-drug regulations without conducting "patient impact studies," notes Stratton Hill, M.D., of M. D. Anderson Hospital, in Houston, Texas. In nine states, a doctor who prescribes any drug that is considered a controlled substance must write the prescription in triplicate form. One copy goes to the "regulatory agency to be used in investigations. The boards base their decisions on biases and misinformation. The result is that patients who need drugs to control their pain are not getting them," adds Hill.[16]

David Joranson, Ph.D., of the Pain Research Group at the University of Wisconsin–Madison, argues that the "Federal Government has laws that clearly recognize legitimate needs, but the states have gone overboard in their zeal for control. Since the boards have no patient input, they do not comprehend much difference between the street addict and the patient in pain. They only think of drugs as abuse."

The Drug Enforcement Administration, a strong advocate of triplicate prescription forms, found that there was at least a *50% drop in doctors' prescribing controlled substances since board implementation of prescription reporting began.*

David Weissman, M.D., of the Medical College of Wisconsin, surveyed Wisconsin physicians and reported that "more than 50% of the physicians would rather reduce drug doses or prescription quantity, reduce the number of refills or choose a less potent drug because of concerns about regulatory scrutiny."[17]

Pharmacies don't want to stock many drugs because of the hassle of state government reporting and fear of theft. Patients who have controlled-substance prescriptions often have trouble finding pharmacies that will fill their prescriptions.

The National Conference of Commissioners on Uniform State Laws (NCCUSL) has prepared a balanced model law, "The Uniform Controlled Substance Act," and has given it to the state legislatures.

The model act would give state laws several new provisions which would recognize that: *(1) Medical use of controlled substances is essential to public health and welfare and must be made available. (2) The ordinary course of professional medical practice includes administering, prescribing, and dispensing of narcotic drugs for the treatment of pain, including intractable pain. (3) Terms such as "addict," "habitual user" or "drug-dependent" should not be used for patients who receive prescribed controlled substances.*[18]

To date, this model act has not been adopted.

How Patients Participate in Poor Pain Control

"Just say no to drugs" can lead patients to think that all drugs are bad. The message left out is "Say yes to drugs when they are legitimately needed for pain."

Patients often think that pain comes with the territory of injury, surgery, or disease. Patients don't know that pain can slow the healing process, possibly impair the immune system, increase physical complications, add length to hospital stays or visits to the doctor. Patients suffer needlessly and incur unnecessary medical bills.

Ronald Melzack, Ph.D., a leader in the neurophysiology of pain for more than thirty-five years, writes, "Prolonged pain destroys the quality of life. It can erode the will to live, at times driving people to suicide. The physical effects are equally profound. Severe, persistent pain can impair sleep and appetite, thereby producing fatigue and reducing availability of nutrients to organs. It may thus impede recovery from illness or injury and, in weakened or elderly patients, may make the difference between life and death."[19]

Some patients suffer in silence because they are trying to be "good patients" or "don't want to bother anyone." Others think that "nothing can be done anyway" or are worried that if they complain the doctors and nurses may not pay attention to their medical problem. Patients who have cancer may fear that pain is a signal that the cancer is progressing. Denial is their method of coping with their fears.[20]

Perhaps one of the greatest problems is that *most patients don't know that they have a right to participate in their own pain management planning and treatment.* They don't know how or whom to ask about pain relief.

In addition, a very serious threat exists for those who cannot act on their own behalf—infants, children, the elderly, and those who do not speak English.[21] This group of patients needs extremely diligent care and assessment, using a variety of methods to help them achieve pain control. Gone are the days when people thought infants and the elderly don't feel pain. They do. Not to treat pain aggressively and compassionately in any patient is bad enough, but not to treat pain in the helpless, such as infants, is "medically unsound as well as barbaric," writes Neil Schechter, M.D., co-director of Children's Pain Service, at the University of Connecticut Health Center.[22]

Suffice it to say, the entire medical, regulatory, and patient approach to pain management must change. Although there are thousands of pain care researchers, doctors, nurses, and other health care professionals—and the U.S. Government—who are trying to change the system, it is not changing fast enough.

The active involvement of patients is the only way to speed the process of making adequate pain care the number one priority in health care. Pain is a nearly universal medical problem in injury, illness, diagnostic procedures, surgery, labor, disease, and cancer treatment. Every patient has a basic human right to adequate pain control. If doctors are unable to address and care for those needs, a patient has the right to seek another doctor who can.

WHAT IS PAIN?

Pain is "an unpleasant sensory and emotional experience associated with actual or potential tissue damage, or described in terms of such damage."[23]

Skin, muscles, and bone contain pain fibers. When there is an injury or disease, what is known as a "noxious stimulation" occurs. The pain fibers send signals to nerves outside the spinal cord. The pain signal is relayed to nerves inside the spinal cord and up to the brain. The message the brain receives is: pain.

There are two types of pain: acute and chronic.

Acute Pain

Acute pain is usually limited to hours, days, or weeks. It is the result of injuries, burns, fractures, surgery, disease, labor, severe headaches, or diagnostic procedures. The number of patients who experience acute pain in one year is staggering. In 1986 the National Center of Health Statistics estimated that in one year Americans experience:

- 64 million injuries, burns, fractures, or wounds
- 50 million heart attacks, labor, dental procedures, etc.
- 23 million surgical procedures

This translates into roughly 136 million days of bed disability and 370 million lost workdays in a single year.

What Happens to the Body in Acute Pain

Acute pain evokes a network of physical, psychological, and emotional distress.

If acute pain is not relieved, the body begins to be stressed by the pain, and a host of serious medical problems can occur. Some of the physical signs of unrelieved pain are:

- Increased heart rate
- Fluid retention
- Increased blood pressure

The patient in acute pain may not breathe deeply, cough, or be able to move freely. This guarding of physical movement can cause fluid to collect in the lungs, which can lead to pneumonia. Blood can begin to pool, causing potentially lethal blood clots, and there can be impairment of normal urinary and bowel function.[24]

Acute pain can cause negative psychological and emotional side effects, such as:

- Anxiety
- Feelings of helplessness
- Anger
- Loss of control
- Depression[25]

How to Tell if a Patient Is in Pain

The American Pain Society states that "pain is always subjective."
Subjective means that *only the patient knows his or her level of pain.
It is not possible to guess or assume what level of pain the patient is
experiencing.* The only method of obtaining that knowledge is the
"patient's self report." A patient who says "I'm in pain" must be
believed.

Some people show a classic expression of pain, such as a furrowed
brow, eyes squeezed shut, and the mouth set in a grimace. However,
not all people show that classic face. Many people are stoic. Although
their faces are calm, they may be experiencing horrible pain. Some
pain victims may even giggle or laugh as a way to cope with the pain.[26]

Assessment and Treatment of Acute Pain

To repeat, *the patient's self-report should be the single most important
indicator of pain.* Hospitalized patients should be asked frequently
about their level of pain. A simple assessment scale that measures pain
on a scale of 0 (no pain) to 10 (the worst pain) can be kept at the
patient's bedside, along with a chart. Pain should be charted like other
vital signs, such as temperature and blood pressure.[27] Nurse Diana
Wilkie, Ph.D., of the University of Washington, says, "We need to
rethink what is adequate pain assessment."[28]

The goal should be steady pain relief. Although it may not be possible to remove all pain, a level of comfort—enough to allow coughing,
breathing deeply, and movement (if appropriate)—should be
achieved.

Doctors often underestimate how much pain a patient is having.
There is too little individual assessment and not enough flexibility in
medication dosage to provide adequate pain control.

A study of fourteen accident and emergency departments manned
by one hundred senior staff doctors found that 50% would either use
the wrong method to administer a drug or wait until a patient was in
severe pain before giving another dose of the analgesic.[29]

Although doctors prescribe pain medication, the order is often written PRN, which means "as needed." Nurses play an active role in when
and how much medication is given. Often, due to poor assessment and
fear of addiction, the nurse will withhold adequate doses. Patients hear
nurses comment, "You don't look like you are in pain," "You shouldn't

be in so much pain," "Can't you wait a while longer?" or "We don't want you to become addicted." There is often little realization that the patient is being led into a potentially dangerous path of medical complications attributable solely to lack of pain control.[30]

The undertreatment of pain has become such a health care crisis that the U.S. Department of Health and Human Services has issued "Federal Guidelines for Acute Pain Management: Operative or Medical Procedures and Trauma," which states:

> 23.3 million operations were performed in 1989 in the United States, and most involved some form of pain management. Unfortunately, clinical surveys continue to indicate that routine orders for intramuscular injections of opioids (morphine-like drugs) "as needed"—the standard practice in many clinical settings—fail to relieve pain in about 50% of postoperative patients. Postoperative pain contributes to patient discomfort, longer recovery periods, and greater use of scarce health care resources, and may compromise patient outcomes. In the past, pain was thought to be inevitable, a harmless though intense discomfort that the patient had to tolerate. Unrelieved pain after surgery or trauma is often unhealthy; fortunately, it is preventable or controllable in an overwhelming majority of cases. Patients have a right to treatment that includes prevention or adequate relief of pain.[31]

"Each patient must be treated as unique. You cannot treat the patient on the average," notes Gary Donaldson, Ph.D., of the Pain and Toxicity Research Program at the Fred Hutchinson Cancer Center.[32] Tony Yaksh, M.D., professor of Anesthesiology at UCSD, comments, "The pain state is complex. All pain is really not the same."[33] Inflexible prescriptions simply don't work.

Doctors need to understand more about pain, the pharmacology of drugs, how long it takes a drug to take effect, and how long it will last. For example, an intramuscular morphine injection can take from thirty to ninety minutes to have a peak effect, due to the individual variables of absorption, metabolic rate, and perhaps genetic differences. In addition, an injection can rapidly lose its potency, for the same reasons. Thus, a patient will likely experience a roller-coaster ride of inadequate pain relief.

Raymond Sinatra, M.D., Ph.D., a professor of Anesthesiology at the

Yale University School of Medicine, depicts the harsh reality of patient suffering. He writes:

> Because pain is not considered an emergency, the length of time patients wait is dependent upon the ward and nursing workload. Once the nurse has responded, he or she usually initiates a "screening" of the complaint to assess whether the patient really needs additional pain medication. Despite published research indicating that psychological dependence occurs in fewer than 0.1% of hospitalized patients, this screening is done presumably in order to avoid opioid abuse. When the level of pain is deemed appropriate and requiring treatment, a long sequence of events occurs before the patient actually receives relief. The nurse must sign out the medication, prepare an injection, and administer the dose. The drug must then be absorbed from the site of administration.

Meanwhile, the patient's pain has returned in full force, and a large dose of opioid is needed, which can leave the patient sedated. Somehow, "the sedation is often equated with a satisfactory analgesic effect," adds Sinatra.[34] At least the patient is not complaining for a while. The goal of trying to achieve continuous pain relief levels, thus reducing the sedation and side effects, is rarely achieved.

No one takes responsibility for the patient's pain management. No one is held accountable. The patient suffers needlessly.

Poor Acute Pain Control Can Result in Chronic Pain

Poor acute pain control can cause a permanent imprinting of pain on pain fibers at the site and into the central nervous system. This imprinting can sometimes lead to ongoing and unnecessary chronic pain. Ronald Dubner, D.D.S., Ph.D., Chief of Neurobiology and Anesthesiology at NIH, states, "Pain is not a passive symptom; it is an aggressive symptom in the central nervous system. To reduce the hyperexcitability of neurons which results from tissue injury, pain-relieving drugs like narcotics or lidocaine should be added to general anesthesia."[35]

Aggressive pain control and a commitment to preventing pain can not only help the patient recover more rapidly, it can lessen complications, shorten the stay in hospital, and therefore reduce the physical, emotional, and financial costs to the patient and his or her family.

John Liebeskind, Ph.D., and Gayle Page, Ph.D., of the University of California, Los Angeles, have found that the stress of untreated surgical pain depresses the immune system of rats with cancer. The cancer grew up to three times as fast in pain-stressed rats than in rats who received morphine. Dr. Liebeskind states: "Pain can kill."[36]

Fear of Addiction Unfounded

The overwhelming fear of addiction on the part of doctors, nurses and patients is unfounded. Opioids are considered the first line of defense against acute pain that is moderate to severe. Clinical studies continue to show that patients rarely become addicted to opioids. Ronald Melzack, Ph.D., writes, "When patients take morphine to combat pain, it is rare to see addiction—which is characterized by a psychological craving for a substance and, when the substance is suddenly removed, by the development of withdrawal symptoms . . . furthermore, patients who take morphine for pain do not develop the rapid physical tolerance to the drug that is often a sign of addiction."[37]

Studies show less than 0.1% of patients who receive opioids become addicted. For example, the Boston University Medical Center reviewed the records of 11,882 patients who received opioids. Only 4 patients out of the 11,882 became addicted while hospitalized.[38]

As a 1989 *Harvard Medical School Health Letter* noted, "Treating pain should be seen as a basic component of treating illness. When pain is severe, giving a narcotic is as appropriate as giving insulin for diabetes."[39]

Chronic Pain

Chronic pain can last for months or years. It can be constant, such as the pain of arthritis, backache, or an old injury. It can be recurrent, such as headache, stomach irritation, or herpes. With chronic pain, a patient does not experience the dramatic physical perils of acute pain. However, chronic pain in its most severe form leaves the patient a shadow of his or her former self, impairing emotional, family, and work relationships. A patient can spend a fortune visiting doctor after doctor in an attempt to find relief.

In 1985 the National Academy of Sciences, the National Academy of Engineering, and the Institute of Medicine identified "Pain and Pain Management as a major health problem that results in discomfort, suffering and disturbs the quality of life and can produce complex and profound alterations in behavior." In spite of these strong views, there were no published data that looked at the extent to which Americans suffer from pain, how it affects them, or how they cope with it.

In 1985 Louis Harris and Associates conducted a national study for Nuprin. The "Nuprin Pain Report" provides the first broadly based systematic study of the frequency, severity, and costs associated with pain. The "Nuprin Pain Report" demonstrates the profound social and economic consequences of pain in the United States. The survey reports:

> Most Americans experience physical pain and most experience three or four different kinds of pain each year. Headaches are the most common type of pain. Almost 3 out of 4 American adults (73%) have suffered from one or more headaches in the last year. Over half have suffered from backaches (56%), muscle pains (53%), or joint pains (51%) in the last twelve months. In addition, over 4 in 10 adults (46%) have experienced stomach pains, and 4 in 10 women (46%) have experienced premenstrual or menstrual pains. Twenty-seven per cent of all American adults have suffered from dental pain in the last twelve months, which represents 47 million Americans. . . . In total, an estimated 4 billion sick days were lost by all adults (approximately 23 days per person). Among the full-time working population, an estimated 550 million days were lost (approximately five days per person) in the previous year. These numbers reflect a massive social cost to the quality of life of Americans and a massive loss of production to the economy.[40]

Patients often experience a complex overlay of biological, social, and psychological factors that affect their world of chronic pain. Sleeplessness, lack of appetite, inactivity, and ongoing impairment of daily life can lead to feelings of loss of control, depression, anger, hostility, and isolation.[41]

The facial expression of chronic pain is often one of depression, exhaustion, sadness, and sometimes no expression at all. Chronic pain can cause depression, but some patients have a history of being depressed before the onset of pain. Margo McCaffery, R.N., writes, "The complicating picture is that the symptoms of chronic pain are somewhat like those of general depression—weight loss or gain, insomnia or hypersomnia, decreased involvement in activities and fatigue. So patients with chronic pain could easily be misdiagnosed as being only depressed."[42]

Patients need extensive medical evaluation. Sometimes there is a very real organic cause. As mentioned, the undertreatment of acute pain can sometimes cause lingering chronic pain. Some patients may respond to various forms of nerve blocks or procedures. Making use of an array of multidisciplinary options such as physical therapy, heat or cold applications, massage, biofeedback, acupuncture, chiropractic, meditation, imagery, and psychological assessment can often be of help. After a patient has failed to respond to these efforts, some experts think that opioids should be employed. "There are clearly some patients who can benefit from opioid [morphine-like drugs] treatment in order to function," says Dr. Portenoy.[43]

Dr. John Bonica writes, "In patients with complex pain problems, effective therapy requires the use of a multimodal approach which is intended not only to reduce or remove the cause of pain, but also to achieve physical, psychologic, and psychosocial rehabilitation of the patient and family."[44]

Patients can often benefit from comprehensive pain treatment centers. Dr. John Loeser, past president of the American Pain Society, warns that not all pain centers provide a multidisciplinary approach. A center should be made up of a team of specialists such as neurologists, physical therapists, occupational therapists, nurses, social workers, psychologists, psychiatrists, and anesthesiologists.[45] Often major hospitals and medical centers have substantial programs for chronic pain. A well-rounded center should include drug therapy as an option if other measures fail.

Chronic Cancer Pain

For patients with the diagnosis of cancer, fear of pain is always present. Dr. Russell Portenoy notes that "Cancer pain is usually associated with a direct effect of the cancer. The course is characterized by fluctuation, typically with the occurrence of frequent breakthrough pains, and gradual progression."[46] Physical pain is a reminder that cancer is present and may mean the progression of disease.

There are a million new cancer cases each year in the United States, with estimates of six million patients who are living with their cancer.[47] More than 50% of chronic cancer patients are undertreated for their pain. Some of the reasons for inadequate cancer pain control are:

- Lack of knowledge of the cancer process
- Poor assessment of pain
- Fear of addiction
- Overattention to trying to cure the cancer

- Fear of side effects of pain drugs
- Poor understanding of the pharmacology of drugs in general
- Not making use of psychological and other alternative approaches such as meditation, biofeedback, music, distraction, and imagery

Jamie Von Roenn, M.D., of Northwestern University, directed a 1989 survey of 1,800 cancer specialists who belong to the Eastern Cooperative Oncology Group. A body of 1,177 doctors who had treated seventy thousand cancer patients within a six-month period responded. The survey indicated that 66% of the doctors said they did not give enough painkillers to patients in need; 60% of the doctors said they do an inadequate job of assessing patients' pain. Fear of side effects was cited as a major reason for undermedicating patients. Poor training and ignoring patient suffering were also factors. Dr. Von Roenn says, "This study is disturbing since these are the doctors who deal with cancer patients. I would have thought they would have known more."[48] Clearly, cancer pain is a low priority.

Assessment of cancer pain is paramount. Diana Wilkie, Ph.D., R.N., says, "Behavior of the patient is critical to accurate pain assessment and pain management." Some patients show the classic signs of a person in pain; others do not. Dr. Wilkie videotaped forty-five lung cancer patients in their homes. The patients used forty-two different behaviors to control their pain. They rocked, changed positions, guarded areas of the body that hurt, moaned, and asked God for help. "The faces of these patients showed little or no facial reaction to pain. They were quite stoic in their expression despite the fact that 53% reported they were in constant pain," reported Wilkie.[49]

Ada Jacox, R.N., writes, "No two people with cancer suffer in the same way since each individual enters the situation with his or her own unique past experiences, his own set of coping behaviors, along with his own type of tumor. For some, a future of total pain relief is nonexistent; thinking about this possibility can, in itself, be a devastating experience. The pain is always there and the only anticipated change is that it will get worse. For others, there is no present pain, but always the fear that there can be in the future if the tumor gets out of control."[50]

Chronic cancer pain is medically, emotionally, and psychologically complicated. Doctors, nurses, and other health care professionals need to learn how to treat cancer pain so patients can live life to the fullest of their capacity and not be condemned to the poorest quality of life known to mankind: suffering.

YOU CAN LEARN ABOUT PAIN

In the following chapters you will learn about pain and begin to understand why pain is being undertreated and how you can avoid undertreatment for yourself and your loved ones. Make a commitment to exercise your basic human right to adequate pain relief. You can change the way your pain is being managed. You, as a consumer, have already had a massive impact on American medicine by asking for and getting better health care. Hundreds of studies show that involved and informed patients have fewer problems, heal faster, and stay well longer.

Seize this moment. Take the information in this book to your doctor's office. Don't ever plan any diagnostic, medical, or surgical procedure without first discussing a "Pain Plan" with your doctor. You need to know how much pain you might have, how long it might last, how it will be treated, and who will be responsible if the pain medication or treatment does not work. You will learn how a pain plan will help you to concentrate on getting well. You don't have to do battle with needless pain.

In this book you will read what the leading pain specialists say about pain and how to control it. Included in the book are your personal pain assessment scale and "The Pain Patient's Bill of Rights" to help you participate in your pain management.

Remember, your doctor has a moral, ethical, and legal obligation to treat your pain. If your pain concerns are not addressed, you should consider a second opinion. Pain control should always be part of your overall "informed consent," as it is with any of your medical or surgical decisions.

If your pain is treated you will heal faster, have fewer medical complications, spend less time in the hospital or at the doctor's office, and enjoy a better quality of family, work, and recreational life. Also important, pain-related costs will be reduced.

You don't have to accept pain. You can say "no" to pain and say "yes" to pain relief!

NOTES

[1]"Acute Pain Management: Operative or Medical Procedures and Trauma," Clinical Practice Guideline. Agency for Health Care Policy and Research, February 1992, iii.

[2]Portenoy, R., personal communication, 1989.

[3]Bonica, J., *The Management of Pain,* second edition (Philadelphia: Lea & Febiger, 1990), vol. 1, 180.

[4]"Acute Pain Management: Operative or Medical Prodedures and Trauma," Clinical Practice Guideline. Agency for Health Care Policy and Research, February 1992, iii.

[5]Cowles, J., *Informed Consent* (New York: Coward, McCann & Geoghegan, 1976), 12–13.

[6]Smith, R., "Current and Emerging Issues in Cancer Pain: Research and Practice." University of Washington, Third Annual Symposium on Pain Research, Bristol Myers-Squibb, July 23–26, 1992.

[7]Evans, W. O., "The Undertreatment of Pain," *Indiana Medicine,* vol. 81, no. 10 (October 1988), 848.

[8]Roark, A., "How Much Pain Killer Is Enough," *Los Angeles Times,* December 10, 1991.
    Angarola, R., Donato, B., "Inappropriate Pain Management Results in High Jury Award," *Journal of Pain and Symptom Management,* vol. 6, no. 7 (October 1991).

[9]Bonica, J., *The Management of Pain,* second edition (Philadelphia: Lea & Febiger, 1990), vol 1, 14.

[10]Portenoy, R., personal communication, 1989.

[11]Ferrell, B., "Pain and the Quality of Life." First International Nursing Research Symposium on Cancer Pain, University of Washington, Seattle, American Cancer Society, July 22, 1992.

[12]McGuire, D., "Psychological Components of Cancer Pain." First International Nursing Research Symposium on Cancer Pain, University of Washington, Seattle, American Cancer Society, July 22, 1992.

[13]Zerwekh, J., "Home Care Issues in Pain Management." First International Nursing Research Symposium on Cancer Pain, University of Washington, Seattle, American Cancer Society, July 22, 1992.

[14]"Acute Pain Management: Operative or Medical Procedures and Trauma," Clinical Practice Guideline. Agency for Health Care Policy and Research, February, 1992, 1–14.

[15]Joranson, D., personal communication, 1993.
    Joranson, D., Cleeland, C., Weissman, A., Gilson, M. S., "Opioid for Chronic Cancer and Non-Cancer Pain: A Survey of State Medical Board Members," *Federation Bulletin: The Journal of Medical Licensure and Discipline,* vol. 79, no. 4 (June 1992), 15–49.

[16]Hill, S., personal communication, 1992.
    Hill S., Ferrell, B., Agency for Health Care Policy Research Panel, "A Federal Proposal for Cancer Pain Management Guidelines." First International Nursing Research Symposium on Cancer Pain, University of Washington, Seattle, American Cancer Society, July 22, 1992.

[17]Weissman, D. E., Joranson, D. E., Hopwood, M. B., "Wisconsin Physicians' Knowledge and Attitudes About Opioid Analgesic Regulations," *Wisconsin Med. Jour.,* December 1991, 671–75.

[18]National Conference of Commissioners on Uniform State Laws, Chicago, personal communication, 1992.

[19]Melzack, R., "The Tragedy of Needless Pain," *Scientific American,* vol. 262, no. 2 (February 1990), 27–33.

[20]Wilkie, D., 'Assessing Cancer Pain Behaviors: Value of Patient's Perspective." First International Nursing Symposium on Cancer Pain, University of Washington, Seattle, American Cancer Society, July 22, 1992.

[21]"Acute Pain Management: Operative or Medical Procedures and Trauma," Clinical Practice Guideline. Agency for Health Care Policy and Research, February 1992, 2.

[22]Schechter, N., Berde, B., Yaster, M., *Pain in Infants, Children, and Adolescents* (Baltimore: Williams & Williams, 1993), vi.

[23]American Pain Society, *Principles of Analgesic Use in the Treatment of Acute Pain and Cancer Pain,* third edition (1992), 2.

[24]"Acute Pain Management: Operative or Medical Procedures and Trauma," Clinical Practice Guideline. Agency for Health Care Policy and Research, February 1992, 2.

[25]"Acute Pain Management: Operative or Medical Procedures and Trauma," Clinical Practice Guideline. Agency for Health Care Policy and Research, February 1992, 3–4.

[26]Bonica, J., *The Management of Pain,* second edition (Philadelphia: Lea & Febiger, 1990), vol. 1, 123.

[27]Portenoy, R., personal communication, 1989.

[28]Wilkie, D., personal communication, 1992.

[29]Reichl, M,. Dodiwala, C. C., "Use of Analgesia in Severe Pain in the Accident and Emergency Department," *Jour. Arch. Emerg. Med.,* vol. 4, no. 1 (March 1987), 25, 31.

[30]Camp, L. D., O'Sullivan, P. S., "Comparison of Medical, Surgical and Oncology Patient's Descriptions of Pain and Nurses' Documentation of Pain Assessment," *J. Adv. Nurs.,* vol. 5 (September 12, 1987), 593–98.

[31]"Acute Pain Management: Operative or Medical Procedures and Trauma," Clinical Practice Guideline. Agency for Health Care Policy and Research, February 1992, 4.

[32]G. Donaldson, "Current and Emerging Issues in Cancer Pain: Research and Practice." University of Washington, Third Annual Symposium on Pain Research, Bristol Myers-Squibb, July 23–26, 1992.

[33]Yaksh, T., American Pain Society, 11th Annual Scientific Meeting, San Diego, October 22–24, 1992.

[34]Sinatra, R. S., "Current Methods of Controlling Post-Operative Pain," *Yale Journal of Biology and Medicine,* vol. 64 (1991), 351–74.

[35]Dubner, R., American Pain Society, 11th Annual Scientific Meeting, San Diego, October 22–25, 1992.

[36]Liebeskind, J., American Pain Society, 11th Annual Scientific Meeting, San Diego, October 22–25, 1992.

[37]Melzack, R., "The Tragedy of Needless Pain," *Scientific American,* vol. 262, no. 2 (February 1990), 27–33.

[38]Porter, J., "Addiction Rare in Patients Treated with Narcotics," *New Eng. Jour. Med.,* vol. 302, no. 2 (1987), 123.

[39]*Harvard Medical School Letter,* vol. 14, no. 8 (June 1989).

[40]"Nuprin Pain Report, A National Study for Nuprin" by Louis Harris & Associates, Inc., September 1985, 7–8.

[41]"Where Does It Hurt, and Why?," University of California, *Berkeley Wellness Letter,* vol. 5, issue 10 (July 1989), 4–6.

[42]McCaffery, M., Beebe, A., *Pain: Clinical Manual for Nursing Practice* (St. Louis: C. V. Mosby Co., 1989), 232–63.

[43]Portenoy, R., personal communication, 1992.

[44]Bonica, J., *The Management of Pain,* second edition (Philadelphia: Lea & Febiger, 1990), vol. 1, 197.

[45]"Pain," *U.S. News & World Report,* June 29, 1989, 57.

[46]Portenoy, R., "Why Do We Care: Pain and Symptom Control." Memorial Sloan-Kettering Cancer Center–European School of Oncology Post-Graduate Course, New York, April 2–4, 1992.

[47]*Cancer Facts and Figures, 1981–1992* (Atlanta: American Cancer Society, 1991–92).

[48]Von Roenn, J., personal communication, 1992.

[49]Wilkie, D., personal communication, 1992.
   Wilkie, D., "Assessing Cancer Pain Behaviors: Value of the Patient's Perspective." First International Nursing Symposium on Cancer Pain, University of Washington, Seattle, American Cancer Society, July 22, 1990.

[50]Jacox, A., *Pain: A Source Book for Nurses and Other Health Professionals* (Boston: Little, Brown, and Co., 1977), 373.

1

PLANNING PAIN MANAGEMENT WITH YOUR DOCTOR

You must discuss pain management with your doctor before any diagnostic, medical, or surgical procedure. Not to do so puts you at risk for pain-related medical complications, longer hospital stays, and days absent from work.

You have a basic human right to adequate pain relief. However, 50% of your acute pain due to injury, trauma, labor, surgery, or disease is undertreated. (Chronic pain and cancer pain will be discussed in later chapters.)

The health care delivery system is not responding to your pain care needs. To help the system reverse this trend of poor pain control, you must take action as a health care consumer. However, to obtain adequate pain management, you have to learn about pain, the language of pain assessment, and the tools of pain management. To change the status quo that results in poor pain control, you and your doctor will have to become partners.

In the Introduction, you read about studies that demonstrate why pain is being undertreated. You now know that you, your doctor, nurses, and other health care providers very likely suffer from a multifaceted overlay of misinformation, myths, and misconceptions about pain and pain relief. Now you know that nothing will change until you become your own advocate for pain control. It will not come easily. Change will take education, patience, diligence, and resolve.

Actually, it is quite surprising that adequate pain management has met with such widespread resistance within the health care system. It does not make sense. Pain is the one physical event that is common to almost all medical problems. It is more common than fever, which is usually treated with concern. Pain complications are legion, but often ignored. Despite thousands of studies over the years that clearly state patients are suffering needlessly by the hundreds of millions, change within the health care profession has come slowly and reluctantly.

The American Pain Society Task Force has concluded that the health care system cannot bring about changes in a timely fashion until the consumer is involved. The American Cancer Society has made 1993 a year in which to focus on educating patients about pain. Their conclusion is also that "the consumer must become involved." Moreover, the World Health Organization has made pain relief a priority on an international scale. As Dr. Betty Ferrell said about the universal undertreatment of pain, "This has to stop. We have to stop the practice of letting humans suffer."[1]

If a patient is suffering from pain-related complications, the stay in the hospital is longer, and dozens of tests must be performed, along with consultations with specialists. If pain causes a patient to have a rapid or irregular heartbeat, an EKG, as well as a battery of other blood and blood gas tests, will be ordered, which must be interpreted by a cardiologist. Unrelieved pain restricts movement, which causes shallow breathing. Secretions may accumulate in the lungs, which could lead to pneumonia; chest x-rays, blood tests, and cultures must be taken and usually evaluated by a pulmonary specialist. If blood clots are suspected in the extremities, clotting times, blood gases, and ultrasound must be ordered and assessed. If blood clots are suspected in the lungs, an avalanche of blood tests, gases, clotting times, and lung scans must be performed and evaluated. Exacerbating the medical picture are other pain-related medical complications, such as lack of normal gastric and bowel function, as well as the overlay of negative emotions such as anxiety, fear, and anger.

Once a pain-related clinical diagnosis is made, it must be documented, treated, and followed. Maybe the patient will have to spend time in intensive care if physical events move downhill too rapidly. In fact, all of the above and more could happen if pain is undermanaged. What started out as medical or surgical treatment for one problem can lead to assessments and treatments for pain-related complications, which could be more serious than the original medical problem.

Poorly managed pain not only causes physical and emotional suffering, it costs a great deal of money. If tests, specialists, and treatments are involved, the cost in dollars rockets into the stratosphere. This is just the medical tip of the pain-related financial-cost iceberg that results from professional reluctance to prevent and treat pain with existing state-of-the-art pain management techniques. And this doesn't factor in the cost of time lost from the workplace.

Aside from the needless suffering, there is the needless and unreasonable financial cost to the patient and the country. At the City of Hope Hospital, a 212-bed hospital in Los Angeles, Dr. Betty Ferrell noted that of the 5,772 scheduled and unscheduled admissions, 255 were for uncontrolled cancer pain. She estimated the pain-related costs to be $20,000 a patient per twelve-day stay, which resulted in more than $5 million for a one-year period![2]

Obviously, you have a vested physical and financial interest in making certain your pain is managed. To overlook the issue simply does not make sense.

When you approach your doctor with the determination to avoid poor pain management, you may find you are charting new waters. Those waters may have been roiled by years of ingrained treatment patterns that fail to relieve pain. You know that your doctor was not taught in medical school about pain and that state-of-the-art pain management programs are not usually available in hospitals.

You may find that your request for change meets with surprise and/or resistance. However, persist and remember the basic fact: *You have a right to adequate pain relief.* Hopefully, your request will be met with the enthusiastic realization that pain control is an idea whose time has come.

If enough patients start making their health care decisions based not only on the treatment of their medical problems but also on the adequate treatment of pain, then medicine will change. It has been proven over the years. In 1975, Informed Consent was not part of the doctor-patient relationship. Patients asked for change. Today Informed Consent is federal law. As recently as 1980, women awoke from a biopsy procedure shocked to find that a cancerous breast had been removed without their knowledge. Women asked for change. Today women have an opportunity to seek a second opinion before any breast cancer procedure is performed. In fact, it is not uncommon for patients to seek second or third opinions for their medical problems. It has become the norm rather than the exception.

Patients' health care choices based on information have changed the way medicine is practiced. They changed when patients began to seek doctors and hospitals that were sensitive to, and acknowledged, their legitimate health concerns. In many instances a partnership was forged between patient and doctor, which resulted in better and safer health care for the patient. It can happen again in pain management.

Now the concern is adequate pain management.

Those involved with pain research and clinical practice know first-hand how harmful unrelieved pain is to the human body. The Surgeon General and the United States Department of Health consider the lack of pain management such a devastating health care crisis that they have issued federal guidelines to doctors and health care providers—as well as mandates to hospitals—to change the practice of undertreatment of pain.

Unfortunately, the message has not reached you, the patient. You must become educated and begin to ask for what is rightfully yours: adequate pain control. If you don't ask, very little will change.

Acute pain and cancer pain will remain largely undertreated and chronic pain management will continue to languish. Medical and nursing schools will continue to teach only token classes on pain; textbooks will continue to ignore pain as part of medical treatment; hospitals will continue not making pain control hospital policy; federal and state medical and pharmacy boards will continue to restrict pain-relieving drugs to those who need them; and you will continue to suffer needless pain.

This lack of pain control does not have to continue. Pain management is available. However, you are going to have to start asking for it. "Health initiatives" commence with you, the consumer.

The following chapters will teach you about pain and pain control measures so that you can make informed choices as part of your overall medical care.

PAIN IS COMPLEX

You have read that pain is an unpleasant sensory and emotional experience arising from actual or potential tissue damage or have heard pain described in terms of such damage. *What you also need to know is how complex and completely individual the pain experience is for every human being.*

Myron Yaster, M.D., of Johns Hopkins Hospital, takes part of the mystery out of pain. He says pain is "much akin to other integrated, complex perceptual functions such as sight and sound. When looking at a painting or listening to music, what makes the image beautiful or the sound pleasing? Why do different people experience the same physical phenomenon and attach completely different values and meanings to it? Similarly, pain is a physical phenomenon that is interpreted uniquely by each person who experiences it."[3]

Physically, following an injury, the pain transmits a message to fibers in the spinal cord, causing an explosion of complicated events to occur simultaneously. Different pain fibers sort out the pain as sharp, dull, or burning, and communicate that message to the brain. At the same moment, hormones (including adrenaline), serotonin, and a dozen other substances flood the body. The heart rate increases and the blood pressure rises. Meanwhile, other fibers attempt to inhibit the pain by releasing what are known as neuropeptides. The most familiar of these is one that is like a naturally occurring morphine.

The pain experience is also colored by dozens of other factors, such as anxiety, fear, helplessness, affect, cultural background, absence of sleep, previous pain experience, age,[4] meaning, and metabolic and possibly genetic factors. This pain moment is filled with millions of combinations that are completely impossible for anyone except the person who is living the pain experience to understand.

Pain is as individual to the human body as a fingerprint. No two are the same. This uniqueness must always be kept in mind by health care professionals when they treat pain. Since pain is different in each person, the treatment of pain must be tailored to each person. It is impossible to cookie-cut pain care. It simply does not work.

There are many avenues that can be taken to help individualize pain treatment. To begin with, your doctor should know about you and your history of pain. The better your doctor knows you, the better the chances are that your pain can be individually managed.

PAIN HISTORY

Your doctor should take a Pain History from you and make it an easily accessible part of your chart.

The Pain History lets your doctor know what illnesses, injuries, or surgical procedures you have experienced that caused you pain, what medications you have taken, which worked for you and which did not. It will help your doctor to discuss future pain medication choices with you.

The Pain History Should Contain the Following Questions:

- How do you react to pain?
- What do you do to handle minor pain? (Take aspirin, sleep, distract yourself, watch TV, etc.)
- Have you had any illness, injury, or surgery for which you have taken pain medications?
- What type and form of pain medication did you take?
- How often do you take pain medication? (One time a day, four times, eight times, etc.)
- How much do you take at one time? (One pill, two pills, six pills, etc.)
- Were there side effects, reactions, or allergies?
- Did you obtain pain relief?
- How long did you take the medication?
- Have you taken opioids (morphine-like drugs) for pain? If so, in what form and for how long?
- Have you taken pain medication for any other reason?
- Do you have chronic pain? If so, what is it? (Backache, headache, arthritis, old injury, etc.)
- How often does it occur? (Daily, weekly, monthly, other)
- Do you take medication when it occurs?
- Are you taking medication now?
- How much do you take and how often? Does it work?
- Does any nondrug therapy help your pain? (Heat, cold, lying down, changing position, etc.)
- Does pain interfere with your home life, job, school, social life?
- Are you depressed, anxious, angry, or experiencing any other negative feelings? If so, why?
- Do you take any other prescription drugs? If so, please name them.
- Do you take over-the-counter drugs, eye drops, vitamins, or other preparations? If so, please name them.
- What, if any, is your choice of over-the-counter or prescription pain medication?
- Is there any medication you don't want? If so, why?

- Is there anything about your past experience with pain or pain medications that you want recorded on your chart?
- Do you have any preconceived ideas or fears about pain, pain medications, opioids, or other drugs?

If your doctor does not ask for a Pain History, write one yourself and request that it be included in your record. Express your concern about adequate pain control. *If your doctor does not feel that your Pain History or pain control is important, you might consider seeking a second opinion from a doctor who considers pain management an integral part of your medical care.*

Remember, pain control is as important to you as your medical or surgical procedure. Pain prevention and relief offset unnecessary pain-related complications. If your doctor is not concerned, you should be.

DIAGNOSTIC PROCEDURES

Diagnostic procedures can sometimes be painful. If your doctor recommends one, ask the following questions:

- Will this procedure be painful?
- Where will I feel the pain?
- What is it like for most people? (Burning, aching, dull, etc.)
- How long might the pain last?
- If you are anxious: Can I have an antianxiety drug before the procedure?
- What pain medication is given during the procedure?
- Might there be pain after the procedure? (If so, ask to have a prescription filled ahead of time to take home.)
- If there is pain, how often may I take medication to achieve a steady level of relief?
- Is there anything I can do at home to lessen pain, like apply heat or cold, massage, meditation, or other suggestions?
- What pain would you consider abnormal?
- What should I do differently if my pain is not relieved?
- Whom can I call if my pain is not relieved?

In addition, if you are especially anxious about the diagnostic procedure, you should let your doctor know. He may be able to explain more details about the test to allay your fears.

WHAT YOU SHOULD KNOW
ABOUT ANESTHETICS

So you will not feel pain during a diagnostic, medical, or surgical procedure, an anesthetic is used. An anesthetic interferes with the pain message transmission. Interference can prevent pain from stamping a pain message into neurons. As a result, you experience less post-invasive pain. There are several forms of anesthetics that can be used.

For sewing up cuts, removing foreign bodies, performing a small biopsy or other minor procedures, your doctor will most likely use:

Topical anesthetic: A substance placed on the skin to numb it.

Subcutaneous anesthetic: A substance (most commonly Lidocaine) injected under the skin to numb the area just beneath the site.

Field block: Injections of anesthetic to numb a large treatment area.

Local nerve block: An injection of local anesthetic around a peripheral nerve to numb the area supplied by the nerve (such as blocking a nerve to the finger).

When the procedure affects an area too large or too deep to use a local anesthetic, another form of anesthesia is used.

Regional blocks cut off the pain message to entire areas. Your doctor can block off large nerves that feed your arm, leg, or more specific areas. These include:

Axillary block: To block the upper extremity for fracture reductions and surgical procedures of the hand and forearm.

Intercostal nerve block: To block the chest and abdominal walls. This can be used for such painful procedures as inserting a chest tube, or it can provide pain relief from rib fractures. A tiny tube can be left at the site for continuous blocking.

Femoral nerve block: This block can be used for fractures of the femur in order to examine, x-ray, and place traction devices.

Epidural Anesthetic

After a local anesthetic is injected to numb the area, a tiny tube is placed near the bony part of the spinal column, but outside the fiber cover of the spinal cord. The anesthetic is injected into the tube in one shot or on a continuous basis. Placing the tube at different levels of the extradural space allows almost any part of the body to be blocked. The anesthetic acts instantly.[5]

You are often given an antianxiety drug to make a procedure easier to handle emotionally. The reaction of "Oh, I don't want to know what is going on" during surgery will be diminished. (Sometimes the doctor may give you a drug that will make you forget that you had a procedure. These drugs are called amnesics.)

An advantage of an epidural is that more anesthetic can be added through the tiny tube. As pointed out, the tube can be left in place to maintain continuous pain relief.

Epidurals are often used for procedures involving the extremities, during labor, childbirth, cesarean section, or orthopedic and urologic procedures, or, in fact, any surgery below the diaphragm.

Recent studies seem to present compelling reasons for using epidurals. *Patients who receive epidurals need less pain medication after surgery than those who are given general anesthesia alone.*

In reviewing records of 929 British patients who had orthopedic surgery, the researchers noted that *patients who had been given local anesthetic blocks didn't request pain medication until more than eight hours after surgery. Those patients who had epidurals combined with opioid premedication and local anesthetic did not need medication for more than nine hours.* These results showed a contrast to those patients who only had general anesthesia for surgery. They needed pain medications less than two hours postsurgery.[6]

Administering small amounts of pain-relieving drugs in the epidural before surgery can prepare and soothe the pain fibers in the spinal cord so there is less pain experienced during surgery. Additional drugs given during surgery keep the pain fibers blocked, lessening postoperative pain.

Phantom limb pain is a well known phenomenon that occurs after the amputation of a limb. The patient can still feel the pain of the missing limb, which is common after amputation and often is self-limiting. "Very few patients have phantom pain," says Peter Koo, Pharm.D., an associate professor of Clinical Pharmacy at the University of California, San Francisco. Possibly an epidural can block the phantom limb pain phenomenon altogether. A study showed that none of the patients who had received a three-day preoperative block experienced pain six months after the amputation. The epidural procedure interrupted the pain message and effectively blocked it.[7]

In 1992 the Hospital for Special Surgery, an orthopedic hospital in New York City, performed 7,208 orthopedic surgical procedures. Epidurals were used 90% of the time. Jeffrey Ngeow, M.D., Chief of the

Pain Service, says, "Whenever possible we try to convince our patients to use regional anesthetics over general. We have the ability to vary the duration of the block from 1 hour to 12 hours by using various drugs."[8]

Nigel Sharrock, M.D., chief of Anesthesiology at the Hospital for Special Surgery, adds, "The big shift away from conventional anesthesia to regional anesthesia can make a vast difference to patients. Since patients are awake, but minimally sedated, anesthesiologists can directly and constantly assess the patient's heart, brain, and lung functions. This enables the physician to safely and deliberately control the patients' blood pressure and their blood flow, and minimize blood loss. Lowered blood loss also results in decreasing the need for blood donors."[9]

In a study of epidural use during total hip replacement surgery, Modig seems to indicate that in addition to the epidural's providing longer pain relief after surgery, the number of postoperative deep vein clots and blood clots to the lungs was decreased significantly.[10]

In addition, women who have epidurals during cesarean section not only enjoy the birth experience, they have fewer postoperative complications, need less pain medication, and have infants who are more responsive than those women who have general anesthesia.[11]

Sometimes epidurals are used for ongoing pain relief. The tiny tube is left at the site and the pain-relieving drug is delivered continuously through a bedside or portable pump the patient can wear at home.

Spinal

A local anesthetic is injected to numb the area where the injection will be given, then a shot of anesthetic passes through the fiber cover that surrounds the spinal cord and directly into the spinal fluid. Continuous doses can be delivered via a bedside or portable pump.

These forms of anesthetics often reduce the grogginess or nausea of general anesthesia, resulting in a quick recovery after surgery.

General Anesthesia

General anesthesia puts you into unconsciousness or, as it is sometimes said, "puts you to sleep". General anesthesia is accomplished by the injection of anesthetics into the blood intravenously, or absorbed into the blood from the lungs following inhalation.

The goal of general anesthesia is to administer the smallest amount of anesthetic that will keep you immobilized during surgery and yet keep you within the margins of safety. You will have a tube inserted down your throat and into your lungs to keep you breathing and prevent you from inhaling secretions.

Although you may be unconscious, your body still experiences pain. You should have opioids administered simultaneously with general anesthesia in order to block the pain message.

General anesthesia should be taken seriously and used when other means of anesthesia or blocks cannot be employed. Of all the anesthesias, this is considered the riskiest, because it depresses the brain function, the lungs, and other vital organs. You must be monitored constantly for any abnormal heart, lung, and blood pressure signs.

It takes longer to prepare a patient for blocks, spinals, and epidurals. Some anesthesiologists use general anesthesia too frequently for procedures that really don't require it. "Convenience, surgical or anesthetic, should not play a significant role in selecting anesthetic agents, especially convenience measured in terms of minutes saved during induction," writes Schwartz in *Principles of Surgery.*[12]

The recovery time from general anesthesia is longer, and the patient has more potential for post-anesthesia complications such as an allergic reaction, vomiting, sore throat, headache, and eye irritation.

CHOOSING YOUR ANESTHESIOLOGIST

It is of extreme importance that you talk to the anesthesiologist well before any diagnostic, medical, or surgical procedure. It is critical that your pain history be taken and that you list any medications you are taking, even vitamins and eye drops.

Always ask for a board-certified attending anesthesiologist to either perform or supervise your anesthesia. Those who are board-certified have passed rigorous tests in this specialty.

Recently the American Society of Anesthesiologists published comprehensive guidelines for safety. The society considers general anesthesia monitoring so important that it has mandated respirator alarms for each patient, a blood pressure check every five minutes, heart monitors to be visible at all times, and an anesthesiologist or anesthetist to follow the patient throughout the procedure.

The incidence of death from *"all forms* of anesthesia, from the most minor to major, is approximately 1 in 1,600," writes Schwartz. He adds, "Failure to recognize that the anesthetic should be tailored to the type of operation has led to inaccurate and dangerous generalizations as to anesthetic selection."[13]

You must carefully investigate your anesthesia options. If the optimum type of anesthesia is selected, your diagnostic or surgical procedure will be less traumatic, decrease the level of pain you experience during and after the procedure, lessen your requirements for pain medications, and help you to recover faster.

If you are not allowed the time to discuss your options, if you are not informed, and if your concerns are not addressed adequately, it would be advisable for you to seek another anesthesiologist to care for you.

YOUR PAIN PLAN

As part of your "pain plan" you will want to discuss in advance postoperative or acute pain management while you are in the hospital.

It has been suggested that you ask about the pain control policy at the hospital to which you plan to be admitted. Obviously, it should concern you if the hospital is not dedicated to pain control, in the same way it would concern you if it is not dedicated to treating illness. It is common knowledge that patients have asked hospitals to be more responsive to their needs in the past in such areas as labor and delivery, child-care, and outpatient procedures, to mention a few. Pain control should be a source of pride of every hospital.

Your pain relief level should allow you to breathe deeply, cough, and move. This will help you recover faster and avoid pain-related complications such as secretion buildup in your lungs that can lead to pneumonia, or blood clots in the extremities that can be life-threatening. *The goal is to achieve an even level of pain-relieving medication in your blood so that you will not experience the roller-coaster effect of a pain–no pain–pain cycle.*

You should be concerned about the following:

- What type of pain you expect to have
- How long the pain may last
- What pain medications you will be given and in what form (oral or intravenous)
- What dose you will be getting

Dosage is important. Find out from your doctor what your dose will be. Write it down. You need to know. Studies have shown that although 50% of patients are underdosed by their doctors, nurses often cut doses even more. If you know how much pain medication you should be getting, you can chart yourself.

Ask what dose you are getting each time it is brought to you. If the nurse is cutting your dose and you are in pain, you need to speak to your doctor.

Dr. Peter Koo says, "Communicate . . . communicate . . . communicate! The patient must ask their doctor 'What one person will be held accountable for my pain management?' The problem lies within the physician's order. A wide range of the dose of pain medication is ordered, and it is often up to the nurse to decide how much to give. Commonly the dose range is too low and the nurse will often pick the lowest dose of the prescribed range."[14]

Reviews of nursing charts repeatedly show that nurses commonly cut their patients' opioid analgesic doses. In a study of 109 patients in five central Illinois hospitals, Felissa Cohen, R.N., writes, "Nurses were overly concerned about the possibility of addiction; choices of analgesic medications seemed irrational; and knowledge of the drugs was inadequate. Moreover, these nurses indicated that complete pain relief after surgery was not their major goal."

Cohen notes, "Much of the responsibility for the patient's pain rests with the nurse. Often the patient's requests for medication are accompanied by increasing doses of disapproval from the nurse along with the analgesia. The statement 'you shouldn't be having so much pain now' is unfortunately a familiar, albeit judgmental one."[15]

Patients who are in pain and ask for more medication often get tagged by nurses as "clock watchers" or "exhibiting addictive behavior," or have their suffering tuned out by overburdened nurses. The reality is that if patients' acute pain is managed adequately, they stop watching the clock, stop begging for medication, and stop suffering.

Betty Ferrell, Ph.D., F.A.A.N., is concerned that "exaggerated fears of addiction among nurses may be increasing." In her recent study of more than two thousand nurses she found that their fears of addiction rose 8.5% in a twenty-month period. She writes, "In view of the increased efforts to reeducate all health professionals about pain control and addiction, this result is indeed discouraging. We wonder if it reflects the success of the 'just say no to drugs' campaign that deals with substance abuse. Ideally, as pain specialists, we should be able to send at least as strong a message to patients, families and caregivers with this statement, 'just say no to pain.' "[16]

As stated in the Introduction, fear of addiction is grossly and wildly exaggerated. *Studies have documented the small risk of addiction in patients who required opioids for pain. In one study, out of 10,000 burn patients, no case of addiction was reported. In another, out of 11,882, only four cases of addiction were reported. Only one was considered serious addiction.*[17]

How often will you receive medication? This is an important question. It is better to get your medication on a *round-the-clock schedule.*

"PRN" equals "as needed." It is a poor choice postoperatively— *"as needed" means that when you "feel pain" you must ask for pain medication.*

When you "feel pain" you will have to call the nurse. The nurse usually has to come to see you, and she may be too busy to bring you your medication when you need it. Another big problem is that the nurse may, as the literature notes, cut your dose.

By that time your pain may be worse. If you have an intramuscular injection, it can take up to ninety minutes to be absorbed, and it may not last. It is better to receive pain medication on a set schedule. This means round-the-clock medication. It has been pointed out that waiting for pain to reappear is illogical and cruel, and perpetuates the memory and fear of pain.

For adequate pain control, regular scheduling is best. If you are on a schedule, there should be an *order left in your chart for "break-through pain"*—which means that if you experience an intense level of pain, you can be given what is known as a *rescue dose.*

If your doctor refuses to put you on a schedule, plan ahead. For example, *if you must ask for medication, don't wait until your pain is severe. Ask for your medication ahead of your pain.* If you know that your pain gets worse every four hours, ask for medication at three and a half hours. That will give the nurse time to get your medication, and you may not have to experience breakthrough pain. Remember, "prevention is the key." Do not wait until you feel severe pain.

Opioids [morphine-like drugs] usually have an analgesic action of three to six hours. (If pain is severe or is not controlled, more analgesic or different time intervals must be considered.) Therefore, the doses should be spaced out evenly over twenty-four hours. This means even during the night. Pain can lead to sleep-deprived nights. If you don't sleep due to pain, then the pain can become worse and you sleep less. It is an unnecessary vicious circle.

Poor pain control can cause loss of mobility, which can lead to poor circulation and blood clots. Poor appetite can also be caused by under-treatment of pain. If you can't breathe deeply or cough, your lungs may fill with secretions, causing infection and possibly pneumonia.

THERE IS NO STANDARD DOSE

As the experience of pain is not the same in all patients, so drugs act differently in each patient. Drug absorption and length of effectiveness are unique to each patient, due to a variety of physical, emotional, biologic, metabolic, and possibly genetic factors.

The correct dose of an opioid, such as morphine, is the dose that provides relief for at least three to four or more hours. However, that may entail a higher drug dose or more frequent administration—even every one to two hours until relief is achieved. The ideal time to begin checking the patient's pain control is after the first dose.

As Raymond Houde, M.D., of Memorial Sloan-Kettering Cancer Center, writes, "The physician's responsibilities are not only to determine and treat the cause of pain, but also to treat the pain itself. There is no predetermined optimal dose for any type of pain; there are merely recommended starting doses from which the optimal dose is determined by titration [adjustment] and the maximal dose limited only by adverse effects."[18]

Dr. Peter Koo says, "A contributing factor to poor pain control is that too often physicians have an archaic view that anyone can manage pain. The reality is not everyone can manage pain without some form of training or re-education. The average physician has little pharmacological training. When we talk about such things as pharmacodynamics and pharmokinetics most M.D.'s have a hard time understanding it. M.D.'s and patients need to access hospital-based and community-based pharmacists to select the right drug, dose, route [intravenous, oral, rectal, etc.] and equivalent doses when going from one route to another such as IV to oral.

"If a patient is having poor pain control or side effects of drugs, the patient should ask the physician to involve the *pharmacist* to help. Hospital-based pharmacists are on salary and are an ideal independent party to assist with pain management." He adds, "Dose requirements vary with the severity of pain, individual response to pain, age, weight and the presence of concomitant diseases. The dose that works is the dose that works."[19]

The addition of other pain-relieving drugs can actually enhance the effectiveness of opioids, so less may be needed. *It is recommended that these "enhancing" drugs be given* at the same time as an opioid *to increase the pain-relieving properties of the opioid:*

- Aspirin
- Acetaminophen (Tylenol)
- Nonsteroidal anti-inflammatory drugs (Advil, Nuprin, Motrin)

In addition, other enhancers include drugs such as antihistamines, tricyclic antidepressants, tranquilizers, and sometimes corticosteroids.

Some doctors and nurses have rigid drug dose limits set in their minds that they will not exceed, even though the patient is still suffering. It is now well documented that cookbook pain management does not work, and can lead a patient directly down the path of severe pain-related complications. Doses must be tailor-made for each patient.

PATIENTS ARE SUFFERING

What is outstanding in the literature is that study after study clearly shows that patients are suffering from unrelieved pain due to under-treatment by doctors and nurses. The following are two studies done fifteen years apart.

In 1973 a classic study of undertreatment of patients' pain in a hospital was performed by Dr. Richard Marks and Dr. Edward Sachar of New York. They reported that of 37 medical inpatients being treated with opioid analgesics for pain, 32% were continuing to experience severe pain and 41% were in moderate pain. Of the 102 staff doctors surveyed, many underestimated the effective dose range, overestimated the duration of pain alleviation, and exaggerated the dangers of addiction for medical inpatients.[20]

In 1987 another study was performed. Fifteen years after the Marks and Sachar research, was there improvement in pain relief? No—it was worse! Dr. Marilee Donovan reported on the pain management of 353 hospitalized patients, 58% of whom had "excruciating pain." Less than 50% of the patients even had a member of the health care team ask them about their pain during their hospitalization. In only 173 of the charts was a patient's pain noted, despite the fact that all 353 patients reported that they had experienced pain in that period. In addition, the dose of opioid was cut by 75% from what the doctor had ordered.[21]

Mitchell Max, M.D., from the National Institutes of Health, writes,

> If the patient reports pain and is given the analgesic that the physician ordered, the medication may be insufficient to relieve it; doctors tend to order doses on the low end of the wide range of individual analgesic requirements. The nurse, who usually lacks authority to change medication orders, may not immediately contact the doctor, who may be preoccupied with a crisis off the ward. Further, there is little to remind caregivers that patients are in pain. Unlike "vital signs," pain isn't displayed in a prominent place on the chart or at a bedside or nursing station. Finally, in cases in which patients remain in pain because of insufficient analgesic treatment, physicians are rarely held accountable. In contrast, routine hospital review procedures query physicians about minor wound infections or failure to sign charts. In a manner of speaking, patients' pain may not intrude into the cognitive world of those persons who write the medication orders.[22]

If you are not getting relief, the Agency for Health Care Policy and Research Acute Pain Guidelines state that *if you are postsurgical, your nurses should be monitoring you every two hours or more frequently until you achieve adequate pain relief.*

PCA: PATIENT-CONTROLLED ANALGESIA

Patient-controlled analgesia is one of the methods of pain control that can decrease the problem of asking for and waiting for pain medication. PCA can be administered intravenously or epidurally.

If it is available in your hospital, *it gives you control over the administration of the predetermined dose of the drug released through a computer lockout mechanism.* If you feel pain, you push a button, and a controlled amount of drug is automatically delivered through the intravenous (IV) line. This method not only gives you control over your pain medications, it decreases the hassle factor of waiting for medication. Studies have shown that patients using PCA often use medication more appropriately when it is needed and experience less anxiety. You should discuss what plans are in place, should the PCA dose of pain medication be too little to control your pain.

Patients and family need education in how to use PCA, but even children can learn to use it. Dr. Myron Yaster writes, "If a child can play Nintendo they can operate PCA." He notes that the only restriction for patients would be "the inability to push the button (weakness or arm restraints), inability to understand how to use the machine, and a patient's desire not to assume responsibility for his or her own care."[23]

"PCA plus" allows the machine to deliver a low-dose continuous infusion of drug along with self-administration of set doses by the patient. This allows patients to sleep through the night, as they receive continuous dosing.

EXTRA PAIN MEDICATION

Sometimes breathing exercises, walking, tests, physical therapy, or dressing changes can also cause pain. The goal is to prevent pain from occurring. Ask for extra medication if you need it.

Pain is more difficult to tame once it has established itself. Plan for extra medication before these events.

The time interval preceding an extra dose depends on how your medication is being administered. For example, if you are taking oral medication, the absorption time is longer (thirty to sixty minutes) than if you receive an intravenous dose. However, you can expect an oral dose to last longer once it has taken effect. The ideal time to perform pain-producing procedures is when the pain medication is at its peak pain-relieving level in your blood. The sooner you can breathe deeply, cough, walk, or are rehabilitated, the sooner you will get out of the hospital.

SIDE EFFECTS OF PAIN MEDICATIONS

Are there any side effects to your pain medication? If so, what plans are in place to offset them, should they occur?

Morphine-like drugs can sometimes cause side effects such as constipation, rash, itching, nausea, vomiting, irritability, mental clouding, or sedation. Most of the side effects can be controlled by planning ahead.

For example, if you are taking an opioid for more than a few days, you should automatically be given a laxative to offset the constipation.

You can have your opioid switched to another opioid. Studies have shown that just because you have a side effect with one opioid does not mean that you will have the same experience with another. Again, this is a result of the unique physical makeup of each patient.

If sedation is a problem, adjusting the dose can often help. In addition, sometimes amphetamines are administered to offset sedation.

Sleeping Problems

Hospitals are uncomfortable places for all patients. Sometimes it is hard to sleep. Ask ahead of time to have a sleep medication order written in your chart, in case you need it. Sleeplessness can make your pain worse. You need sleep to cope with pain.

PAIN ASSESSMENT

Research has shown that the most common reason for unrelieved pain in U.S. hospitals is the failure of the staff to routinely assess pain and pain relief.

Dr. Rollin Oden writes, "One cannot determine for the individual patient how much pain occurs in response to tissue damage, nor infer from the surgery performed, body surface burned or the number and types of bones broken how much pain the patient 'should' have. One has to rely on the expressions of the patient to accurately measure the subjective nature of pain."[24]

When you are not believed, you not only experience the physical pain, you experience the negative emotional pain of anxiety, helplessness, fear, and sometimes hopelessness.

Pain Is What You Say It Is

Pain is what you say it is and not what the doctor or nurse expects it to be or thinks it should be.

A simple method of communicating your pain level is to use the *0–10 Numeric Pain Intensity Scale.* You can take it with you to the hospital. Tell your doctor or nurse that this is one method you will use to tell them about your pain level. You can use it verbally if you are too weak to write.

The chart is based on a scale of 0 = no pain to 10 = worst pain.

0–10 Numeric Pain Intensity Scale

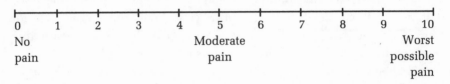

Ask the nurse to chart your pain along with your vital signs of blood pressure and temperature.

The research literature shows that nurses rarely chart patients' pain levels before or after medication. That is poor charting practice. Pain management is as important as your medical or surgical procedure. Your pain scores should be part of your chart.

When you are experiencing severe pain, you should be monitored and assessed every two hours, or more frequently if the pain escalates or is not relieved. The goal, along with treatment for your illness, should be prevention of pain and adequate pain control.

The following is a simple *Patient's Personal Daily Pain Chart* that you can photocopy and take to the hospital for you or a member of your family to use for tracking your pain. It will help you, your doctor, and nurses and other health care professionals to work together to keep your pain managed adequately.

You or a family member should keep your personal pain chart at your bedside to note pain, when it is better, when it is not, what your dose should be, and in what form it is given.

As you now know, unrelieved pain can be harmful in its own right, causing unnecessary medical complications.

Asking About Your Pain

Your doctor or nurse should say to you, *"Tell me about your pain."* This open-ended request will allow you to do so. As you have read, it is often extremely difficult to tell if patients are in pain just by looking at them.

A patient can be in horrible pain and not show it.

Patients may be reluctant to tell anyone they are in pain because they think pain is normal as a result of surgery or illness; they may want to be seen as "good patients"; they don't want to bother or worry anyone; they have misconceptions about addiction; or they are afraid that if

Patient's Personal Daily Pain Chart

Name_____Date_____

Doctor_____

Medication(s)?_____

How often?_____What form? (IV, oral, etc.)_____

What dose?_____

0 = No pain   10 = Worst pain

0	1	2	3	4	5	6	7	8	9	10
No pain					Moderate pain					Worst possible pain

Time A.M./P.M.	Pain Score 0–10	Dose Received	Pain Score 30 mins. IV or 60 mins. oral	Comments

Describe your pain in your own words_____

_____

_____

they mention pain their illness may not be treated as a priority. It is important to your healing process to keep your pain in control.

Describing Your Pain

Just saying "I'm in pain" when you are in pain is a start. However, it will help you and those who care for you if you learn how to describe your pain.

Ronald Melzack, Ph.D., and W. S. Torgerson, Ph.D., write:

> To describe pain solely in terms of intensity, however, is like specifying the visual world in terms of light flux only, without regard to pattern, color, texture and the many other dimensions of visual experience.
>
> There is convincing evidence that a multitude of nerve impulse patterns is transmitted centrally from the skin as a result of tactile, thermal, and chemical stimulation. The classification of these patterns into a smaller number of "modalities" is a function of the capacity of the central nervous system to select and abstract from the total information it receives. The word "pain" in this formulation refers not to a specific sensation which can vary only in intensity, but to an endless variety of qualities that are categorized under a single linguistic label. There are the pains of a scalded hand, a stomach ulcer, a sprained ankle; there are headaches and toothaches. Each has unique qualities. The pain of a toothache is obviously different from that of a pin prick, just as the pain of a coronary occlusion is uniquely different from the pain of a broken leg.[25]

The authors categorize pain into three major classes, with thirteen subclasses. The classes were:

1. Words that describe *sensory qualities,* in terms of temporal, spatial, pressure, thermal, and other properties.
   Temporal: Beating, pounding, throbbing, pulsing, etc.
   Spatial: Radiating, shooting, spreading, etc.
   Pressure: Piercing, stabbing, penetrating, etc.
   Thermal: Burning, searing, scalding, etc.
2. Words that describe *affective qualities,* in terms of tension, fear, and autonomic (nervous system) properties that are part of the pain experience.
   Tension: Dragging, tiring, fatiguing, etc.

Fear: Terrifying, dreadful, fearful, etc.

Autonomic: Sickening, nauseating, suffocating, etc.

3. *Evaluative words* that describe the subjective overall intensity of the total experience of pain: Unbearable, excruciating, horrible, etc.

"Pain, like vision and hearing, is a complex perceptual experience," adds Melzack.[26]

Since pain is so uniquely multidimensional, the more you describe your pain in detail, the better chance you have of obtaining relief. Some of the characteristics of your pain that you should describe are:

- *Site(s):* Where is the pain (or pains)? Does it stay in one place? Does it spread or radiate?
- *Timing:* When did you notice it? How long ago? Is it constant? Does it come and go? Is there a set time between pains?
- *Describe:* Give your description—stabbing, burning, aching, sharp, or other—in your own words. What makes it worse?
- *Movement* (sitting, standing, walking, etc.): What makes it better? (Lying, sleeping, doing something special, heat, cold, etc.)
- *Sleep:* Can you sleep? How many hours? Not at all? Does pain wake you?
- *Emotions:* Are you anxious, angry, depressed, feeling helpless?
- *Treatment:* Have you had relief at any time? What has worked or not worked for you?

If you are specific about your pain and can communicate with your doctor and nurse, they will have a better understanding of it.

An assessment tool that can provide the caregiver more information about your pain is the *McGill Pain Questionnaire* (on pages 42–44). This questionnaire is to be filled out describing "your present pain."

You have read that your pain is as unique as you are, for a variety of physical, emotional, biologic, and possibly genetic reasons. Part of your experience of pain has to do with how your pain affects you.

Biobehavioral Pain Profile

Jo Anne Dalton, Ed.D., R.N., F.A.A.N., is an associate professor of the School of Nursing at the University of North Carolina. She is interested in why patients with the same diagnosis experience different pain. Her emphasis is on what makes up these differences from a behavioral point of view. Dr. Dalton notes that health care providers need to know

McGill Pain Questionnaire

1. WHERE IS YOUR PAIN?
   Please mark, on the drawings below, the areas where you feel pain.
   Put E if external, or I if internal, near the areas which you mark. Put
   EI if both external and internal.

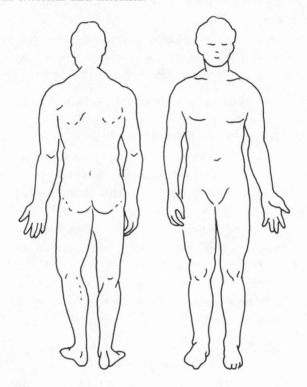

2. WHAT DOES YOUR PAIN FEEL LIKE?
   Some of the words on page 43 describe your *present* pain. Circle
   ONLY those words that best describe it. Leave out any category that
   is not suitable. Use only a single word in each appropriate category—
   the one that applies best.

Sensory: 1–8   *Evaluative:* 16
Affective: 9–15   *Miscellaneous:* 17–20

1	2	3	4
Flickering	Jumping	Pricking	Sharp
Quivering	Flashing	Boring	Cutting
Pulsing	Shooting	Drilling	Lacerating
Throbbing		Stabbing	
Beating		Lancing	
Pounding			

5	6	7	8
Pinching	Tugging	Hot	Tingling
Pressing	Pulling	Burning	Itchy
Gnawing	Wrenching	Scalding	Smarting
Cramping		Searing	Stinging
Crushing			

9	10	11	12
Dull	Tender	Tiring	Sickening
Sore	Taut	Exhausting	Suffocating
Hurting	Rasping		
Aching	Splitting		
Heavy			

13	14	15	16
Fearful	Punishing	Wretched	Annoying
Frightful	Gruelling	Blinding	Troublesome
Terrifying	Cruel		Miserable
	Vicious		Intense
	Killing		Unbearable

17	18	19	20
Spreading	Tight	Cool	Nagging
Radiating	Numb	Cold	Nauseating
Penetrating	Drawing	Freezing	Agonizing
Piercing	Squeezing		Dreadful
	Tearing		Torturing

3. How Does Your Pain Change With Time?
   a. Which word or words would you use to describe the *pattern* of your pain?

1	2	3
Continuous	Rhythmic	Brief
Steady	Periodic	Momentary
Constant	Intermittent	Transient

   b. What kind of things *relieve* your pain?
   c. What kind of things *increase* your pain?

4. How Strong Is Your Pain?
   People agree that the following 5 words represent pain of increasing intensity. They are:

1	2	3	4	5
Mild	Discomforting	Distressing	Horrible	Excruciating

To answer each question below, write the number of the most appropriate word in the space beside the question.

1. Which word describes your pain right now?　＿＿＿＿＿＿
2. Which word describes it at its worst?　＿＿＿＿＿＿
3. Which word describes it when it is least?　＿＿＿＿＿＿
4. Which word describes the worst toothache you
   ever had?　＿＿＿＿＿＿
5. Which word describes the worst headache you
   ever had?　＿＿＿＿＿＿
6. Which word describes the worst stomachache
   you ever had?　＿＿＿＿＿＿

The McGill Pain Questionnaire © 1993. Permission granted by R. Melzack.

more about patients and their attitudes. If more is known, then it is possible to know more what to do about pain. It is not just a simple issue of "pain/no pain."

The *Biobehavioral Pain Profile* is a simple assessment tool developed by Dr. Dalton. The questions can give doctors and nurses an in-depth look at how pain is *affecting* a patient. It adds dimension and shades impossible to understand when a patient simply says, "I'm in pain." Most doctors and nurses are unfamiliar with these forms of assessment. However, you can help those who care for you by filling out a profile questionnaire (see Chapter 5). Some items may not apply to you, but if you are in pain, most will.

If you feel your pain is not being managed adequately, you can request a visit from the "pain team," if your hospital has one. If it does not, requesting a consultation from a neurologist, psychiatrist, psychologist, anesthesiologist, or pharmacist may yield a different approach to solving your pain problems.

It is important to remind yourself and your family of the following:

- Pain can harm you and slow your recovery.
- Pain does not come with the territory of illness.
- You will not be a better person if you suffer pain silently.
- Pain management is part of your overall medical treatment.

ATTITUDES COMMUNICATED BY NURSES

McCaffery and Beebe note "The Important Attitudes Communicated by the Nurse to the Patient and Family." They should be:

1. I care.
2. I believe you about your pain.
3. I respect the way you are reacting to the pain.
4. I want to explore with you what you think will help to relieve your pain.
5. I want to discuss with you what your pain means to you.
6. I am willing to stay with you even if I fail to help control your pain.
7. If you cannot relate to me, I will try to find someone else for you.

Included in their instruction is a "Summary of Guidelines for Using and Individualizing Pain Control Measures":

1. Use a variety of pain control measures.
2. Use pain control measures before pain becomes severe.
3. Include what the patient believes will be effective.
4. Consider the patient's ability or willingness to be active or passive in the application of pain control measures.
5. Institute and modify pain control measures on the basis of patient response.
6. If the pain control measure is ineffective the first time it is used, consider encouraging the patient to try it again.
7. Keep trying.
8. Do no harm.[27]*

*McCaffery, M., Beebe, A., *Pain: Clinical Manual for Nursing Practice* (St. Louis: C. V. Mosby Co., 1989), 40. Reprinted by permission.

PAIN CONTROL METHODS

How Drugs Are Administered

Most patients and many doctors and nurses may be unaware of the various modes in which pain-relieving drugs can be administered.

- *Oral:* The preferred route of administration because of convenience, cost, and blood levels produced.
- *Tablets/capsules:* Delay in absorption time (thirty to sixty minutes), and 20% to 30% of the dose may not be absorbed. Peak effect occurs one to two hours after dose. Some come in long-acting timed-release doses.
- *Liquid:* Helpful for those patients who have trouble with tablets. Can be combined with other medications if necessary.
- *Mucosal:* Dissolving tablets on gumline. One to two hours' dissolving time.
- *Nose spray:* For patients who cannot take medication orally, or prefer this system. Takes about fifteen to twenty minutes to be absorbed.
- *Patch:* An adhesive patch worn for forty-eight to seventy-two hours. Contains a measured dose of pain medication that provides forty-eight hour relief. (If patients are on other oral or intravenous pain medications, there is a period of time during which both should be used until the medication in the patch is absorbed to a peak level in the blood.) Can be worn for widespread pain control. It is called "transdermal" when the drug is delivered across the skin.
- *Rectal:* This route provides slow but good absorption.
- *Intramuscular:* A single dose injected into muscle. The injection is painful. There are huge differences in how long it takes the drug to be absorbed by the muscle and how long relief lasts.
- *Intravenous:* Single dose injected into a vein. An intravenous line (IV) may be left in place for single, multiple, or continuous (PCA) doses of medication. Takes effect in ten to fifteen minutes. Peak effect is similar.
- *Subcutaneous:* Injected under the skin. For patients who cannot take oral medication or whose veins cannot be used. Can also use PCA at the bedside or through portable pumps.
- *Epidural:* Tiny tube placed outside the spinal column. Can be used

for a single, multiple, or continuous infusion of drug. Can use PCA at bedside or a portable pump.
- *Spinal:* Injected directly into the spinal space. Can be single, multiple, or continuous infusion of drug. Can use PCA at bedside or a special implantable pump, which requires a special procedure.

Types of Pain Medications

It is important to remember that each person not only has an individual response to pain, but has an individual response to how drugs are absorbed and metabolized. In addition, there may be genetic differences that account for varied responses. There is no set dose that will be the same for everyone.

NSAIDs

Aspirin:
- The original NSAID (nonsteroidal anti-inflammatory drug).
- Most commonly used for mild to moderate pain.
- Nonnarcotic.
- Some patients are sensitive to this and/or can develop gastric distress or bleeding.
- Has anticoagulant action, should not be used if the patient is taking anticoagulants.
- Should not be used in children under twelve with viral illness, due to risk of Reye's syndrome.
- Takes about thirty to sixty minutes to work.

Acetaminophen (such as Tylenol):
- For mild to moderate pain.
- No anti-inflammatory effect.
- Does not irritate stomach.
- Patients suffering from chronic alcoholism and liver disease must be followed carefully.
- Takes thirty to sixty minutes to work.

The nonsteroidal anti-inflammatory drugs are for mild to moderate pain. If one NSAID does not work, another can be tried. They can decrease levels of inflammation at the site of tissue injury. They do not cause sedation and respiratory depression, or impair bowel or bladder function.

Many patients are familiar with ibuprofens, such as Nuprin, Motrin, and Advil, or other NSAIDs: Indocin, Naprosyn, Clinoril, Feldene, etc. Patients vary in their individual response to NSAIDs.

Do not use if anticoagulants are being used. Some patients may have gastric distress. (Trilisate is not associated with gastric distress and bleeding.)

It is suggested that NSAIDs be used in concert with opioids to increase analgesia, lessen the need for the opioid, and reduce opioid side effects. There is an analgesic ceiling with the above medications when used alone for pain relief. Beyond a certain point there will be no further analgesic effect.

Opioid Analgesics

These are for moderate to severe acute pain. Remember, the brain naturally produces its own opioids in response to pain. There are areas in the brain, the spinal cord, and other sites in the body that are receptors for opioids.

When you are given an opioid, such as morphine, it rushes to these special opiate receptor sites like a homing pigeon flying to its perch. The binding between the receptor and the opioid relieves and inhibits pain.

Codeine:
- Considered a "weak" opioid.
- For moderate to moderately severe pain.
- Can cause constipation, itching, or nausea.
- Considered the "most frequently prescribed and underprescribed drug," notes Dr. Koo.

Morphine:
- Considered a "strong" opioid.
- For moderately to very severe pain.
- Comes in many forms and doses, including long-acting (e.g., MS Contin); a long-acting rectal form is in production.
- Can cause constipation, itching, or nausea.
- Using other drugs to counteract the side effects and/or adjusting the dose can reduce side effects.
- If there are too many side effects or morphine is ineffective, other opioids are available.
- Morphine is considered the "gold standard" for acute pain relief.
- Effective for about four hours.

- Rarely addictive when used for acute or cancer pain.
- Can be also be injected into a site, such as through an arthroscope into the knee after arthroscopy, to provide pain relief.

Drug tolerance takes place when the dose does not relieve pain or larger doses are needed to achieve the same level of relief. This can happen with certain cancer patients (see Chapter 5).

Physical dependence can take place after a period of treatment with opioids. Just as no doctor would suddenly withdraw many medications such as those for controlling blood pressure, he would not suddenly withdraw pain-relieving opioids. This problem is solved by tapering off the drug slowly.

Dilaudid:

- A derivative of morphine.
- Can be a good answer for those who cannot take morphine because of nausea.
- Effective for about four hours.
- There are multiple ways to administer the drug.
- Available as a suppository.

Methadone:

- A synthetic with similar action to morphine.
- Less gastric distress.
- Effective for about six hours.
- It is a very long-acting drug and it is most difficult to use by untrained clinicians.[28]

Demerol:

- Potent for severe pain.
- Can cause side effects that result in an irritable mood.
- Produces analgesia for only two and a half to three hours.
- Used when other drugs cannot be tolerated.
- Usually not used for chronic cancer pain because of side effects.
- Commonly underdosed and administered on too infrequent a schedule for acute pain.

Fentanyl:

- Commonly used in anesthesia.
- Can be used IV.
- Rapid onset, short duration of effect.
- Used in forty-eight-hour pain patch.

Oxymorphone:
- Very rapid onset, similar to morphine in action, and also available in suppository form.

Levorphanol:
- Longer-acting than morphine.
- Similar duration to methadone and good oral absorption.

Adjunctive Drugs

Adjunctive drugs are used to provide additional pain relief, reduce side effects, or lessen anxiety.

Tricyclic antidepressants:
- On their own, can provide analgesic effect in a few days.
- Helpful for chronic or cancer pain.

Amphetamines:
- Helpful in reducing opioid dose and/or sedation.
- Have pain-relieving qualities.

Antihistamines:
- Have sedating and pain-relieving qualities.

Sedatives, tranquilizers, hypnotics:
- Used for anxiety and also for pain.

SITE-SPECIFIC PAIN CONTROL[29]*

Head and Neck Surgery

Dental Surgery

Most dental surgery is brief and noninvasive, such as extractions, periodontal work, etc.

Anxiety often is a dominant feeling. Antianxiety drugs and/or behavioral modification can be helpful. Mild pain can usually be well managed by NSAIDs such as aspirin, or ibuprofens such as Nuprin, Motrin, or Advil.

More serious dental procedures, such as surgery for impactions and periodontal surgery, can produce severe pain. The pain onset can be delayed by *preoperative* treatment with ibuprofen and/or the application of long-acting local anesthetic during the procedure. Postoperative

*Adapted from the Agency for Health Care Policy and Research, Guideline for Acute Pain Management: Operative or Medical Procedures and Trauma, February 1992. Call (800) 358-9295 to get a copy.

pain often requires the addition of a weak opioid such as codeine, dihydrocodeine, or oxycodone combined with aspirin or acetaminophen.

Some procedures performed on the oral cavity such as wiring the mouth closed after jaw fracture) make oral medication impossible to take. NSAIDs in rectal form can be given or opioids administered in the variety of routes mentioned in this chapter.

Pain that does not respond to treatment may be the result of infection, peripheral nerve injury, or the beginning manifestations of emotional and behavioral changes that might indicate a chronic pain syndrome.

Radical Head and Neck Surgery

These procedures often restrict the patient's oral intake for long periods of time. Prolonged preoperative pain due to radiation therapy and chemotherapy is often present.

Painful swallowing after head and neck, ear, nose, throat, and endocrine surgical procedures may require liquid forms of pain medication and topical anesthetics such as a gel-like Lidocaine. NSAIDs are not recommended for such procedures as thyroid surgery, due to the possibility of postoperative bleeding or compromised airway.

Neurosurgery

Central nervous system patients must be carefully followed for abnormal neurologic signs and symptoms during the postoperative period. Opioid analgesics must be closely monitored.

Pain control should not interfere with the assessment of motor and sensory function and level of consciousness after spinal cord surgery. The use of opioids may be contraindicated, so it falls to the clinician's judgment to balance analgesia and the need to assess neurologic function.

As mentioned earlier, NSAIDs may be contraindicated in this setting.

Epidural and/or local anesthetics can minimize the need for systemic opioids and allow more accurate monitoring. However, this method must be judged carefully and be used by those proficient in administration of this route.

Chest and Chest Wall Surgery

Chest Noncardiac Surgery

Sites include the heart, esophagus, lungs, ribs, chest wall, and breast. Pain can come from surgery and drains or chest tubes. Drains or chest tubes can cause intense irritation and pain at entry sites or deeper. NSAIDs can be used in suppository form to reduce inflammation. For pain related to the surgical procedure, epidural or neural blocks can be used; they must be monitored carefully for side effects.

An example of a coordinated approach to postoperative analgesia is the placement of an epidural catheter prior to anesthesia, which is used to deliver local anesthesia, either alone or mixed with an opioid for analgesia during surgery, and then left in place after the operation for ongoing diluted analgesic. Monitoring and care of these patients must be carried out by specially trained professionals until the patient is switched over to oral analgesics. Epidural PCA can be used in this setting.

Cardiac Surgery

Most cardiac surgery involves opening the sternum and the use of high doses of opioids such as morphine. Close observation is required to distinguish between pain from surgery and pain that may signal cardiac pain, which could indicate a cardiac emergency.

Abdominal and Perineal Surgery

Upper Abdominal Surgery

Gallbladder, biliary system, stomach, intestine, or vascular surgery in the upper abdomen fall into this category.

Operations on the upper abdomen compromise pulmonary function and mobility. As mentioned earlier, decreased ability to move, breathe deeply, or cough can cause life threatening pain-related complications such as buildup of lung secretions that can lead to infection or pneumonia and/or blood clots in the extremities that can cause embolisms.

These patients should receive round-the-clock opioids, either infused or continuously by vein or epidural until they can be switched over to an oral route. PCA is a choice. If health care professionals are untrained in the above techniques, scheduled injections can be given.

Lower Abdominal Surgery

This includes abdominal hysterectomy, cesarean section, hernia repair, episiotomy, urological and gynecological procedures, and hemorrhoidectomy.

The pain management plan is the same as for patients undergoing upper abdominal procedures. Suppression of pain and surgical stress response is more complete with epidural local anesthetic after lower abdominal surgery than upper abdominal surgery.

Many obstetrical or urological procedures are performed using spinal or epidural anesthesia, and the addition of low doses of opioid to a local spinal anesthetic appears to lengthen the duration of pain relief after the local anesthetic effect has subsided.

Patients in active labor must be approached with special expertise in order to monitor the mother for hypotension and to ensure fetal well-being. PCA can be used. After birth, mothers and infants must be monitored for sedation.

Pain after hemorrhoidectomy can be intense and severe. Local anesthetic suppositories can be used for pain control.

Back Surgery

Operations on the spine are frequently performed on patients who have experienced chronic pain. These patients can have an overlay of depression, anxiety, and irritability. They may have a tolerance to opioid medication. Therefore, the dose must be adjusted to fit their needs. In addition, muscle relaxants can offset muscle spasms associated with these operations.

Operations on the spinal cord may include opening the dura around the spinal cord and limit the role of epidural and spinal delivery of pain medications. These patients need to be monitored for neurologic, sensory, motor, and autonomic functioning.

Surgery on Extremities (Orthopedic and Vascular)

The majority of operative procedures on the extremities produce moderate pain. However, some fractures can cause severe pain. The high degree of potential blood clot formation must be considered.

Pain control postoperatively should allow early ambulation and movement. Supplementing opioids with epidural infusion of a local anesthetic can be of benefit for establishing early mobility and lessening the potential for blood clot formation.

Monitoring of orthopedic patients who have external fixation devices or casts for swelling or neurological symptoms is a must.

Soft Tissue Surgery

Surgical procedures involving soft tissue surgery are often done in the outpatient setting. These patients require careful education before and after the procedure. Anxiety can be present due to the unknown outcome of a surgical biopsy (for example, the feared results of a breast biopsy) and may require antianxiety drugs or behavioral assistance. The education and support of these patients is supremely important.

AT-HOME CARE

Too often both inpatients and outpatients are sent home without medication in hand from the hospital pharmacy, or any written form of a pain management plan to follow. Sometimes a doctor writes a pain management plan to follow. Sometimes a doctor writes a prescription for an opioid [morphine-like drug] that is unavailable in a local pharmacy. This can cause unecessary pain and suffering for patients and is poor medical practice.

Proper pain management for patients at home should include:

- At least a twenty-four-hour dose of medication to take home from the hospital pharmacy so that patients have an opportunity to fill a written prescription at their local pharmacy at their convenience. It can be difficult to get a prescription filled and cope with pain at the same time.
- Instructions about the drugs to be taken and how often. This should include any information on side effects and any restrictions about taking medication with or without food, other drugs, alcohol, etc.

If the prescription is for a strong opioid, the doctor should call the pharmacy of the patient's choice to make certain that the drug is available. There have been many reports of patients denied prescriptions by pharmacists who refused to stock strong opioids, due to fear of excessive federal or state regulation and/or theft.

The patient should also be informed of any alternative nondrug treatments for pain control, such as heat, cold, massage, etc.

The doctor or nurse in charge should always give the patient the name and phone number of the doctor or other health care professional who can be contacted, should pain not be adequately managed.

NONDRUG ALTERNATIVES

There are other helpful measures that can be taken to ease your pain. A simple technique is slow rhythmic *breathing* for relaxation.

1. Breathe in slowly and deeply.
2. Breathe in and out slowly and regularly, at whatever rate is comfortable for you. You may wish to try abdominal breathing. If you do not know how to do abdominal breathing, ask your nurse for help.
3. To help focus on your breathing, breathe slowly and rhythmically: Breathe in as you say silently, "In two, three"; breathe out as you say silently, "Out, two, three"—or each time you breathe out, say silently a word such as "peace" or "relax."
4. You may imagine that you are doing this in a place that is very calming and relaxing for you, such as lying in the sun at the beach.
5. Do steps 1 through 3 only once, or repeat steps 2 and 3 for up to twenty minutes.
6. End with a slow deep breath. As you breathe out, say to yourself, "I feel alert and relaxed."

If you intend to do this for more than a few seconds, try to get into a comfortable position in a quiet place. You may close your eyes or focus on an object. This breathing exercise may be used for only a few seconds or for up to twenty minutes.[30]*

Other nondrug pain-relieving techniques include:

- *Massage:* Can help to relieve tension causing pain, relaxing muscles and imparting a sense of well-being.
- *Biofeedback:* A behavioral technique to control and modify emotional, nervous, and muscular responses by altering blood pressure and pulse. Must be taught by a professional.
- *Guided imagery:* Going to another setting created in the mind. For example, remembering a happy event or a visit to the beach, or imagining a setting.
- *Education/instruction:* Informing patients about what will take place, how much pain they may expect, and what type of pain-relieving techniques may lessen anxiety.
- *Prayer:* Some data show that some patients benefit from prayer.
- *Music:* Tapes of music you enjoy can help distract from pain and painful procedures and tests.
- *Video:* Players are small enough today to bring to a hospital room so you can watch distracting movies or tapes.
- *Books:* Sometimes overlooked as a way to escape for a little while.

*Adapted from McCaffery, M., Beebe, A., *Pain: Clinical Manual for Nursing Practice* (St. Louis: C. V. Mosby Co., 1989). Reprinted by permission.

Physical Relief Techniques

- *Heat:* Heat packs or dry/moist heating pads may help to relieve your pain.
- *Cold:* Cold packs or ice help to ease pain, lessen edema, and limit muscle spasm. A rubber glove or ziplock bags can be filled with water and alcohol and put in the freezer. The alcohol keeps the ice mushy, so it can be formed around a body part or small area. Even a bag of frozen peas can be used.

  For some painful areas, ice placed directly on the skin can provide fast pain relief.

  Sometimes alternating heat and cold can provide relief.
- *Cryoanalgesia* (extreme cold): Used to destroy peripheral nerves for long-term relief of pain.
- *Mobilization:* Stretching or strength-building exercises can aid in pain relief. Special compression devices are used to reduce swelling of the extremities.
- *Counterirritant:* A substance that causes irritation in one area to decrease pain in that area or in another, distant area. Also, rubbing, pressure, vibration, etc.
- *TENS* (transcutaneous electrical nerve stimulation): Can provide patient with analgesia at various sites using electrodes.
- *Nerve block:* Transmission of pain can be interrupted using local analgesias. Relief can be temporary or long-acting.

  Sometimes alcohol or other agents are used to attempt permanent relief.
- *Neurosurgery:* Rare, and used only when all other measures have failed.

SUMMARY

You must become your own advocate for pain control in order to change the medical care system. Learn about why pain is a completely different experience in each human being, and therefore should be treated uniquely. Discuss your pain history with your doctor. If you are to undergo a diagnostic procedure, ask if you should expect pain and for how long, and what medication you will be given. Never be subjected to any diagnostic, medical, or surgical procedure without a pain plan worked out between you and your doctor. If your doctor refuses to acknowledge treatment of pain as part of your overall medical care plan, seek a second opinion.

Learn about anesthetics, anesthesias, pain medications, and forms of pain-relief delivery.

Take a pain assessment chart with you to the hospital. Chart your own medications and assessment, using the *Patient's Personal Daily Pain Chart* on page 39.

Become familiar with the Pain Patient's Bill of Rights. *You have a basic human right to adequate pain control.*

Pain Patient's Bill of Rights

You have a right to:

- Have your pain prevented or controlled adequately
- Have your pain and pain medication history taken
- Ask how much pain to expect and how long it might last
- Have your pain questions answered freely
- Develop a pain plan with your doctor
- Know what medication, treatment, or anesthesia will be given
- Know the risks, benefits, and side effects of treatment
- Know what alternative pain treatments may be available
- Sign a statement of informed consent before any treatment
- Be believed when you say you have pain
- Have your pain assessed on an individual basis
- Have your pain assessed using the 0 = no pain, 10 = worst pain scale
- Ask for changes in treatments if your pain persists
- Compassionate and sympathetic care
- Receive pain medication on a timely basis
- Refuse treatment without prejudice from your doctor
- Seek a second opinion or request a pain care specialist
- Your records upon request
- Include family in decision making
- Remind those who care for you that pain management is part of your diagnostic, medical, or surgical care

© 1992 Jane Cowles, Ph.D.

NOTES

[1]Ferrell, B., personal communication, 1992.

[2]Ferrell, B., personal communication, 1992.
Ferrell, B. "Is Pain Adequately Controlled in Patients with Cancer?," *Oncology Nursing Bulletin,* May 1992, 9.

[3]Yaster, M., Bean, J.D., Tremlett, M., Nichols, E., Rogers, M.C., *Textbook of Pediatric Intensive Care* (Baltimore: Williams & Wilkins, 1992), 1518–42.

[4]Yaster, M., Bean, J.D., Tremlett, M., Nichols, E., Rogers, M.C., *Textbook of Pediatric Intensive Care* (Baltimore: Williams & Wilkins, 1992), 1518–42.

[5]Bonica, J., "Management of Pain with Regional Analgesia," *Postgrad Med.J.,* vol. 60, no. 70 (December 1984), 903.

[6]McQuay, H. J., Carroll, D., Moore, R. A., "Postoperative Orthopedic Pain—The Effect of Opiate Premedication and Local Anesthetic Blocks," *Pain,* 33 (1988), 291–95.

[7]Wall, P. D., "The Prevention of Postoperative Pain," *Pain,* 33 (1988), 289–90.

[8]Ngeow, J., personal communication, 1992.

[9]*Horizon,* Hospital for Special Surgery, Winter 1992, 15–16.

[10]Modig, J., Borg, T., Karlstrom, T., et al., "Thrombembolism After Total Hip Replacement: Role of Epidural and General Anesthesia," *Anesthesia and Analgesia,* 62 (1983), 174.

[11]Juul, J., Lie, B., Friberg Nielson, S., "Epidural Analgesia vs. General Anesthesia for Cesarean Section," *Acta Obstetricia et Gynecologica Scandinavica,* 67 (1988), 203–206.

[12]Schwartz, S. I., *Principles of Surgery,* fourth edition (New York: McGraw-Hill, 1984).

[13]Schwartz, S. I., *Principles of Surgery,* fourth edition (New York: McGraw-Hill, 1984).

[14]Koo, P., personal communication, 1993.

[15]Cohen, F., "Postsurgical Pain Relief: Patients' Status and Nurses' Medication Choices," *Pain,* 9 (1980), 265–74.

[16]McCaffery, M., Ferrell, B., "Addiction Fear Increasing Among Nurses," letter, *Journal of Pain and Symptom Management,* vol. 6, no. 6 (August 1991), 351.

[17]Porter, J., Jick, H., "Addiction Rate in Patients Treated with Narcotics," *New Engl. J. Med.,* 302 (1980), 123.
Perry, S., Heidrich, G., "Management of Pain During Debridement: A Survey of US Burn Units," *Pain,* 13 (1982) 267–80.

[18]Houde, R., Kosterlitz, H. W., Terenius, C. Y., Dahlem Konferenzen 1980 (Weinheim: Verlag Chemie), 396.

[19]Koo, P., personal communication, 1992.
Koo, P., "Managing Cancer and HIV-Related Pain: Current Concepts and Future Directions." University of California, San Francisco, School of Medicine, Pharmacological Management of Pain, December 3, 1992.

[20]Marks, R., Sachar, J., "Undertreatment of Medical Inpatients with Narcotic Analgesics," *Annals of Internal Medicine,* vol. 78, no. 2 (February 1973), 173–81.

[21]Donovan, M., Dillon, P., McGuire, L., "Incidence and Characteristics of Pain in a Sample of Medical-Surgical Inpatients," *Pain,* 30 (1987), 69–78.

[22]Max, M., "Improving Outcomes of Analgesic Treatment: Is Education Enough?," *Perspective, Annals of Internal Medicine* 113 (1990), 885–89.

[23]Yaster, M., Bean, J., Tremlett, E., Nicholas, E., Rogers, M., *Surgical and Anesthetic Considerations, Pain, Sedation, and Postoperative Anesthesia in the Pediatric Intensive Care Unit,* 1533.

[24]Oden, R., "Acute Postoperative Pain: Incidence, Severity, and the Etiology of Inadequate Treatment," *Anesthesiology Clinics of North America,* vol. 7, no. 1 (March 1989), 1–15.

[25]Melzack, R., Torgerson, W. S., "On the Language of Pain," *Anesthesiology,* vol. 34, no. 1 (1971), 50–59.

[26]Melzack R., Torgerson, W. S., "On the Language of Pain," *Anesthesiology,* vol. 34, no. 1 (1971), 50–59.

[27]McCaffery, M., Beebe, A., *Pain: Clinical Manual for Nursing Practice* (St. Louis: C. V. Mosby Co., 1989), 40. Reprinted by permission.

[28]Koo, P., personal communication, 1993.

[29]Adapted from the Agency for Health Care Policy and Research, Guideline for Acute Pain Management: Operative or Medical Procedures and Trauma, February 1992. Call (800) 358-9295 to get a copy.

[30]Adapted from McCaffery, M., Beebe, A., *Pain: Clinical Manual for Nursing Practice* (St. Louis: C. V. Mosby Co., 1989). Reprinted by permission.

2

CHRONIC NONMALIGNANT PAIN

Imagine living a life defined by pain.

Normally, pain from a headache, muscle strain, cut, injury, or illness disappears with over-the-counter medications and/or medical or surgical treatment. But what if the pain recurs often or never goes away?

What if your headache returns daily or weekly, with such blinding force that you must stay in bed with the curtains closed for hours or days? What if the pulled muscle remains constantly sore, despite heat, ice, medication, and physical therapy? What if your lower back keeps aching, the pain waking you at night? What if nerves burn under an old incision site on your hand, or the ankle you fractured years ago never stops hurting? Perhaps you have ongoing, intermittent, or continuous pain as a result of arthritis, nerve damage, or other medical problems.

After visits to the doctor, tests, x-rays, blood workups, physical therapy, and prescribed pain-relieving medications, nothing relieves the pain. You are convinced that something must be wrong—how can anything hurt so much and not be wrong?

You seek a second opinion from a neurologist or orthopedic specialist and hear a variation of the same tune. More tests and more drugs. Maybe you hear "We don't understand why you still have pain," "You shouldn't be having this much pain," "It's all in your head," or "You'll just have to learn to live with the pain."

Because your doctors can't provide the instant cure that Americans have always believed possible, you begin to get angry and depressed and even hostile to the doctors who can't give you what you need: pain relief.

Because of the pain, you have difficulty getting to school or work all the time. You curtail your social activities and stop exercising. Maybe your spouse or your children find that a once-normal home life is now filled with a mantra: "I don't feel very good," or "Don't bother Daddy [or Mommy] right now."

You begin to feel guilty because you cannot be a whole, functioning person. You feel resentful when you realize that your pain has taken on a life of its own, and the lives of others revolve around your pain. You don't sleep well, and you feel fatigued, depressed, and alone.

The diagnosis is chronic, nonmalignant pain. Its trademark is pain that interferes with normal life. The theme is suffering. The number of patients affected is staggering.

CHRONIC PAIN AFFECTS MILLIONS

"In 1989, chronic pain syndromes afflicted ⅓ (over 80 million) of the American population. Over 50 million were partially or totally disabled for periods ranging from a few days (e.g., recurrent headaches) to months, and some were disabled permanently. In most patients with back disorders, arthritis, headache and many other chronic painful conditions, it is not the underlying pathology but the pain that is usually the primary factor that prevents the patient from carrying on a productive life. On the basis of the data acquired, it was estimated that in 1989, as a result of chronic pain, well over 550 million work days were lost," writes Dr. John Bonica.[1] Together with health care costs and payments for compensation, litigation, and quackery, Dr. Louis Sullivan, former Secretary of Health and Human Services, notes, in 1992 the cost of chronic pain approached $100 million or more.[2] Aside from the cost in dollars, chronic pain costs patients and their families untold human suffering.

Chronic pain has become so widespread that it is now considered to be epidemic.

DEFINITION OF CHRONIC PAIN

The American Pain Society defines chronic pain as:

> ... persisting beyond the expected healing time and often [it] cannot be ascribed to the effects of a specific injury. Chronic pain may or may not have a well-defined temporal onset, and by definition has not

responded to treatments directed at the etiology of pain. The cause of chronic pain due to non-malignant diseases may be difficult to elucidate, and in contrast to acute pain, there are no signs of autonomic nervous system activity (sweating, increased heart rate, pupil dilation). Because the physician has few objectives which serve to substantiate the complaint of pain, this may sometimes prompt the inexperienced clinician to say that the patient does not "look" like he is in pain. Furthermore, chronic pain may be associated with changes in personality, lifestyle and functional ability and may be associated with symptoms and signs of depression-hopelessness, helplessness, loss of libido and weight and sleep disturbance.[3]

Dr. M. B. Bond writes, "Severe pain, whether acute or chronic, leads to increased self-concern, withdrawal from social contacts, and to reduction in tolerance for external stimuli such as light or sound." He adds:

> Severe or persistent pain alters personality . . . especially tendencies to anxiousness, depression, or preoccupation with health. . . . There has been debate about the extent to which severe and persistent pain alters personality. . . . When pain is severe and intractable without clear prospects of relief, a different range of emotions is aroused. Anger and resentment about failure to gain relief are common, especially amongst those who regard their pain as "meaningless." . . . When pain becomes chronic, an interesting phenomenological change may be observed. Patients begin to talk of pain as alien, as unwelcome though often commanding total attention, as invasive, malign, almost tangible, and coming from without the self.[4]

There is massive disagreement within the health care profession about what *causes* chronic pain. The only agreement is that it is recurring or constant, and that it can be devastating to the sufferer and often mystifying and frustrating for the clinician to treat. Chronic pain is complex in nature. It is often misdiagnosed and often inappropriately treated.

TYPES OF CHRONIC PAIN

In some patients, chronic pain may be linked to *"injuries to the peripheral or central nervous system,"* writes John D. Loeser, M.D., Director of the Multidisciplinary Pain Center at the University of Washington

School of Medicine. He adds, "This type of pain at no time was associated with tissue damage in the part of the body that hurts; although an injury to the nervous system 'heals' by passing from acute changes to those recognized as stable endpoints, the functions of the neurons and axons [nerve cells] lost in the injury are not restored with healing, unlike skin or bone. A chronic alteration of neurological function results."[5]

"Abnormal pain is crazy pain," says Dr. Gary Bennett, a pain expert at the neurobiology and anesthesiology branch of the National Institute of Dental Research in Bethesda. The injury can be the result of an amputation of a limb, mastectomy, diabetes, herpes zoster, shingles, other surgery, or a minor injury such as a brick dropped on an ankle or even a bee sting.[6] Whatever the original cause, the pain results in burning, aching, or flashes of pain that feel like electrical shocks. For some patients, a drop in temperature, a breeze, or a gentle touch on the skin can lead to excruciating pain. The condition is mysterious and responds poorly to conventional treatment.

"Another type of chronic pain is seen in association with *degenerative changes in joints.* Here, there are pathological changes in the parts that hurt, but restoration to normal tissues may not occur. Both acute inflammatory changes and chronic degenerative changes can co-exist. . . . Many patients with arthritis have significant pain, but they usually have measurable impairment as well as disability," notes Dr. Loeser. He adds:

> *Finally, most of the patients with chronic pain have no pathological mechanism known today.* Chronic pain is [the pain of] any patient in whom the persistence of the complaint of pain has exceeded healing time of a recognizable injury. It is not a matter of a stated number of weeks or months or years of pain complaints. The diagnosis of chronic pain of unknown origin should be made as soon as the physician is confronted with pain complaints that have exceeded expectations based upon the injury. Either the wrong diagnosis has been made or something other than the original injury is perpetuating the pain complaints.[7]

LACK OF EDUCATION IN PAIN MANAGEMENT

As mentioned earlier, doctors, nurses, and health care professionals receive little education about pain or pain management in professional schools and hospital residency programs. Hospitals do not make pain management a priority. Compounding the problem for chronic pain sufferers, doctors have been trained to treat pain in the "acute pain model." This means that they look for disease or injury as a cause of the pain, and treat it. However, there is often no disease or injury that can be clearly defined to explain chronic pain. Even if there is an ongoing disease or degenerative process such as arthritis, pain often remains difficult to treat. For the patients who have no clear, definable reason for their pain, life can become intolerable because of the pain, and because they are often treated by the medical community with skepticism that their pain is real.

Rarely is the time taken to perform in-depth psychological evaluations or exhaustive physical tests of patients in chronic pain.

"The inability (or unwillingness) of many health care professionals to spend several hours in the initial work-up of the patient is probably due to the pressure of their clinical practice and lack of interest in, and knowledge of, chronic pain syndrome. Consequently, a correct diagnosis is not made and the patient is started on a course of empirical [nonscientific] therapy which usually ends up in drug toxicity and other iatrogenic [doctor-caused] complications, or in an endless series of hopefulness, disappointment, frustration and hopelessness," writes Dr. Bonica.[8]

Says Dr. Gerald Aronoff, former Director of the Boston Pain Center, who has consulted on more than nine thousand pain patients:

> One of the major criticisms of modern medical practice arises out of what might also be perceived as one of its major strengths. As technology has flourished, physicians have become more highly specialized. With specialization has come the tendency for physicians to treat organ systems, rather than the whole patient. I can say that this is frequently the patient's perception. It is unfortunate that as highly trained as most physicians are, there is often overuse of sophisticated diagnostic equipment and invasive procedures in treating chronic pain syndrome patients. These procedures have not made an appreciable impact on chronic pain syndromes nor alleviated the suffering of such patients.[9]

CONFLICT BETWEEN DOCTOR AND PATIENT

An unfortunate, misinformed, and destructive standoff often takes place between the patient and the medical community. It is easier for health care professionals to be sympathetic to those patients with pain that results from progressive disease, but when it comes to patients who have no apparent medical reason for their pain, sympathy can diminish. McCaffery and Beebe report:

> . . . remarks heard about patients with chronic nonmalignant pain seem angry and derogatory. Many were no doubt born out of the frustration of seeing so many efforts fail, and not knowing what else to do. The following are examples of some of the statements that have appeared in the literature, and have been heard in clinical settings about people who suffer chronic nonmalignant pain:
> Uses his pain
> Addicted
> Enjoys his drugs
> Drug-dependent
> A "crock"
> Plays pain games
> Uncooperative
> Malingering
> Exaggerates his pain
> Controls others with his pain
> Imagines his pain
> Has psychological pain
> Not willing to learn to live with his pain
> Doesn't want to get better
> A pain-prone person
> Etc.[10]

The authors note that the above remarks *"serve no useful purpose in the relationship with the patient. . . .* It is increasingly recognized that collaborating and working with the patient with chronic nonmalignant pain has the potential for far superior results than does being in an adversarial position and waging war with the patient."[11] In addition, they point out that a patient who returns again and again to doctors' offices or emergency rooms with reports of severe pain, but presents with no clear medical findings to explain the pain, elicits negative feelings from the medical staff. Some patients appear not to "look as if they are in pain," despite verbal statements of pain. The staff tends to disbelieve the patient. Many health care professionals view the chronic pain patient who is familiar with the names and doses of his or her drugs with disapproval, while patients who know the dose and type of drug they are taking for heart disease or diabetes are looked upon with favor.[12]

Patients view the medical profession with anger, frustration, and hostility. They feel "If doctors really cared about my pain they'd do something about it," or "There are drugs that can cure pain," or they suffer from self-recrimination: "If the doctors can't figure out a reason for my pain, it must be all in my head," "If I'm in this much pain I must have done something wrong," "If I just ignore it, the pain will go away."[13] The doctor–patient health care relationship often results in an emotional, unproductive pitched battle. The patient says he has pain and the medical community discounts his pain. The patient remains in pain and often "doctor-shops," looking for a doctor who will believe him and provide him with the elusive magic cure.

Patrick D. Wall, M.A., D.M., puts pain in excellent perspective. He writes, *"So long as one person remains in pain and we cannot help, our knowledge of pain remains inadequate."*[14]

The Patient Must Be Believed

As discussed in Chapter 1, the patient is the only authority about his or her pain. *When patients say they are in pain, they must be believed. There is absolutely no way that another person can know or guess what kind of pain the patient is experiencing. Each patient's pain is as unique as his fingerprint. There is no explanation for why the same injury suffered by two people can result in such dramatically different pain experiences.* As discussed earlier, what is known is that there are complex physical, emotional, metabolic, cultural, social, familial, and possibly genetic factors that influence the individual's perception of his pain.

THE MEANING OF PAIN TO PATIENTS

Drs. Donald Price and Stephen Harkins, of the departments of Anesthesiology and Gerontology, Medical College of Virginia, recently wrote about the pain-related affect that involves an elaborate meaning directed toward the implications of having pain. They note, "These meanings are likely to relate to perceptions of how pain will interfere with different aspects of one's life, a reflection of how difficult it is to endure the pain over time, and concern for the long-term consequences of having pain. Persistent pain can be experienced as a serious threat to freedom, significance of life, and ultimately self-esteem." They add, "Pain is often experienced not only as an immediate threat to body, comfort, or activity, but also to well-being and life in general. It is, then, the cognitions and accompanying negative emotions related to the meanings of how pain influences life activities and future that constitute much of the second stage of pain-related affect, a stage that may be thought of as suffering."[15]

Dennis Turk, Ph.D., and Justin Nash, Ph.D., of the Pain Evaluation and Treatment Institute at the University of Pittsburgh School of Medicine, write:

> The person who has a chronic pain condition resides in a complex and costly world that is populated not only by the large number of sufferers but also by their family members, health care providers, employers, and third-party payers (insurance companies, government). Family members feel increasingly hopeless and frustrated as medical costs, disability and emotional suffering increase while income and available treatment options decrease. Health care providers grow increasingly frustrated as available medical treatment options are exhausted while the pain condition worsens. Employers, who are already resentful of growing Workers' Compensation costs, pay higher costs while productivity suffers because the employee frequently calls in sick. Third party insurance payers watch as health care costs soar with repeated diagnostic testing for the same chronic pain condition.[16]

CHRONIC PAIN IS COMPLEX

In the acute pain model, the patient is examined and tested and treated for the medical or surgical problem. The result is usually successful, and the patient goes on with his life. However, as has been pointed out in this chapter, chronic pain does not go away. In addition, much more is happening to the individual than the physical pain. Because of pain, the patient begins to alter the way he approaches life in general. School, job, family, and spouse are affected by the patient's pain.

Drs. Turk and Nash write:

> Like currently available diagnostic approaches, conventional medical treatments are often limited in what they can offer to chronic pain sufferers. Long-term relief is rarely possible, even in cases where the source can be identified. The conventional medical approach, which is very effective in relieving acute pain and pain associated with cancer, relies upon the use of pain relieving medications combined with brief periods of rest to promote healing or to prevent further tissue damage. However, applying this approach to a chronic noncancer pain problem often is ineffective and can even result in additional physical and emotional problems.[17]

Wayne O. Evans, Ph.D., of the Rehabilitation Center for Pain, Community Hospital of Indianapolis, writes, "Most treatment approaches to the problem of chronic pain have been based on a dichotomy between physiological and psychological causes. This dualistic view of the patient greatly reduces the available treatments. It reinforces the tendency to isolate the symptoms from the individual experiencing the pain and to focus treatment on target organs. . . . It is a disservice to the patient not to appreciate the complexities of pain. It is clear that no single theory adequately describes the entire experience of pain involving sensations, affects and meanings." He adds, "Physiological findings demonstrate that there is no possible simple correlation between the degree of tissue damage and the degree of suffering and disability that is experienced by the patient."[18]

Deconditioning of the Body

Persistent pain has an erosive effect upon the patient's life. A vicious circle takes place. The more the patient tries to protect the area of pain by guarding, splinting, limping, or holding a part of the body in strange positions to ward off pain, the more deconditioned and weak the site becomes. Other areas of the body become overdependent and overused. As Dr. Turk points out, "If someone is limping, the leg that gets little use causes loss of muscle strength, flexibility, and endurance. The result is much like a leg that has been in a cast for a long time. When the cast is taken off the muscle is atrophied, which usually requires rebuilding the muscle mass and tone. The other leg, which has the majority of weight on it, becomes strained and overused. Pain may be generated in both legs and/or in other areas."[19] The very method a patient uses to protect a painful area not only results in deconditioning of the area, but makes it vulnerable to muscle spasm, muscle fatigue, and injury due to weakness.

The more a patient restricts physical activity, the more isolated he becomes from the interaction of once-enjoyed exercise, hobbies, friends, family affairs, job, school, parenting, and intimacy.

"Pain often provokes emotions and moods that themselves can exacerbate pain. The fear of the problem's worsening often leads to withdrawal from any involvements. Once a pain problem becomes chronic, psychological factors are of increasing importance in the understanding and management of pain,"[20] writes Clare Philips, Ph.D., of Vancouver, Canada.

The psychological aspects of pain go back to the explanation of Melzack and Wall's "gate control" theory of pain in the central nervous system. As mentioned in Chapter 1, when there is an injury, the brain is flooded with messages. Is the pain sharp, dull, or burning? At the same pain moment, naturally occurring pain-inhibiting (morphine-like compounds) are released, along with pain-related stress hormones that cause the heart rate to increase, the pulse to quicken, and a host of other events to take place. The gate opens and closes, to let the pain message get through to the brain or to restrict it. Other information—such as "How bad is the injury?," "What does it mean?," and "How much sleep has the person had?"—added to individualized psychological, emotional, cultural, and other factors, also affect the ultimate perception of pain.

When a person is anxious, angry, depressed, or feeling helpless or hopeless, the gate is opened, allowing the perception of pain to increase. Dr. Turk points out, "It is likely that psychological factors can *directly* influence physiological responses [for example, muscle tension, blood flow, brain chemicals] that play an important role in the production of pain. Second, psychological factors can *indirectly* influence pain through coping styles that can help maintain the pain disorder, decrease physical conditioning and increase disability." He adds:

> When directly influencing pain-producing physiological responses, psychological factors can either trigger a pain episode (for example, headache) or aggravate an ongoing pain experience (for

example, persistent low back pain). The psychological factors that commonly trigger or worsen pain are thoughts and feelings occurring in response to common life stressors such as family conflict or work pressures. These thoughts and feelings can result from distorted perceptions ("It is my fault if my husband feels angry") and unrealistic expectations ("I must complete all of the day's tasks before the day ends").[21]

A study of the direct effect of thoughts on the physiological pain response was conducted by Turk et al. Muscle tension sensors were placed on the lower back, forearm, and forehead of patients with back disorders, patients with other disorders, and those with no disorders. Patients were asked to describe their pain, state when they last experienced it, and state the last time they were extremely stressed. Just by describing their pain or stress, the back disorder patients had significantly elevated muscle tension in their backs, but none in the forearm or forehead. The other patients had none. Another study, of patients with TMJ (temporal mandibular joint, which causes severe jaw and head pain), demonstrated similar results.[22]

Polypharmacy

Another significant problem that affects many chronic pain patients is the unskilled use of various drugs meant to relieve their pain. It has been pointed out that opioids (morphine-like drugs) are extremely effective for relieving acute pain and chronic cancer pain, and often are underprescribed. However, for some chronic pain patients the use of opioids and tranquilizers on a long-term basis can be inappropriate. Sometimes the drugs prescribed for chronic pain are the wrong drugs, such as those prescribed for pain states associated with injuries to the nervous system. Notes Dr. Loeser, "Other drugs that are specific to neuron function are needed, such as antidepressants, anticonvulsants, or intraspinal opiates."[23]

Some patients desperate for someone or something to relieve their pain will consume a vast array of medications, often with no rhyme or reason, and on a random schedule that further impedes their goal— pain relief.

As McCaffery and Beebe point out, *"Although the term 'drug abuse' may appear in the patient's record, the fact that a person has used narcotics for pain relief for a long time does not necessarily mean he is abusing them."*

Most chronic pain patients take drugs to relieve pain. There is rarely any relationship to the street addict who takes drugs to get high. In addition, "There is some acute pain which can last for months or is recurrent, e.g. weekly or monthly episodes for a few days, or is an exacerbation of chronic nonmalignant pain. Examples of acute pain that may be erroneously treated as chronic nonmalignant pain are sickle cell crisis, burn pain that lasts for weeks or months, weeks or months of pain related to orthopedic injuries following an accident (e.g. unhealed fractures, infected wounds), exacerbation of neck pain from excessive strain, or postoperative pain from a laminectomy performed on a patient for chronic low back pain."[24]

In addition, there are a number of patients with chronic pain who have no history of drug abuse, have not been able to achieve relief, and might be considered as candidates for opioids, notes Russell Portenoy, M.D.

Psychological Factors

"It is becoming increasingly apparent that the understanding and clinical management of pain relies heavily on the appreciation that psychological factors play an important role," note Dr. Lindsey Edwards et al., of University College, London. They add that "there are a number of questionnaires designed to measure specific psychological aspects of the pain experience." The researchers are concerned with the "emotional, cognitive, behavioural and social consequences of long-term pain. In general, negative pain-related cognitions and passive pain-coping strategies have been associated with greater pain intensity, behavioural disruption, heightened distress, poor adjustments and negative affect. . . . As pain persists, pain behaviours and emotions associated with the experience of pain are likely to reinforce the notion of illness and the sick role, thus inhibiting coping and reducing the probability of effective treatment."[25]

The more *passively* a patient copes with chronic pain (feeling overwhelmed, helpless, that nothing can be done to control the pain, etc.), the worse the pain becomes and the higher the level of suffering overall.

"It appears that patients employ a wide variety of strategies for coping with their pain," write Drs. Gregory Brown and Perry Nicassio of the departments of Psychology and Psychiatry at Vanderbilt University. The researchers studied 361 rheumatoid arthritis patients using a self-report questionnaire that assessed the patients' active or passive coping strategies. "While Active Coping was associated with reports of less pain, less depression, less functional impairment, and higher general self-efficacy, Passive Coping was correlated with reports of greater depression, greater pain and flare-up activity, greater functional impairment, and lower general self-efficacy." They add:

> We propose that, irrespective of their type, coping strategies may be classified as adaptive or maladaptive based on their relationship to indices of pain and psychosocial functioning. Specifically, patients may use active or adaptive pain coping strategies when attempting to control their pain or to function in spite of their pain. Alternatively, patients may use passive or maladaptive pain coping strategies when relinquishing control of their pain to others, or when allowing other areas of their life to be adversely affected by pain. Patients who assume a more active role in dealing with their pain also may be less likely to be depressed or helpless than patients who are less active, or passive, in coping with pain.[26]

The Family

"The pain" may become the main focus of a patient's life. The result is that the patient ultimately cannot communicate on any subject but pain. If the patient accepts pain as the main dimension in his or her life, the family is held captive to how well or poorly the patient feels on a given day. The family is like a hanging mobile. One part is out of kilter and forces the rest of the mobile to revolve around the off-balance piece.

Dr. Ranjan Roy, of the Department of Psychiatry, University of Manitoba, Winnipeg, Canada, writes, "The word 'family' in contemporary society calls for precise definition, as there are numerous types of families ranging from the traditional nuclear to the emerging reconstituted and single-parent families to more nontraditional homosexual families."[27]

Lynne Rustad, Ph.D., of the Veterans' Administration Medical Center in Cleveland, notes the effects of chronic disability on families in midlife:

> Although there has been a traditional bias in clinical research toward the study of "the patient" with relative inattention to the

implication of illness for the family, there is now a growing body of clinical and research data which suggests that chronic disease and disability may have a profound effect on the able-bodied spouse. Spouses of patients with chronic pain reported significantly decreased marital adjustment following the onset of pain. The wife of the disabled man must often adjust to significant changes in role and life-style. If she was a dependent person prior to the onset of her husband's illness and tended to see him in a strong, dominant and protective role, the reversal brought about by illness which suddenly places her in the position of caretaker may severely challenge her ability to cope. On the other hand, the wife, forced, with some resentment, into a dependent, passive role before illness, may welcome the opportunity to gain control and "take charge" even when this is detrimental to her husband's rehabilitation and self-esteem. The wife must also cope with anxiety about her spouse's health, and she may live in constant fear that she will do something that will harm him. She may even be afraid to express anger or her own feelings of helplessness, lest she upset her husband. Changes in sexual functioning following illness or disability may further threaten the integrity of the relationship.

The husband of the disabled woman has been relatively neglected by clinicians and researchers alike. In addition to performing his usual work, the husband may be expected to assume additional responsibilities in the home. He may have to devote significantly more time to the physical and emotional care of their children as well as assisting with homemaking tasks. Medical care bills can pose a severe financial burden.[28]

Children of disabled parents appear to suffer from the same lack of professional attention. They may be neglected by the healthy parent or deprived of normal interaction with the disabled parent, may not understand what has happened, and may suffer from anxiety and loss of the role structure of the family.[29]

Turk notes that although psychological factors may influence the perception of pain, they are *not the cause* of the pain. Individuals who feel they have some control over how they cope with pain feel less helpless and hopeless.

EVALUATION OF CHRONIC PAIN

Although many chronic pain patients have visited numerous doctors in their quest for relief, most do not explore their problem in a disciplined fashion. Because the goal is usually the magic single pill or cure, they are set up for failure. Visits to doctors are often made for relief of symptoms, and rarely include the results of scans or tests, a drug history, or discussion about job, family situation, psychological impact, and the level of impairment in their lives. Whether the chronic pain consultation commences with a community doctor who truly understands the complex issues surrounding chronic pain or in a pain clinic setting (see Chapter 11), there are certain assessments that usually should be made by the health professional, depending on the severity of the pain.

Drs. Turk and Melzack provide a note of caution. When health care professionals evaluate pain, they write, "In clinical areas there should be some relation between the instruments selected and treatment. It is unfair to ask patients to complete a lengthy assessment battery or to submit to a large number of laboratory tests if the information collected is simply entered in the patient's file but has no impact on treatment. Insufficient attention has been devoted to customizing treatments to important characteristics of patients."[30]

Wesley Kinney, M.D., and Edward Brin, M.D., of the Department of Anesthesiology at Vanderbilt University School of Medicine, note that the aging population in the United States will continue to contribute to the prevalence of chronic pain patients seen by doctors. They write:

> A fundamental goal shared between the physician and patient—the elimination of incapacitating chronic pain, or the perception of such, whenever possible—is such a crucial task that it should be, and is, addressed in all manner of practice settings. Certain essential elements of the evaluation of the patient with chronic pain must be properly addressed to facilitate an optimal patient outcome, whether the initial patient evaluation occurs in the office of the general or family practitioner, the internist, surgeon, or by a consultant pain specialist in a pain clinic or hospital. The importance of a thorough, accurate evaluation before implementing a well organized, comprehensive treatment for chronic pain patients cannot be over-emphasized, as many of these patients have already

spent considerable time and resources seeking relief, only to receive inadequate results, repeated disappointments, and chronic frustration. Adequate assessment of the patient complaining of chronic pain depends on the solid foundation of a thorough history and a careful physical examination, supplemented as needed with appropriate laboratory, radiological and other ancillary tests. Of particular importance is the thorough assessment and management of any associated psychological, social, or economic or vocational factors, which are common to most chronic pain patients. For many patients these often are a strong contributory cause of their complaints and suffering, if not the predominant cause.[31]

Dr. Loeser writes that suffering "is a personal, private, internal event whose existence can only be inferred." He adds that pain behavior is anything the patient does or does not do because of pain or suffering. "Pain behaviors include such things as talking about pain, moaning, taking pills, going to doctors, lying down, refusing to work, or collecting compensation payments. Like all other forms of behavior, pain behaviors are always real and always measurable."[32]

It is critical to make the distinction between impairment and disability, notes Dr. Loeser. It is clear that the evaluation of chronic pain is multifocal and requires time, attention to detail, and knowledge of the complex physical and psychological factors that make up the tapestry of the chronic pain patient.

Drs. C. Richard Chapman and Karen L. Syrjala, of the Fred Hutchinson Cancer Research Center in Seattle, write:

> The ability to quantify the relevant dimensions of chronic pain is critical for successful patient management because (a) chronic problems are characterized by a relatively stable baseline and the effects of interventions can be rigorously assessed; (b) the dangers of overmedication and repeated surgery can be minimized if treatment effects can be evaluated; and (c) when there is a poor fit between organic diseases and pain behavior, treatment of chronic pain is often a process of rehabilitation that requires documentable increases in activity level and functional capacity if it is to be effective. Furthermore, some patients or some types of problems are better suited for certain types of interventions than for others. Optimal matching of patient and treatment strategy depends on accurate and comprehensive assessment of the pain problem.[33]

Drs. Kinney and Brin suggest the following approach to patient evaluation:[34]

- *Medical history:* Time must be taken to review the patient's history. A careful history tangibly demonstrates to the patient that the physician is committed to being involved and concerned with the patient.

  Such histories can often be lengthy and repetitive. It is important to delineate the cardinal features of the pain, such as time and nature of its onset, the location of the pain, whether or not it radiates, duration of the pain (persistent versus intermittent), any factors that make the pain worse or better, and all relevant characteristics of any associated symptoms. It is important to determine if the patient is in the middle of any workers' compensation case or litigation.

- *Psychological background:* A multitude of internal and external factors may influence how pain is perceived and how pain may influence behavior. These include ethnic, cultural, social, and religious values; personality; learned attitudes; socioeconomic environment; integrity or disruption of physical systems; perception and communication; and prior experiences with pain and its treatment.

- *Availability and appropriateness of support* from significant others, medical professionals, and community resources. These factors impact directly on the perception, severity, and duration of the patient's pain, coping behavior, and motivation and potential for recovery and rehabilitation.

- *An assessment of the patient's pain state:* Severity and chronicity of pain, sensory and emotional components of pain behaviors, and personality and functional capacity.

- *An in-depth history* that includes a life profile and an assessment of family dynamics. (Psychometric evaluations should be reviewed.)

- *Polypharmacy:* Chronic pain patients often take many different medications prescribed by many different doctors. (Patients may be using medications on a hit-or-miss basis, based on misinformation, myths, or misuse. The result may be little pain relief combined with impairment of function, complex side effects, and sometimes drug dependency, tolerance, and depression.) A meticulous inventory of drugs the patient is currently using is crucial in order to discontinue or change medication or alter the schedule.

- *Physical examination:* Essential to the evaluation and treatment of chronic pain is a comprehensive and accurate physical examination. In addition to cataloguing all findings relative to the chronic pain, it is also critical for detecting serious coexisting medical conditions such as vascular, heart, lung, liver, or gastrointestinal disease, nerve disorders, or diabetes. The presence and degree of such disorders or diseases must be taken into account in planning drug therapy, nerve block treatments, and exercise regimens.
- *Neurological examination:* Should include a general impression, as well as specific attention to any area of apparent dysfunction, such as level of consciousness, memory, social interaction, emotional expressiveness, language, dressing ability, and others.

    Any mental status deficit which would preclude the patient's participation in history taking, treatment, etc., should be noted.
- *Cranial nerve deficits:* For example, facial herpes zoster.
- *Motor dysfunction:* Movement, gait, weakness, hand grasp, walking, rising from a chair, dressing or undressing, strength and muscle, and others.
- *Skin sensation testing:* Pinprick, skin changes.
- *Muscle stretch reflexes:* Biceps, triceps, quadriceps, etc.
- *Musculoskeletal examination:* Noting of any joint abnormalities, pain with motion, restriction of range of motion, etc.
- *Trigger point:* A localized area of muscle that is firmer than normal and/or an area which, when tapped, elicits a pain response from the patient.
- *Other findings:* Localized edema (swelling), tenderness, trigger points, which can occur anywhere in the skeletal muscle. (It is suggested that trigger points not be overlooked.)
- *Cutaneous examination:* Characteristic skin changes that cause warm, red skin, sometimes punctuated by periods of intense vasoconstriction, could indicate reflex sympathetic dystrophy. Once established, RSD manifests itself with smooth, glossy skin of the affected extremity, tenderness, swelling, and thickening.
- *Subjective pain behavior:* Moaning, groaning, writhing, crying, or shouting out. This behavior can vary with each patient and with

cultural or ethnic background. Anxiety and depression may markedly increase subjective pain behavior.

- *Objective signs of pain:* These are involuntary. They may include rapid heartbeat, sweating, elevation of blood pressure, or muscle spasm when painful area is stimulated.
- *Abnormal findings:* Muscle atrophy, trigger points, skin temperature. These may indicate that definite physical states underlie the patient's pain.

Other Diagnostic Procedures

MRI (magnetic resonance imaging), CT (computerized tomography), and ultrasonography are the most widely used diagnostic tools. These are noninvasive techniques that display the internal structure of the body with little or no radiation.

- *Myelography:* X-ray of the spinal cord after injection of a contrast medium. Can visualize the contents of the entire spinal canal.
- *Electrodiagnostic studies:* Such as the electromyelogram (EMG), which records the electrical properties of muscle. Ideally, it is used during the first few days following an injury or the onset of symptoms.
- *Nerve blocks:* Can be useful diagnostic tools. The patient is given injections of different concentrations of local anesthetic agents.
- *Thermography:* Involves the identification and analysis of thermal energy patterns in the body. It is safe, accurate, and relatively inexpensive.

Tools for Assessment

John Reeves, Ph.D., a medical psychologist from the Pain Center at Cedars-Sinai Medical Center in Los Angeles, notes that the "0–10 Numeric Pain Intensity Scale and the McGill Pain Questionnaire [see Chapter 1] should be used as part of a basic evaluation process."[35]

Chapman and Syrjala point out their concern that "some testing or instruments demand more of certain patients than they can provide. For example, the McGill Pain Questionnaire uses a vocabulary that is too complex for poorly educated patients. Other tests are not useful with patients from certain cultural subgroups because the tests presume that patients engage in activities that they never perform. Still others are too great a burden for very sick or heavily medicated patients."[36]

The Minnesota Multiphasic Personality Inventory is the instrument that is most commonly used to evaluate the psychological status of chronic pain patients. However, Laurence Bradley, Ph.D., Julie McDonald Haile, B.S., and Theresa Jaworski, Ph.D., note that there are "some problems with this instrument, such as its length and inconsistency of predicting treatment outcome."[37]

The *Survey of Pain Attitudes* is a self-report measuring the following dimensions of pain beliefs: (1) pain control, (2) solicitude, (3) medical cure, (4) disability, (5) medication, and (6) emotion.

Survey of Pain Attitudes

Instructions: Please indicate how much you agree with each of the following statements about your pain problem by using the following scale:

0 = This is very untrue for me.
1 = This is somewhat untrue for me.
2 = This is neither true nor untrue for me (or it does not apply to me).
3 = This is somewhat true for me.
4 = This is very true for me.

1. There are many times when I can influence the amount of pain I feel   0 1 2 3 4
2. The pain I usually experience is a signal that damage is being done   0 1 2 3 4
3. I do not consider my pain to be a disability   0 1 2 3 4
4. Nothing but my pain really bothers me   0 1 2 3 4
5. Pain is a signal that I have not been exercising enough   0 1 2 3 4
6. My family does not understand how much pain I am in   0 1 2 3 4
7. I count more on my doctors to decrease my pain than I do on myself   0 1 2 3 4
8. I will probably always have to take pain medications   0 1 2 3 4
9. When I hurt, I want my family to treat me better   0 1 2 3 4
10. If my pain continues at its present level, I will be unable to work   0 1 2 3 4

11. The amount of pain I feel is completely out of my control	0	1	2	3	4
12. I do not expect a medical cure for my pain	0	1	2	3	4
13. Pain does not necessarily mean that my body is being harmed	0	1	2	3	4
14. I have had the most relief from the pain with the use of medications	0	1	2	3	4
15. Anxiety increases the pain I feel	0	1	2	3	4
16. There is little that I or anyone can do to ease the pain I feel	0	1	2	3	4
17. When I am hurting, people should treat me with care and concern	0	1	2	3	4
18. I pay doctors so they will cure me of my pain	0	1	2	3	4
19. My pain problem does not need to interfere with my activity level	0	1	2	3	4
20. My pain is not emotional, it is purely physical	0	1	2	3	4
21. I have given up my search for the complete elimination of my pain through the work of the medical profession	0	1	2	3	4
22. It is the responsibility of my loved ones to help me when I feel pain	0	1	2	3	4
23. Stress in my life increases my pain	0	1	2	3	4
24. Exercise and movement are good for my pain problem	0	1	2	3	4
25. Just by concentrating or relaxing, I can "take the edge" off my pain	0	1	2	3	4
26. I will get a job to earn money regardless of how much pain I feel	0	1	2	3	4
27. Medicine is one of the best treatments for chronic pain	0	1	2	3	4
28. I am unable to control a significant amount of pain	0	1	2	3	4
29. A doctor's job is to find effective pain treatments	0	1	2	3	4
30. My family needs to learn how to take better care of me when I am in pain	0	1	2	3	4
31. Depression increases the pain I feel	0	1	2	3	4
32. If I exercise, I could make my pain problem much worse	0	1	2	3	4
33. I believe that I can control how much pain I feel by changing my thoughts	0	1	2	3	4
34. Often I need more tender loving care than I am now getting when I am in pain	0	1	2	3	4

35. I consider myself to be disabled   0   1   2   3   4

36. I wish my doctor would stop prescribing pain medications for me   0   1   2   3   4

37. My pain is mostly emotional, and not so much a physical problem   0   1   2   3   4

38. Something is wrong with my body which prevents much movement or exercise   0   1   2   3   4

39. I have learned to control my pain   0   1   2   3   4

40. I trust that the medical profession can cure my pain   0   1   2   3   4

41. I know for sure I can learn to manage my pain   0   1   2   3   4

42. My pain does not stop me from leading a physically active life   0   1   2   3   4

43. My physical pain will never be cured   0   1   2   3   4

44. There is a strong connection between my emotions and my pain level   0   1   2   3   4

45. I can do nearly everything as well as I could before I had a pain problem   0   1   2   3   4

46. If I do not exercise regularly, my pain problem will continue to get worse   0   1   2   3   4

47. I am not in control of my pain   0   1   2   3   4

48. No matter how I feel emotionally, my pain stays the same   0   1   2   3   4

49. Pain will never stop me from doing what I really want to do   0   1   2   3   4

50. When I find the right doctor, he or she will know how to reduce my pain   0   1   2   3   4

51. If my doctor prescribed pain medications for me, I would throw them away   0   1   2   3   4

52. Whether or not a person is disabled by pain depends more on your attitude than the pain itself   0   1   2   3   4

53. I have noticed that if I can change my emotions, I can influence my pain   0   1   2   3   4

54. I will never take pain medications again   0   1   2   3   4

55. Exercise can decrease the amount of pain I experience   0   1   2   3   4

56. I'm convinced that there is no medical procedure that will help my pain   0   1   2   3   4

57. My pain would stop anyone from leading an active life   0   1   2   3   4

As you may remember from Chapter 1, assessment of pain should encourage you to impart as much information about your pain as possible to your doctor and other health care professionals. The more they know about your pain and how it affects you, the better they will be able to individualize your care.

At the Pain and Evaluation and Treatment Institute at the University of Pittsburgh Medical Center,

> . . . [a] central emphasis is placed on individuals and their inter-
> pretation and understanding of their problem, their fears, beliefs
> and attitudes about their symptoms, treatment and the health
> care system. These cognitive variables are important as they will
> influence how patients present their symptoms to families,
> friends, employers, as well as health care providers, respond to
> explanations provided, motivation for treatment and adherence
> to recommendations. It is useful to ask patients about what they
> think is wrong with them, what worries them, what they have
> been told about their symptoms, what problems the symptoms
> have caused them, and how they think their pain should be
> treated. Once a rationale for the persistent pain is presented, it is
> helpful to ask patients and their family members if the explana-
> tion makes sense to them. Similarly, once a treatment has been
> prescribed, the therapist should ask how credible the treatment
> seems and whether they feel it will be effective for them.[38]

There are many instruments designed to measure pain beliefs and coping abilities. It is important for evaluation to understand what patients believe about their pain, what they know about their pain, how pain impacts their life, and how they cope with pain.

One of the many instruments is the *West Haven–Yale Multidimensional Pain Inventory* (MPI), an assessment tool developed by Drs. Kerns, Turk, and Rudy. It measures the impact of pain from the patient's perspective. It is reproduced here at the suggestion of Dr. Robert Kerns, Director of the West Haven Comprehensive Pain Management Center and associate professor of Psychiatry, Neurology, and Psychology at Yale University. Dr. Kerns notes that their center spends "a great deal of effort up front to assess patients as thoroughly as possible to individualize treatment to each patient."[39]

Drs. Kerns and Jacob write, "The West Haven–Yale Multidimensional Pain Inventory is designed to assess the broad domain of psychosocial variables relevant to the chronic pain experience." They add,

"We encourage its use in the context of a multimodal and multidimensional assessment regimen."[40] The pain inventory is divided into three sections. Section 1 evaluates vocational, social/recreational, and family/marital functioning; support and concern from significant others; pain severity; life control with regard to activities of daily living and daily problems; and affective distress. Section 2 assesses patients' perceptions of the responses of others to their demonstrations and complaints of pain. Section 3 assesses patients' reports of their participation in four categories of common daily activities: household chores, outdoor work, activities away from home, and social activities.

Dr. Kerns notes that a videotape and questions precede the main body of the inventory. He adds, "The reader will *not* be able to score this inventory, but it will enable you to review it and think about how the questions apply to you."[41] You may be able to find a health professional in your community or pain clinic to administer the complete test to you and help you to assess and define your pain.

The West Haven–Yale Multidimensional Pain Inventory

SECTION 1
In the following 20 questions, you will be asked to describe your pain and how it affects your life. Under each question is a scale to record your answer. Read each question carefully and then *circle* a number on the scale under that question to indicate how that specific question applies to you.

1. Rate the level of your pain at the present moment.

   | 0 | 1 | 2 | 3 | 4 | 5 | 6 |
   No pain   Very intense pain

2. In general, how much does your pain problem interfere with your day to day activities?

   | 0 | 1 | 2 | 3 | 4 | 5 | 6 |
   No interference   Extreme interference

3. Since the time you developed a pain problem, how much has your pain changed your ability to work?

   | 0 | 1 | 2 | 3 | 4 | 5 | 6 |
   No change   Extreme change

   ____Check here, if you have retired for reasons other than your pain problem.

4. How much has your pain changed the amount of satisfaction or enjoyment you get from participating in social and recreational activities?

| 0 | 1 | 2 | 3 | 4 | 5 | 6 |
No change   Extreme change

5. How supportive or helpful is your spouse (significant other) to you in relation to your pain?

| 0 | 1 | 2 | 3 | 4 | 5 | 6 |
Not at all   Extremely
supportive   supportive

6. Rate your overall mood during the *past week.*

| 0 | 1 | 2 | 3 | 4 | 5 | 6 |
Extremely   Extremely
low mood   high mood

7. On the average, how severe has your pain been during the *last week?*

| 0 | 1 | 2 | 3 | 4 | 5 | 6 |
Not at all   Extremely
severe   severe

8. How much has your pain changed your ability to participate in recreational and other social activities?

| 0 | 1 | 2 | 3 | 4 | 5 | 6 |
No change   Extreme change

9. How much has your pain changed the amount of satisfaction you get from family-related activities?

| 0 | 1 | 2 | 3 | 4 | 5 | 6 |
No change   Extreme change

10. How worried is your spouse (significant other) about you in relation to your pain problems?

| 0 | 1 | 2 | 3 | 4 | 5 | 6 |
Not at all   Extremely
worried   worried

11. During the *past week* how much control do you feel that you have had over your life?

| 0 | 1 | 2 | 3 | 4 | 5 | 6 |
Not at all   Extremely
in control   in control

12. How much *suffering* do you experience because of your pain?

| 0 | 1 | 2 | 3 | 4 | 5 | 6 |
No suffering   Extreme suffering

13. How much has your pain changed your marriage and other family relationships?

| 0 | 1 | 2 | 3 | 4 | 5 | 6 |
No change   Extreme change

14. How much has your pain changed the amount of satisfaction or enjoyment you get from work?

0	1	2	3	4	5	6

    No change   Extreme change
    ____Check here, if you are not presently working.

15. How attentive is your spouse (significant other) to your pain problem?

0	1	2	3	4	5	6

    Not at all   Extremely
    attentive   attentive

16. During the *past week* how much do you feel that you've been able to deal with your problems?

0	1	2	3	4	5	6

    Not at all   Extremely well

17. How much has your pain changed your ability to do household chores?

0	1	2	3	4	5	6

    No change   Extreme change

18. During the past week how irritable have you been?

0	1	2	3	4	5	6

    Not at all   Extremely
    irritable   irritable

19. How much has your pain changed your friendships with people other than your family?

0	1	2	3	4	5	6

    No change   Extreme change

20. During the past week how tense or anxious have you been?

0	1	2	3	4	5	6

    Not at all   Extremely
    tense or anxious   tense or anxious

SECTION 2

In this section, we are interested in knowing how your spouse (or significant other) responds to you when he or she knows that you are in pain. On the scale listed below each question, *circle* a number to indicate *how often* your spouse (or significant other) generally responds to you in that particular way *when you are in pain*. Please answer *all* of the 14 questions.

***Please identify the relationship between you and the person you are thinking of. _____

1. Ignores me.

0	1	2	3	4	5	6

    Never   Very often

2. Asks me what he/she can do to help.

0	1	2	3	4	5	6
Never						Very often

3. Reads to me.

0	1	2	3	4	5	6
Never						Very often

4. Expresses irritation at me.

0	1	2	3	4	5	6
Never						Very often

5. Takes over my jobs or duties.

0	1	2	3	4	5	6
Never						Very often

6. Talks to me about something else to take my mind off the pain.

0	1	2	3	4	5	6
Never						Very often

7. Expresses frustration at me.

0	1	2	3	4	5	6
Never						Very often

8. Tries to get me to rest.

0	1	2	3	4	5	6
Never						Very often

9. Tries to involve me in some activity.

0	1	2	3	4	5	6
Never						Very often

10. Expresses anger at me.

0	1	2	3	4	5	6
Never						Very often

11. Gets me some pain medications.

0	1	2	3	4	5	6
Never						Very often

12. Encourages me to work on a hobby.

0	1	2	3	4	5	6
Never						Very often

13. Gets me something to eat or drink.

0	1	2	3	4	5	6
Never						Very often

14. Turns on the T.V. to take my mind off my pain.

0	1	2	3	4	5	6
Never						Very often

SECTION 3

Listed below are 18 common daily activities. Please indicate *how often* you do each of these activities by *circling* a number on the scale listed below each activity. Please complete *all* 18 questions.

1. Wash dishes.
   0   1   2   3   4   5   6
   Never   Very often

2. Mow the law.
   0   1   2   3   4   5   6
   Never   Very often

3. Go out to eat.
   0   1   2   3   4   5   6
   Never   Very often

4. Play cards or other games.
   0   1   2   3   4   5   6
   Never   Very often

5. Go grocery shopping.
   0   1   2   3   4   5   6
   Never   Very often

6. Work in the garden.
   0   1   2   3   4   5   6
   Never   Very often

7. Go to a movie.
   0   1   2   3   4   5   6
   Never   Very often

8. Visit friends.
   0   1   2   3   4   5   6
   Never   Very often

9. Help with the house cleaning.
   0   1   2   3   4   5   6
   Never   Very often

10. Work on the car.
    0   1   2   3   4   5   6
    Never   Very often

11. Take a ride in a car.
    0   1   2   3   4   5   6
    Never   Very often

12. Visit relatives.
    0   1   2   3   4   5   6
    Never   Very often

13. Prepare a meal.

0	1	2	3	4	5	6
Never						Very often

14. Wash the car.

0	1	2	3	4	5	6
Never						Very often

15. Take a trip.

0	1	2	3	4	5	6
Never						Very often

16. Go to a park or beach.

0	1	2	3	4	5	6
Never						Very often

17. Do a load of laundry.

0	1	2	3	4	5	6
Never						Very often

18. Work on a needed house repair.

0	1	2	3	4	5	6
Never						Very often

Pain Diary

An important part of the assessment is for the patient to keep a *Pain Diary* for two weeks prior to treatment. As has been suggested in other parts of the book, it can be a valuable tool. The patient won't have to rely on memory about when the pain occurred, what caused it to worsen, what kind of stress was present, what was happening with the family, job, or school, how the patient felt emotionally, how many hours he or she slept, what medication was taken, etc. The patient should include the use of the *0–10 Numeric Pain Intensity Scale* in the daily log to rate pain.

The *Pain Diary* should be kept on a twenty-four-hour basis and be as detailed as possible. The patient should not rely on memory. If it isn't filled in frequently, entries can be made at mealtime, but if it isn't filled out on a daily basis, it will be of little help in assessing pain. The following is an example of a diary from the University of Washington Multidisciplinary Pain Center, Seattle.

In addition, a *Family Member/Significant Other Pain Diary* can be most useful to chart the pain of loved ones. As mentioned in this

Chronic Pain Diary

When filling out each daily diary, please keep track of time by rounding off to the nearest 15, 30, 45, or 60 minutes.

Please record the amount and type of medications taken in the application time slot.

Record the intensity of the pain for each hour you are aware of. Use a scale of 0–10 (0 = no pain, 10 = unbearable).

Day _____ Date _____

	SITTING		WALKING AND STANDING		RECLINING		MEDICATIONS		PAIN LEVEL
	Major Activity	*Time*	*Major Activity*	*Time*	*Activity*	*Time*	*Amount*	*Type*	*(0–10)*
12–1 A.M.									
1–2 A.M.									
2–3 A.M.									
3–4 A.M.									
4–5 A.M.									
5–6 A.M.									
6–7 A.M.									
7–8 A.M.									
8–9 A.M.									
9–10 A.M.									
10–11 A.M.									
11–12 A.M.									
12–1 P.M.									
1–2 P.M.									
2–3 P.M.									
3–4 P.M.									
4–5 P.M.									
5–6 P.M.									
6–7 P.M.									
7–8 P.M.									
8–9 P.M.									
9–10 P.M.									
10–11 P.M.									
11–12 P.M.									

TOTAL
HOURS   SITTING_____ WALKING_____ RECLINING___

Pain Scale:
  0 = no pain
  10 = unbearable

(Hours Sitting + Hours Walking + Hours Reclining = 24 Hours)

From Bonica, J., *The Management of Pain,* second edition (Philadelphia: Lea & Febiger, 1990). Reprinted by permission.

chapter and in Chapter 3, the caregivers can often offer valuable information about the impact of pain within the home setting and make
observations of what they think causes their loved ones to have pain
and at what level. They too can make use of the *0–10 Numeric Pain
Intensity Scale.*

TREATMENT

Once the assessment of the physical, emotional, psychological, and
familial measurements have been made, there are certain standard
short-term, mid-term, and long-term goals to be set.

Some patients may need to enter special treatment programs to
deal with dependence on drugs or alcohol. Other patients will need
to be slowly weaned from excessive use of certain prescription
drugs. Others will need changes in medications or how they are administered.

It is suggested that a trained pharmacist with knowledge of
chronic pain management lend his expertise. Only one doctor
should be prescribing drugs for the patient. Medications of various
types may be continued, reintroduced, changed, or added, if appropriate, at a later date.

Psychological Techniques
to Reduce Pain Perception

As mentioned, relaxation techniques can help lessen the perception of
pain, keep stress at bay, and perhaps affect blood flow and muscle
tension. (For the basic relaxation exercise, see page 55.)

Some of the techniques are:

- *Biofeedback:* These techniques can teach control over specific
  body functions—muscle tension, blood flow, and heart rate.
- *Imagery:* Using the basic relaxation techniques, the patient can
  imagine being at the site of a pleasant memory (for example, the
  beach) or create a special scene he can imagine himself being in.
- *Hypnotherapy:* Used by a psychotherapist, it provides intense concentration on a single idea and a suggestion made over and over
  —for example, "I am relaxed, calm, and free of pain."
- *Music:* Can distract the patient from the pain.

Exercise

As mentioned earlier, inactivity can lead to loss of muscle tone and strength and cause stiffness or weakness. The exercise plan must be individualized and initiated only after a complete physical evaluation. The prescription for exercise should take into account the goals for each patient, given his or her diagnosis, age, and ability. Even the most impaired individual can benefit from gentle exercise (e.g., while seated in a chair).

Most chronic pain patients have curtailed activity and therefore suffer from overall deconditioning, weakness, and loss of muscle tone. The goal is to begin gentle stretching and exercises with a *physical therapist.*

Jamie Wilensky, M.D., of Tufts University School of Medicine and Director of Rehabilitation Medicine at Whittier Rehabilitation Hospital in Haverhill, Massachusetts, writes that the objectives of therapeutic exercise may be listed as follows:

1. Develop a sense of good body alignment.
2. Relax unneeded musculature to permit smooth, coordinated, efficient motion.
3. Increase muscular strength as needed to attain and maintain good alignment and function.
4. Achieve flexibility within a normal range.
5. Maintain and increase range of motion.

Exercises are categorized as passive, active, active-assisted, and resisted and resistive. The principles of relaxation and the appropriate exercises are prescribed for patients with persistent muscle guarding and spasm and persistently tense muscles. The learning of relaxation skills constitutes a major treatment modality for pain reduction.

Most of the exercises for soft tissue pain condition involve mobilizing and stretching exercises. After 25 years of age, there is a general and steady loss of flexibility, which is the ability to yield to passive stretch and then to relax. Flexibility helps to facilitate action with minimal resistance to the tissue. Stretching exercises designed to produce a greater range of motion have resulted in significant improvement in flexibility. Lack of flexibility may lead to muscle "brittleness" and soft tissue complaints.

In the treatment of muscle spasms or muscle pain, as a follow-up to heat therapy, a deep sedative massage often enhances the subjective well-being of the patient.

Therapeutic Heat

1. Increases the elasticity of collagen tissue
2. Decreases joint stiffness
3. Produces pain relief
4. Relieves muscle spasm
5. Assists in the resolution of edema, or inflammatory processes. Heat application is not for everyone and must be tailored to each patient.

Therapeutic exercise can be overdone. Pain may result from improper performance, improper diagnosis, or too vigorous a program. Probably the most important adjunct to physical therapy is the relationship developed between the therapist and the patient. A therapy program achieves success only after proper evaluation, the establishment of reasonable goals, individualization of the exercise program, and last and most importantly, motivation of the patient to diligently perform the exercise plan.[42]*

Swimming and aqua-therapy are easy on the body, have no impact, and can be performed by almost anyone. Other exercises that are low-impact could be walking, biking, rowing, and light weight work, depending on the prescription.

Other Techniques

Pain-relieving techniques could include:

- *Occupational therapy:* Patients can learn to regain physical independence on the job and in the home. Learning to increase skills can restore their faith in their ability to perform tasks without fear.
- *Individual, group, or family therapy:* Therapy can help patients feel that they are not alone. They learn how to cope with the mental or emotional factors that lead to increased pain response.

  If family therapy is involved, the patient and family can work together to understand pain and how it affects their lives, how

*Wilensky, J., "Physiatric Approach to Chronic Pain," *Evaluation and Treatment of Chronic Pain,* second edition, ed. Aronoff, G. (Baltimore: Williams & Wilkins, 1992), 176–201.

to reduce stress, and how to change longstanding patterns of reaction to pain.
- *Becoming active:* Distract away from pain. Revisit or start activities, hobbies, volunteering, etc.

Physical

- *Cold therapy:* Can relieve pain by reducing swelling, spasms, and inflammation. Can be used as a counterirritant. Use ice directly on the skin, a mixture of ice/water/alcohol in a bag, ice packs, cold wet packs, or evaporative cold spray.

   Sometimes a combination of heat and cold therapy can relieve pain.
- *Acupuncture:* A therapeutic practice of Chinese origin, consisting of the introduction of fine needles at certain points in the skin along vital "lines of force," where the pain is suffered.

Neurostimulation

- *TENS* (Transcutaneous Electrical Nerve Stimulation): A small, portable electrical charger can be worn on a belt to transmit an electrical signal to an underlying nerve through external electrodes placed on the skin. The signal acts to prevent the pain message from being transmitted to the brain.
- *Peripheral nerve stimulation:* Direct application of an electrode around a major peripheral nerve with the use of an implanted stimulator.
- *Dorsal column stimulation* (spinal cord stimulation): Implanting an electrode directly over the spinal cord.

Other

- *Massage:* Can relax the body, reduce tension, and improve circulation to muscles.
- *Pacing oneself:* Setting realistic goals for work, home, exercise, etc. Make goal charts for one week, one month, six months, for your life, work, hobbies, exercise, etc. Keep a goal diary.
- See Chapter 1 for regional analgesias, local anesthetics, blocks, etc.

Contact some of the chronic pain resources listed at the end of this chapter or at the end of the book.

Specific problems involving chronic pain call for particular approaches to treatment.

HEADACHE

Writes Donald J. Dalessio, Chairman of the Department of Medicine at Scripps Clinic and Research Foundation in La Jolla, California:

> Headache has been called the most common medical complaint of civilized man; yet severe and especially chronic headache is caused only infrequently by organic disease. Hence it may be inferred that chronic headache, for the most part, represents an inability of the individual to deal in some measure with the uncertainties of life, a symptom of an underlying disorder of thought or behavior rather than structural disease of the nervous system. Nonetheless, headache may also be the presenting complaint of catastrophic illness such as brain tumor, cerebral hemorrhage, or meningitis, and to ignore the symptom in this context is to risk the life of the patients. Headache may be equally intense whether its source is benign or malignant.[43]

Recurrent headache affects people of all age groups. Up to 57% of male and 76% of female adolescents and young adults experienced one or more headache episodes within the past month, notes Frank Andrasik, Ph.D., of the Department of Psychology at the University of West Florida. He adds, "The Nuprin Pain Report [discussed in the Introduction] ascertained that up to 157 million days of productive work activity are lost to headache each year for full-time employees. In 1984, headache accounted for about 18 million outpatient physician visits."[44]

Dr. Dalessio notes that "the most common headaches are those associated with mood disorders, particularly depression, anxiety, and emotional tension. Next most commonly encountered are vascular headaches of the migraine type and associated variants including cluster headache. The headaches provoked by fever and septicemia probably rank next in frequency, and then come those due to nasal, and paranasal, ear, tooth, and eye disease. The headaches of meningitis, intracranial aneurysm, brain tumor, and brain abscess, though very important and singularly dramatic, are less common."[45]

The National Headache Foundation estimates that of the forty-five million Americans who suffer from chronic headaches, sixteen to eighteen million have migraines.

Evaluation

Headache History

The history is the most important part of the evaluation of headache patients. Dr. Dalessio writes, "Remember that the diagnosis of headache often depends on the patient's description of his or her symptoms. There are *no* precise clinical tests."[46]

Dr. John Bonica suggests, "In taking the history of headache, the same sequence should be followed as that used to obtain information about pain elsewhere in the body."[47] Some questions he suggests are:[48]

- Is it acute? Sudden? Minutes? Hours?
- Is it subacute? Days, weeks, months?
- Is it chronic? Years?
- What is its period? Constant? Intermittent? Recurrent? Regular? Irregular?

Because frequency and duration are two facts that define the pattern of a headache and help in its diagnosis, care must be exercised to obtain information as to how often the patient has headaches and how long they last.

- In the case of recurrent attacks, how has the frequency and character changed over the years?
- Has the character of the headache changed recently?

Once a general pattern has been established, it is important to focus on a detailed description of each episode.

- Are there warning symptoms, such as feelings of well-being? Depression? Irritability?
- Where is the headache located? Is it unilateral or bilateral? Is it at the front of the head? Is it at the temples? The eyes?
- What is its quality? Pulsating? Pressing? Radiating?
- Is the discomfort felt as sharp? Dull?
- How severe is the headache?
- Is the discomfort mild? Moderate? Severe? Excruciating?

- Is it associated with visual disturbances? Nausea? Vomiting? Generalized malaise? Hyperirritation? Photophobia (abnormal reaction to light)? Phonophobia (abnormal reaction to sound)?
- Are there any other symptoms, such as numbness? Tingling? Paresis (muscle weakness or partial paralysis)? Speech difficulty? Personality changes? Dizziness? Somnolence (sleepiness)? Poor memory?
- Does the headache usually start at a certain time of day? In association with the menstrual cycle?
- Is it abrupt or slow in onset?
- Is it related to social factors? Work? Family? Gatherings with friends?
- What factors bring on the headache? Work? Emotional upset? Stress? Poor sleep? Certain foods? Certain drinks? Strong lights? A change in weather?
- What factors relieve a headache? Lying down? Pacing?
- What forms of therapy has the patient received previously?
- If medication has been prescribed, what is the medication? What is the dose? Has it been effective? What side effects have been experienced?

General History

Information about the general health of the patient and the health of the family should be obtained, including any family history of headache or psychiatric disease. A general medical history should be taken, and the patient should be asked about any injuries and illness involving the head and neck.

In evaluating headache, as with any other chronic pain problem, it is essential to carry out a psychological and psychosocial evaluation. Information should be obtained about the consumption of alcohol, coffee, tea, cigarettes, headache pills, and psychotropic drugs.

Information about the patient's total workload on the job and/or at home should be obtained to determine whether there are interpersonal conflicts in these environments.

The emotional state of the patient should be assessed, including anxiety, depression, and neurotic tendencies.

Each patient must have a careful physical examination and a brief neurologic assessment and any laboratory tests the doctor deems necessary for evaluation.

Quality of Life Function

In addition, a quality of life function and functional impairment assessment should be made. It should include such items as:

- *Social avoidance:* Avoiding social events, sex, travel, etc.
- *Housework activities:* Shopping, housework, cooking, etc.
- *Daily mobility avoidance:* Avoiding lifting, carrying, bending, climbing stairs, etc.
- *Activities avoidance:* Avoiding gardening, hobbies, etc.
- *Daily exercise avoidance:* Standing, walking, other exercise
- *Stimulation avoidance:* Avoiding loud noise, lights, work, etc.
- *Nonverbal complaint:* Grimace, frown, sigh, rubbing the site of pain, etc.
- *Verbal complaint:* Telling a friend, someone in the family, etc.
- *Self-help strategies:* Drinking alcohol, sitting on a hard chair, having back massaged, applying heat, etc.
- *Medication:* Taking a prescribed or unprescribed pill
- *Crying*
- *Distraction:* Distracting yourself by reading, etc.[49]*

Headache Diary/Log

Dr. Andrasik writes, "Pain is a private event and no method yet exists that can reliably objectify any headache parameters. By default, subjective ratings of head pain, sampled throughout the day, have come to be regarded as the 'gold standard.' "[50]

The following (on page 98) is an example of a *Headache Diary,* a patient's self-report of the headache, its duration and intensity, and medication consumption.

Migraine Headache

Of the most common chronic headaches, the two basic types of migraine are classic migraine, which is preceded by an aura and advance warning, and common migraine, which has no aura or advance warning.

Classic Migraine (Migraine with Aura)

A classic migraine is a recurring disorder manifesting with attacks of neurological symptoms, that gradually develop over five to twenty

*Adapted from Phillips and Jahanshahi (Pergamon Press, 1986), 120.

Headache Diary

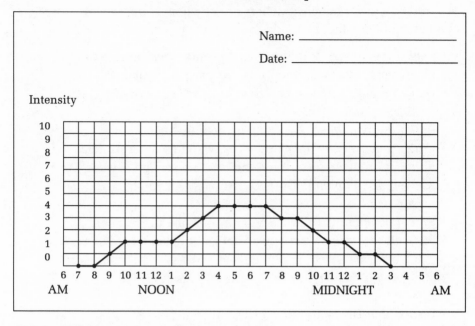

Name: _____

Date: _____

Intensity

6   7   8   9   10 11 12 1   2   3   4   5   6   7   8   9   10 11 12 1   2   3   4   5   6
AM   NOON   MIDNIGHT   AM

 0 No Headache.
 2 Slightly painful—I only notice it when I focus my attention on it.
 4 Midly painful—I can ignore it most of the time.
 6 Moderately painful—I continually notice it but I can continue what I am doing.
 8 Very painful—I can only perform tasks which require little concentration.
10 Extremely painful—it makes it virtually impossible to do anything.

Medication: Each time medication is taken for headache please indicate amount, type, and dosage level.
              Example: 1. Valium, 5 mg.

1. _____   3. _____   5. _____

2. _____   4. _____   6. _____

From Andrasik, F., Burke, E. J., "Assessment of Headaches." Reprinted by authors' permission, 1993. [51]

minutes and usually last less than sixty minutes. It includes headache, nausea, and/or vomiting.

Light or sound phobia, or a combination of these, usually directly follows aura symptoms (a change in visual and sensory perceptions such as flashing lights or dark spots) or occur after a free interval of less than an hour.

The headache usually lasts four to seventy-two hours, but may be completely absent.

A typical classic attack would follow this sequence: warning, aura, headache phase (with symptoms), resolution.

Common Migraine (Migraine without Aura)

This is a recurring headache disorder manifesting with attacks lasting four to seventy-two hours. Typical characteristics are its one-sided location, pulsating quality, moderate to severe intensity, and aggravation by routine physical activity. It is usually associated with nausea and sensitivity to light and sound. Vomiting, diarrhea or abdominal cramps may also occur.

Common migraine is the source of more disability from headache than any other type.

About 25% of patients report a vague, prolonged prodrome (early warning symptom) that precedes the painful phase by hours or a day rather than several minutes. The warning may cause symptoms such as deep fatigue, depression, euphoria, and cravings for certain foods, unusual thirst, etc. The patient usually wants to be in a dark and quiet room.

Exceptionally Severe Migraine

Certain types of migraine can be so severe and painful that the patient seeks help in a doctor's office or an emergency room. Strong opioids, antinausea drugs, tranquilizers, and other medications may have to be injected.

Causes

Migraine attacks may be precipitated by the external environment, including such factors as hot, muggy weather or extreme changes in weather; sudden changes in barometric pressure; smoke-filled rooms; carbon monoxide in cars, houses, or garages; toxic fumes; strong smells; bright flickering lights; or loud noise.

Certain patients may be affected by foods, such as chocolate; aged cheeses; wine, beer, or alcohol in any form; fermented foods; cured meats; pickled herring; some citrus fruits; or Chinese or other food containing monosodium glutamate.

Attacks may be precipitated by physiological factors, such as sleeping late, sleeping too little, missing or postponing meals, menstrual periods, ovulation, taking oral contraceptives, prolonged mental strain, excessive physical exercise, or extreme changes in the pace of living.

Psychological factors may cause an attack—for example, anger, anxiety, fear, guilt, depression, or combinations of some of the above.

Family history may be a factor.

A psychologist or psychiatrist may be able to help patients modify behavior that could cause headaches. Biofeedback, behavioral therapy, meditation, relaxation techniques, and hypnosis may also be helpful.

Prevention

Prevention is the goal in managing migraine. Being aware of what causes attacks and how to avoid them can be important for the patient.

Medications

Seymour Solomon, M.D., of the Montefiore Medical Center Headache Unit, Bronx, New York, says, "Just as there is not a uniformly effective medication, so, too, there is no standard dose. Common errors, made by doctors and patients, are not sticking with a given medication long enough and using too small a dose."[52]

Some of the medications used for migraine to prevent or stop an acute attack are:

Aspirin **(Empirin, Bufferin, Bayer, etc.):**
- Aspirin with caffeine (Anacin)
- Aspirin with acetaminophen and caffeine (Excedrin)
  Some research indicates that aspirin may help prevent migraine.

Acetaminophen **(Tylenol)**

Ibuprofen **(Advil, Motril, Nuprin)**

Prescription pain relievers include:

Beta blockers:
- Propranolol (Inderal)
- Metoprolol (Lo-pressor)

Calcium-Channel Blockers:
- Verapamil (Isoptin, Calan)
- Diltiazem (Cardizem)
- Nifedipine (Procardia)

Anticonvulsants:
- Extended phenytoin sodium capsules (Dilantin)
- Primidone (Mysoline)
- Carbamazepine (Tegretol)

Antihistamines:
- Diphenhydramine hydrochloride (Benadryl)

NSAIDs (**nonsteroidal anti-inflammatory drugs**):
- Naproxen (Naprosyn)
- Indomethacin (Indocin)
- Phenylbutazone (Butazolidin)
- Meclofenamate (Meclomen)

Ergotamine products:
- Cafergot (pill and suppository)
- Wigraine (pill and suppository)
- Migral (pill)
- Bellergal (with phenobarbital)
- Medihaler ergotamine (inhalant)

    It is not advisable to use ergotamine more than two or three times a week, as it can cause rebound headaches.

Other Ergotamines
- Dihydroergotamine (injection)

Antidepressants:
- Imipramine (Tofranil)
- Amitriptyline (Elavil, Endep)
- Doxepin (Sinequan, Adapin)
- Nortriptyline (Pamelor, Aventyl)

Antianxiety:
- Chlordiazepoxide (Librium)

Antinausea:
- Metoclopramide (Reglan)
- Trimethobenzamide (Tigan)

- Hydroxyzine (Vistaril)
- Thiethylperazine (Torcan, Norzine)
- Promethazine (Phenergan)
- Prochlorperazine (Compazine)

Weak Opioids:
- Codeine (Tylenol with codeine)
- Dihydrocodeine acetaminophen and caffeine (DHC Plus)

Others:
- Aspirin, butalbital, caffeine (Fiorinal)
- Acetaminophen, butalbital, caffeine (Fioricet)
- Sumatriptan (Imitrex), auto-injection for migraines.
- Butorphanol (Stadol), nasal spray for migraines.

Other Treatment

Mark Friedman, D.D.S., of Mt. Vernon, New York, is making use of an experimental cold laser technique on the trigeminal nerve for migraines, cluster headaches, and TMJ. He believes it improves circulation to the nerve.[53]

The trigeminal nerve is complex network of nerves that supplies sensation to the face, scalp, nose, teeth, lining of the mouth, upper eyelid, sinuses, and two-thirds of the tongue; controls saliva production and tears; and stimulates the contraction of the jaw muscles used for chewing. Thus far, he has treated ninety patients whose symptoms have not returned.

Cluster Headache

Cluster headaches are attacks of severe, strictly unilateral pain around the eye, temple, or forehead or a combination of these, lasting fifteen minutes to three hours and occurring in frequency from once every other day to eight times a day. They are among the most painful of headaches. There is no warning of an oncoming headache.

They are associated with one or more of the following: nasal congestion, forehead and facial sweating, eyelid edema, constriction of the pupil, drooping of the upper eyelid, and tearing.

Attacks occur in a series lasting weeks or months (so-called cluster periods), separated by remission periods that usually last months or years. About 10% of cluster headache patients have chronic symptoms. Approximately 90% of cluster headache patients are male.

During attacks, patients tend to pace the floor, bang on the wall, cry for help, resist help, or go into a trancelike state. Lying still seems to make the headache worse.

In general, cluster headache patients do not respond as well to psychotherapy as they do to a medical approach.

Some of the treatments for cluster headaches are:

- The use of very hot or very cold applications
- A period of five to ten minutes of violent exercise
- Breathing 100% oxygen (8 to 10 liters/min. for ten to fifteen minutes)
- The prompt use of ergotamine in a readily accessible form, such as two whiffs from an inhaler or an oral, sublingual, rectal, or injectable dose.

In a hospital setting, for extreme cases, some of the other medications used for cluster headaches are:

Intravenous Pentobarbital (Nembutal)

Intravenous Diazepam (Valium)

Steroid Therapy:
- Prednisone
  Should not be continued for more than one month. Use with caution.

Lithium Carbonate:
- Lithium (Eskalith, Lithane, Lithobid)

Calcium-Channel Blockers:
- Verapamil (Isoptin, Calan)

Others:
- Beta blockers, tricylic antidepressants, tranquilizers, NSAIDs, anticonvulsants

Other Treatment

Dr. Seymour Solomon, Director of the Montefiore Headache Clinic in New York, is conducting studies on cluster headaches using topical capsaicin (Zostrix) applied on swabs and inserted into the nasal passage.

Tension Headache or Muscle-Contraction Headache

This form of headache is described as a tight band, pressure, viselike compression, or a cap applied tightly to the head and neck. When the pressure is severe, it becomes pain.

The tension headache often occurs before, during, or after stress. Some headaches may occur in separate attacks, lasting until tension has been relieved However, in some patients the attacks may continue for weeks or months or years.

The factors leading to this state may be physical in nature, such as maintaining a fixed position of the head and neck during such activities as typing, reading, and driving.

Analgesic over-the-counter drugs are helpful in relieving these headaches.

Ergotamine is not helpful unless the condition is part of a combined headache.

The *constant* use of analgesic agents, especially those containing phenacetin and acetaminophen, may perpetuate the headache.

Caffeine intake and tranquilizing drugs should be kept to a minimum.

Antidepressant drugs of the tricyclic type may, after three to four weeks, relieve headaches of this type. Relaxation techniques, biofeedback, and hypnosis may help. Psychotherapy or counseling may help patients gain insights into their tension levels.

See also "Myofascial Pain," below.

Combined Headache ("Mixed Headache")

This type of headache is characterized by throbbing and pounding in conjunction with the viselike pressure of a tension headache. It may be associated with nausea and vomiting in severe attacks, similar to migraine. It may wake the patient from sleep. It may be bilateral or allover head pain. It may occur at the time of menstruation.

Drugs effective in treating migraine symptomatically and prophylactically (in advance of the onset of symptoms) may be helpful for some patients.

Modification of life-style and habits and solution of family and work problems may be helpful. These patients tend to accumulate many drugs and may use them to excess.[54]*

*Definitions and treatments of headaches adapted from Graham, J. R., Bana, D. S., "Headache," *Evaluation and Treatment of Chronic Pain,* second edition, ed. Aronoff, G. (Baltimore: Williams & Wilkins, 1992).

Relative Potency of Headache Drugs on a Seven-Point Scale

1	1 (cont.)	2	3	4	5	6	7
APC	Actifed	Darvon	Cafergot (Cafregon)	Codeine	Demerol	Dilaudid	Morphine
Alka Seltzer	Phenilin	Fiorinal	Cynergen	Empirin Compound with Codeine #3			
Anacin	Motrin	Darvocet N	Flexeril	Leratine			
Aspirin	Idenal	Dolene	Librium	Ponstel			
Bufferin	Dimetapp	Soma	Valium	Talwin			
Cope	Sudafed		Triavil	Percodan			
Empirin	Percogesic		Inderal	Tylenol III (with Codeine)			
Excedrin	Rondec		Tranxene	Empracet			
Midrin			Ergostat	Tylenol IV (with Codeine)			
Nervine			Tofranil				
Norgesic			Elavil				
Parafon			Propranol				
Persistin			Sansert				
Phenaphen			Ergottar				
Robaxisal			Zomax				
Sinutab			Dilantin				
Tylenol			Sinequan				
Vanquish			Endep				
Coricidin D			Seconal				
Corincider							
Arthritic							
Ascriptin							

© Frank Andrasik, Ph.D. Permission granted, 1993.

In addition, some patients can find some relief from some headaches by using heat/cold therapy and gentle stretching exercises prescribed by a physical therapist, or sleep.

Myofascial Pain

Head and neck myofascial pain as a result of tension headache originates from the muscles and the tissues surrounding them. Myofascial pain involves extremely tender or sore spots, which are known as trigger points. Myofascial pain can take place in any part of the body.

Steven B. Graff-Radford, D.D.S., of the Pain Center at Cedars-Sinai Medical Center in Los Angeles, writes, "Orofascial pain is a complex and often puzzling problem that clinicians are faced with day to day."[55]

The Pain Center at Cedars-Sinai Medical Center provides a comprehensive program for treatment of head and neck pain. The following is adapted from their program:

- The myofascial trigger points, extremely tender spots or "knots" in tight shortened muscles, can be active or latent. When trigger spots are active they cause pain to be felt in areas distant from them. This pain is called referred pain and can be reproduced if the trigger point is pressed.
- Stress, strain, and other factors may act upon normal muscle, causing it to become shortened or tight. There will be one or more spots in the muscle that are harder and tighter than the rest of the muscle.
- Muscle shortening and the development of trigger points may occur for many different reasons. Most adults, and even children, have latent or nonpainful trigger points in their muscles from previous strains and stresses. These include physical and psychosocial factors.
- Physical stressors include trauma or accidents—for example, whiplash or a fall—and poor body mechanics or poor postural habits, such as generally poor posture, holding the phone on your shoulder while you talk, watching TV in an awkward position, or sleeping on your stomach.
- Dental problems can play a part: ill-fitting dentures, missing teeth, poor bite, grinding or clenching the teeth.
- Psychosocial stressors are the stress of daily living and interpersonal interactions.

- Stress can cause tension in shoulders and clenching or grinding of the teeth. If it continues, the muscles become sore and tender, resulting in trigger points.
- Although the pain may be in a cheek or over the eyes, the trigger point is typically in a muscle elsewhere.

Treatment

The goals of treatment are to reduce myofascial pain and decrease the trigger point size and activity.

Muscle rehabilitation involves interrupting trigger point activity to allow stretching of the shortened muscle without causing an increase in referred pain. This is important because long-term reduction of the trigger point depends on restoring the muscle to its original length.

Temporary interruption in trigger point can be achieved by a technique known as "spray and stretch." This involves the application of a cold spray to the skin. The cold spray acts to distract the muscle and seems to stop reflex nerve responses that prolong the trigger point activity. This technique will allow the trigger point to let go momentarily, and permit the muscle to stretch out. Trigger point activity can also be stopped by injecting the trigger point directly with local anesthetic or normal saline (salt) solution. Acupuncture, or dry needle insertion, into the trigger points is effective in some cases.

The second step is stretching the muscle out to its original resting length. While the cold spray or trigger point injection lasts, the muscle must be stretched and exercised. Long-term relief can be achieved only if the muscle is restored to its normal length. This reduces the size and sensitivity of the trigger points and thus reduces the amount of referred pain. The patient is sent home with a program of daily exercises to perform.

Prevention

To prevent the trigger points from developing again, contributing physical factors must be changed. This means improving body mechanics —improving poor postural habits (holding the telephone in a hand or using a headset, watching TV in an easy chair instead of on a couch, sleeping on the back rather than the stomach), and having appropriate dental work done—and learning to manage daily stressors through relaxation techniques, biofeedback, or self-hypnosis.

Dr. Graff-Radford, John Reeves, Ph.D., and Bernadette Jaeger, D.D.S., evaluated "25 chronic myofascial head and neck pain patients in a systematic musculoskeletal rehabilitation program. The program emphasized the acquisition of self-management skills through a highly structured interdisciplinary format. Physical and cognitive behavioral therapies were aimed at reducing the factors which perpetuate myofascial pain. The results immediately following treatment, and at three, six and twelve months post-treatment when compared to pretreatment scores, showed highly reliable reductions in self-reports of pain and medication intake."[56]

The National Headache Foundation publishes a chart (beginning on page 109) which explains the symptoms of the majority of headaches.

LOW BACK PAIN

It is estimated that back pain will be experienced by four out of five Americans at some point. It has been reported that back pain is second only to colds as the cause of days missed from work.

Most back pain resolves itself. However, it is estimated that more than eleven million Americans are impaired by back pain.

Complicating the back pain problem is that back pain in many patients has no specific medical cause. Conversely, many individuals who have abnormal scans of their back report no pain. Exactly why some people have back pain and others do not remains a mystery.

John Frymoyer, M.D., and William Cats-Baril, Ph.D., of the University of Vermont, reviewed the literature in more than six hundred publications for the prevalence, incidence, risk factors, and natural history of low back pain and sciatica. They noted an epidemic of low back pain affecting industrialized societies, particularly in the Western hemisphere. Of note is their discovery:

> Despite the incidence and prevalence of low back pain and sciatica, the major factor responsible for its societal impact relates to disability. There is little information to suggest mankind has had more back symptoms or impairments during the past 20 or more years. What has changed is the resultant disability. During that time interval, the number entering the permanently low back disabled has grown at a rate that far exceeds the population growth and virtually all other chronic health conditions. At the present time, the

The Complete Headache Chart

Type	Symptoms	Precipitating Factors	Treatment	Prevention
Hangover Headaches	Migrainelike symptoms of throbbing pain and nausea.	Alcohol, which causes dilation and irritation of the blood vessels of the brain and surrounding tissue.	Liquids (including broth). Consumption of fructose (honey, tomato juice are good sources) to help burn alcohol.	Drink only in moderation.
Allergy Headaches	Nasal congestion, watery eyes.	Seasonal allergens, such as pollen, molds. Allergies to food are *not* usually a factor.	Antihistamine medication or desensitization injections.	Desensitization.
Caffeine-Withdrawal Headaches	Throbbing headache caused by rebound dilation of the blood vessels several hours after consumption of large quantities of caffeine.	Caffeine.	Stop caffeine consumption.	Avoidance of excess caffeine.

© National Headache Foundation. Reprinted by permission, 1993.

The Complete Headache Chart (continued)

Type	Symptoms	Precipitating Factors	Treatment	Prevention
Exertion Headaches	Generalized head pain during or following physical exertion (as in running, jumping, or sexual intercourse) or passive exertion (sneezing, coughing, moving one's bowels, etc.).	Organic diseases, such as aneurysms, tumors, or blood-vessel malformation, are the precipitating factor in about 10% of exertion headaches. The rest are usually related to migraine or cluster headaches already in progress. Cause *must* be accurately determined.	Most commonly aspirin, indomethacin, or propranolol. Surgery to correct organic disease is occasionally indicated.	None.
Trauma Headaches	Localized or generalized pain, can mimic migraine symptoms. Headaches usually occur on daily basis and are frequently resistant to treatment.	Pain can occur after relatively minor trauma. Cause of pain is often difficult to diagnose.	Possible help from anti-inflammatory drugs, propranolol, or biofeedback.	Standard precautions against trauma.
Hunger Headaches	Pain, which strikes just before mealtime, caused by muscle tension, low blood sugar, and rebound dilation of the blood vessels.	Strenuous dieting or skipping meals.	Regular, nourishing meals containing adequate protein and complex carbohydrates.	Same as treatment.

The Complete Headache Chart (continued)

Type	Symptoms	Precipitating Factors	Treatment	Prevention
Temporomandibular Joint (TMJ) Headaches	A muscle-contraction type of pain, sometimes accompanied by a "clicking" sound on opening the jaw. Infrequent cause of headache.	Malocclusion (poor bite), stress, and jaw clenching.	Relaxation, biofeedback, use of bite plate. In extreme cases correction of malocclusion.	Same as treatment.
Tic Douloureux Headaches	Short, jablike pain in facial area, often around the mouth or jaw. Pain lasts from several seconds to several months. Can occur many times a day. Relatively rare disease of the neural impulses; more common in women after age 55.	Cause unknown. Pain brought on by chewing, cold air, even touching face. If condition occurs under age 55, neurological disease, such as MS, may be a factor.	Anticonvulsants and muscle relaxants. Neurosurgery.	None.
Fever Headaches	Generalized head pain that develops with fever. Caused by inflammation of the blood vessels of the head.	Infection.	Aspirin, acetaminophen, antibiotics.	None.
Arthritis Headache	Pain at back of head or neck. Intensifies on movement. Inflammation of joints and muscles.	Unknown.	Anti-inflammatory drugs. Muscle relaxants.	None.

The Complete Headache Chart (continued)

Type	Symptoms	Precipitating Factors	Treatment	Prevention
Eyestrain Headaches	Usually frontal, bilateral pain, directly related to using eyes. Rare cause of headache.	Muscle imbalance. Uncorrected vision, astigmatism.	Correction of vision.	Same as treatment.
Temporal Arteritis	A boring, burning, or jabbing pain caused by inflammation of the temporal arteries. Pain, often around ear, on chewing. Weight loss, problems with eyesight. Rare: affects people over 50.	Cause unknown. May be due to immune disorder.	Steroids.	None.
Tumor Headache	Symptoms include pain that becomes progressively worse; projectile vomiting; possible visual disturbances; speech or personality changes; problems with equilibrium, gait, or coordination; seizures. Condition is extremely rare.	Usually unknown.	Surgery and/or radiation.	None.

The Complete Headache Chart (continued)

Type	Symptoms	Precipitating Factors	Treatment	Prevention
Tension Headaches	Dull, nonthrobbing pain, frequently bilateral, associated with tightness of scalp or neck. Degree of severity remains constant.	Emotional stress. Hidden depression.	Rest, aspirin, acetaminophen, ice packs, muscle relaxants. Antidepressants if appropriate, biofeedback, psychotherapy. If necessary, *temporary* use of stronger analgesics.	Avoidance of stress. Use of biofeedback, relaxation techniques or antidepressant medication.
Common Migraine	Severe, one-sided throbbing pain, often accompanied by nausea, vomiting, cold hands, tremor, dizziness, sensitivity to sound and light.	Certain foods. Use of the Pill or menopausal hormones. Excessive hunger, change in altitude or weather. Bright or flashing lights. Excessive smoking, emotional stress. Hereditary component.	Ice packs. Analgesics such as aspirin, acetaminophen, or ibuprofen. Medications known as vasoconstrictors, such as ergotamine, which constrict the blood vessels. The nonsteroidal anti-inflammatory agents (NSAIDs) may also be helpful. For prolonged attacks, steroids may be helpful.	Avoidance of precipitating factors. Biofeedback. Propranolol. The calcium channel blockers and the NSAIDs may help prevent migraine headaches.

The Complete Headache Chart (continued)

Type	Symptoms	Precipitating Factors	Treatment	Prevention
Classic Migraine	Same as for common migraine, except victim develops warning symptoms. These may include visual disturbances, numbness in arm or leg, the smelling of strange odors, hallucinations. Preliminary reaction subsides within one-half hour and is followed by severe pain.	Same as for common migraine.	At earliest onset of symptoms use of biofeedback or vasoconstrictors can ward off attack. Once pain has begun, treatment is the same as for common migraine.	Same as for common migraine.
Cluster Headaches	Excruciating pain around or behind one eye. Tearing of eye, congestion of nose, flushing of face. Pain frequently develops during sleep and may last for several hours. Attacks occur every day for weeks or months, then disappear for up to a year. 90% of cluster patients are male, most between ages 20 and 30.	Alcoholic beverages, excessive smoking.	Ergotamine or oxygen inhalation.	Steroids ergotamine, methysergide. Small regular doses of lithium carbonate for chronic cluster headaches.

The Complete Headache Chart (continued)

Type	Symptoms	Precipitating Factors	Treatment	Prevention
Menstrual Headaches	Migraine-type pain that occurs shortly before, during, or after menstruation or mid-cycle, at time of ovulation.	Variance in estrogen levels.	Same as for migraine.	Small doses of vasoconstrictors before and during menstrual period. Anti-inflammatory drugs during menstruation may also help. Hysterectomy does not cure menstrual headaches.
Hypertension Headaches	Generalized or "hatband" type pain, most severe in morning. Diminishes as day goes on.	Severe hypertension: over 200 systolic and 110 diastolic.	Appropriate blood-pressure medication.	Keep blood pressure under control.
Aneurysm	Early symptoms may mimic frequent migraine or cluster headaches. Cause is balloonlike weakness or bulge in blood-vessel wall. May rupture or allow blood to leak slowly. A ruptured aneurysm (stroke) results in sudden, unbearable headache, double vision, rigid neck. Victim rapidly becomes unconscious.	Congenital tendency. Extreme hypertension.	If uncovered early, surgery.	Keep blood pressure under control. If aneurysm is severe, surgery may be indicated.

The Complete Headache Chart (continued)

Type	Symptoms	Precipitating Factors	Treatment	Prevention
Sinus Headache	A gnawing pain over nasal area, often increasing in severity as day goes on. Caused by acute infection, usually with fever, producing blockage of sinus ducts and preventing normal drainage. Sinus headaches are rare—migraine and cluster headaches are often misdiagnosed as sinus in origin.	Infection, nasal polyps, anatomical deformities, such as deviated septum, that block the sinus ducts.	Antibiotics, decongestants, surgical drainage if necessary.	None.

estimate is that there are 5.2 million low back disabled Americans; of that number, one half or 2.6 million are thought to be permanently disabled. The resultant socioeconomic impact probably accounts for a very significant component of the direct health care and indirect costs of low back disorders. Most studies demonstrate that between 70% and 90% of the total costs relate to those with disability, either temporary or permanent.

They note the direct costs of services and goods for the delivery of medical care and indirect costs of lost workdays and transfer payments.

Hospital inpatient	$ 6,780,462,000
Outpatient and emergency room	387,980,000
Outpatient diagnostic and therapeutic	2,000,000,000
Physician inpatient	1,707,080,000
Physician office outpatient and emergency room	2,411,690,000
Other practitioner	3,825,119,000
Drugs	191,697,000
Nursing home	4,952,394,000
Prepayment	615,080,000
Non-health-sector goods and services	1,564,651,000
Total direct costs	$24,336,153,000

The researchers report that an estimated 16 million patient visits were made to medical doctors for "sprains, strains, and lumbar disorders in 1990." Also to be taken into account are more than 50 million visits to chiropractors for low back disorders and more than 2 million visits to physical and occupational therapists. More than 4.3 million visits were made to psychiatrists and neurologists. The non-health-sector costs for attorneys related to low back disabilities in the nation as a whole could approach $5 billion.

"The indirect costs for workers' lost wages and homemakers' potential lost earnings could be calculated at $3.6 billion dollars. Based on all analyses, it is quite possible to inflate the total costs of low back disorders into the $75 to $100 billion range."[57]

It is clear that low back pain elicits a huge cost to the patient, the health care system, and the overall economy.

"The feature that distinguishes low back pain from other pain complaints and from most other health issues is the number of days of disability it causes in those of working age,"[58] note Loeser et al.

Peter Polatin, M.D., and Tom Mayer, M.D., of the University of Texas at Southwestern Medical Center, Dallas, note that research shows "50% of low back pain resolves itself in two weeks and 90% resolves within 3 months, and those patients who remain symptomatic after that period have the poorest prognosis and cost the most in health dollars. Surgery may be of benefit for only 1% or 2% of patients with low back episode. It therefore falls within the province of conservative care to manage the majority of these patients."[59]

Deconditioning, discussed earlier, is a result of disuse. Polatin and Mayer point out that low back patients experience

> . . . repetitive microtrauma, spinal soft tissue disruption, and perhaps have surgically precipitated scarring, that has been accompanied by immobilization and inactivity. Muscle atrophy is not as easily discernible in the low back as it is in a dysfunctional extremity, which is readily compared to the unimpaired side. Nevertheless, atrophy of the abdominal flexor and trunk extensor muscle groups have been identified even at a relatively early stage of immobilization. The lumbar facet joints typically involved in back extension become immobilized with inactivity, causing progressive loss of joint function and range of motion. With disuse, cardiovascular fitness and neuromuscular coordination deteriorate. These changes themselves have therefore exacerbated and perpetuated a state of physical disability.[60]

The patient who experiences acute low back pain is usually seen by a family physician. After serious injury is ruled out, a few days of bed rest seem to have the best outcome for low back patients.

"Treatments for acute back pain that do seem to be effective include the following: 'back school,' brief (under 3 days) bed rest, endurance training, and, in very carefully selected patients, diskectomy. Few proven therapies exist for chronic low back pain. Therefore management strategies should not impair the natural healing process," note Loeser et al.[61] In addition, the authors point out that pain-relieving medications and tranquilizers should be used in the acute phase. They point out that some patients have a misconception that drugs heal the tissues, when in fact the drugs block the feeling of pain but do not heal the tissues.

John Sarno, M.D., a professor of Clinical Rehabilitation Medicine at the New York University School of Medicine, has been treating back pain since 1965. His philosophy of the cause of low back pain is unique. Sarno doesn't believe that pain in the back and buttocks (or neck and shoulders), in a majority of cases, is a result of structural abnormalities, arthritis, disk disorders, or the vague group of muscle conditions thought to be due to poor posture, weakness, overexertion, nerve involvements, etc. Sarno believes "that tension affects the circulation of blood to the involved area and that when muscles and their associated nerves are deprived of their normal supply of blood, the result is pain in the back and/or limbs. Specifically, a reduction in local blood supply results in reduced oxygen to the muscles and nerves, which appear to be the direct cause of muscle and nerve pain."[62] He adds that "my studies and clinical experience suggest that these types of pains are brought on by tension. Among most victims of back pain, tension leads to a physical process involving the muscles and nerves of the neck, shoulders, and back. I call this condition the *tension myositis syndrome* (TMS). . . . TMS is generally a harmless physical disorder brought on by tension. Tension, in turn, is primarily the result of certain personality characteristics and is often increased by real life situations."

Dr. Sarno surveyed 100 TMS patients with regard to how their pain started. "Up to 60% said it did not start with a physical incident."

How Pain Began in 100 Patients with TMS

1. Gradual (no physical incident)	60%
2. Accident or injury	40%
3. Strain, lift, push, pull	18%
4. Twist or bend	10%
5. Other	4%

There is probably no other medical condition which is treated in so many different ways and by such a variety of practitioners as back pain. Though the conclusion may be uncomfortable, the medical community must bear the responsibility for this, for it has been distressingly narrow in its approach to the problem. It has been trapped by a diagnostic bias of ancient vintage and, most uncharacteristically, has uncritically accepted an unproven concept, that structural abnormalities are the cause of back pain. . . . Sir William Osler, often referred to as the father of modern medicine, frequently pointed out the importance of emotional factors in physical illness.

... All doctors should be practitioners of holistic medicine in the sense that they recognize the interaction between mind and body. To leave the emotional dimension out of the study of illness demonstrates a bias and is, therefore, poor science.[63]

Evaluation

Patient evaluation of chronic low back pain is the same as that suggested for chronic pain earlier in the chapter. It includes:

Information about the injury
Past medical history
Family history
A complete physical evaluation
Socioeconomic information
Employment data
A pain diary, which includes activity, medication, impairment, etc.
A psychological evaluation

Questionnaires

Some of the low back questionnaires can help the doctor understand the level of impairment. The *Roland and Morris Disability Questionnaire* can help in evaluating how back pain affects your life. Follow the directions on how you think of yourself *today.*

The *Fear-Avoidance Beliefs Questionnaire* asks you about how much physical activities, such as bending, lifting, walking, or driving, affect or might affect your back pain. Follow the directions at the top of the questionnaire.

When all disease and other abnormalities are ruled out, and no definite cause of low back pain can be established, a treatment program must be devised. It is important for patients to know that surgery for low back pain when no clear diagnosis can be made is generally not successful, and may lead to pain as a result of surgery. The advice "Let your pain be your guide to activity" often works against the patient, by providing him or her with a life of inactivity, deconditioning, and ongoing pain.

Roland and Morris Disability Questionnaire

When your back hurts, you may find it difficult to do some of the things you normally do.

These are some sentences that people have used to describe themselves when they have back pain. When you read them, you may find that some stand out because they describe you *today*. As you read the list, think of yourself *today*. When you read a sentence that describes you today circle YES. If that sentence does not describe you today circle NO. Remember, only answer YES if you are sure that the sentence describes you today.

1. I stay at home most of the time because of my back. YES/NO
2. I change position frequently to try and get my back comfortable. YES/NO
3. I walk more slowly than usual because of my back. YES/NO
4. Because of my back I am not doing any of the jobs that I usually do around the house. YES/NO
5. Because of my back, I use a handrail to get upstairs. YES/NO
6. Because of my back, I lie down to rest more often. YES/NO
7. Because of my back, I have to hold on to something to get out of an easy chair. YES/NO
8. Because of my back, I try to get other people to do things for me. YES/NO
9. I get dressed more slowly than usual because of my back. YES/NO
10. I only stand up for short periods of time because of my back. YES/NO
11. Because of my back, I try not to bend or kneel down. YES/NO
12. I find it difficult to get out of a chair because of my back. YES/NO
13. My back is painful almost all the time. YES/NO
14. I find it difficult to turn over in bed because of my back. YES/NO
15. My appetite is not very good because of my back pain. YES/NO
16. I have trouble putting on my socks (or stockings) because of the pain in my back. YES/NO
17. I only walk short distances because of my back pain. YES/NO
18. I sleep less well because of my back. YES/NO
19. Because of my back pain, I get dressed with help from someone else. YES/NO
20. I sit down for most of the day because of my back. YES/NO
21. I avoid heavy jobs around the house because of my back. YES/NO
22. Because of my back pain, I am more irritable and bad tempered with people than usual. YES/NO

23. Because of my back, I go upstairs more slowly than usual.   YES/NO
24. I stay in bed most of the time because of my back.   YES/NO

Score: Total of all items answered YES.

© M. Roland and J. B. Lippincott Co., from *Spine*, 1983. Reprinted with permission, 1993.

Fear-Avoidance Beliefs Questionnaire

Here are some of the things which other patients have told us about their pain. For each statement please circle any number from 0 to 6 to say how much physical activities, such as bending, lifting, walking or driving, affect or would affect *your* back pain.

	Completely Disagree		Unsure		Completely Agree		
1. My pain was caused by physical activity	0	1	2	3	4	5	6
2. Physical activity makes my pain worse	0	1	2	3	4	5	6
3. Physical activity might harm my back	0	1	2	3	4	5	6
4. I should not do physical activities which (might) make my pain worse	0	1	2	3	4	5	6
5. I cannot do physical activities which (might) make my pain worse	0	1	2	3	4	5	6

The following statements are about how your normal work affects or would affect your back pain.

	Completely Disagree		Unsure		Completely Agree		
6. My pain was caused by my work or by an accident at work	0	1	2	3	4	5	6
7. My work aggravated my pain	0	1	2	3	4	5	6
8. I have a claim for compensation for my pain	0	1	2	3	4	5	6
9. My work is too heavy for me	0	1	2	3	4	5	6
10. My work makes or would make my pain worse	0	1	2	3	4	5	6

11. My work might harm my back   0   1   2   3   4   5   6
12. I should not do my normal
    work with my present pain   0   1   2   3   4   5   6
13. I cannot do my normal work
    with my present pain   0   1   2   3   4   5   6
14. I cannot do my normal work
    till my pain is treated   0   1   2   3   4   5   6
15. I do not think that I will be
    back to my normal work
    within 3 months   0   1   2   3   4   5   6
16. I do not think that I will ever
    be able to go back to that work   0   1   2   3   4   5   6

From the *Handbook of Pain Assessment* (New York: Guilford Publications). Permission granted, 1993.

Treatment[64]*

To control symptoms, use ibuprofin, such as Advil, Nuprin, Motrin; acetaminophen, such as Tylenol; aspirin; nonacetylated salicylates, such as Trilisate; or a combination of some of these. Drugs should usually be taken on a scheduled basis, not hit-or-miss.

Understand stress to the back:

- If incapacitated by back symptoms, avoid sitting. Sitting can stress the back mechanically.
- Resume walking as soon as possible, to limit deconditioning.
- Eat and rest standing up.
- Avoid weight gain.

Use other measures at home, such as heat, cold, massage, or ice massage.

To restore function, walk twenty to thirty minutes for every three hours spent lying down during the day.

Build and/or maintain endurance to speed recovery and protect against future injury. (Even patients with the most severe symptoms can be started on standing and walking activities by the third day after the onset of symptoms.) Put a minimal load on the spine. Exercise may include walking, speed walking, swimming, arm-supported stationary cycling, or jogging (for younger patients).

*Adapted from Loeser, J., Bigos, S., Fordyce, W., Volinn, E., "Low Back Pain," *The Management of Pain*, vol. 2, ed. Bonica, J. (Philadelphia: Lea & Febiger, 1990).

Exercise a minimum of five times a week until the symptoms resolve, or for six weeks before starting activities that are more stressful.

The basis for symptom control and physical restoration is the provision of guidelines for safely increasing the overall activity level.

Patients should also be aware of symptom control while attempting to perform lifting or other strenuous work. Patients should learn the proper body movements for good posture—how to rise, sit, etc.

Most importantly, patients with chronic low back pain need to understand that passive treatments do not work. Too much rest and overmedication often can be linked to depression. The goal for chronic low back pain is to be able to tolerate the normal activities of daily living.

"If the risk factors for low back disability are analyzed, it becomes clear that this is not a medical problem. Factors that are important are dominantly psychosocial and include poor health habits, job dissatisfaction, less appealing work environments, poor ratings by supervisor, psychologic disturbances, compensatory injury and history of prior disability,"[65] note Drs. Frymoyer and Cats-Baril.

When those factors affect the patient's life, the use of relaxation techniques, biofeedback, meditation, etc., may be of help when psychological and/or illness behaviors continue to keep the patient incapacitated. Psychological counseling and/or family therapy can also play a role.

New Technique

Epidural endoscopy is a new technique that may shed light on back pain of unknown origin. A tubelike instrument with lenses and a light source attached allows internal examination of the spinal cord and into the brain. Dr. Lloyd Saberski, Director of the Center for Pain Management at Yale, found that some patients who have pain but show no abnormalities actually have hidden inflammation, scars, or injury that can be seen through the endoscope. He then treats the specific area with steriods, saline, or other drugs.

Dr. Saberski does not stop looking for a patient's pain. For example, he asks patients to bring in the shoes they wear regularly. He says, "Many times when scans do not show anything the doctors throw in the towel and tell the patient that 'nothing can be done.'" Dr. Saberski maps a patient's pain using a fluoroscopy technique. It is akin to how a dentist probes teeth for pain. He wants to identify the pain so that rehabilitation can take place.[66]

ARTHRITIS

"Arthritis. The very word evokes a specter of fear and pain. People think of getting old, being unable to get around, and of becoming more dependent upon others. More so than with any other disease, the word *arthritis* carries with it a sense of hopelessness and futility. But the very opposite should be true. All arthritis can be helped," write Kate Lorig, R.N., Dr.P.H., and James F. Fries, M.D., of the Stanford University School of Medicine.[67]

"Arthritis" literally means "inflammation of the joint." There are more than a hundred kinds of arthritis. The most common are osteoarthritis and rheumatoid arthritis.

Arthritis affects more than thirty-five million Americans and stands out as the nation's most crippling disease.

The most common forms of arthritis are:

Osteoarthritis

This is a degenerative joint disease. It is often known as the arthritis that everyone gets as they age.

The tissue that is involved with osteoarthritis is cartilage, found at the ends of bones. A cartilage breakdown can be the result of wear and tear due to the aging process and/or overuse. Weight-bearing and frequently used joints are most affected. The disease is either primary, with no predisposing factors, or secondary, which is associated with trauma, metabolic disorder, or congenital abnormality.[68]

Areas Affected

- The mildest form causes knobby enlargement of finger joints. The ends of the fingers become bony. Other finger joints may become involved. Sometimes there is stiffness, but generally the result is the appearance of the fingers.
- Degenerative joint disease affects the spine in the neck and low back area. Bony growths appear, involving the disks rather than the cartilage at the ends of bones. Usually there is no pain unless nerves in the back are involved.
- Weight-bearing joints are affected—usually the knees and hips.

There can be pain on one side or both. Walking may become impaired.

The condition can commence with deep aching pain that is generalized. Pain can occur during or after using a joint. Joints may be stiff in the morning for a short period of time and/or after resting.

Diagnostic x-rays may show a narrowing of the joint space, the presence of bony spurs, or damaged cartilage.

Most sufferers can obtain pain relief with:

- Aspirin (nonacetylated salicylates)
- NSAIDs (such as Nuprin, Motrin, Advil)
- Acetaminophen (such as Tylenol)
- Indomethacin (Indocin) and other anti-inflammatory drugs listed in the next section (can help some patients)
- Injections of corticosteroids (occasionally helpful)
- Removal of excess fluid from a joint (may help)

Caution should be used with these procedures, as the injections may have an unwanted side effect of actually damaging the cartilage and bone.*

Physical Therapy

As mentioned earlier, deconditioning is the patient's enemy. Loss of mobility, strength, and function from disuse can further impair the patient's life. In addition, favoring a joint such as a knee or hip can weaken the muscles and result in injuries. If the opposite knee or hip is forced into a position of overuse, pain can be generated on the "good" side.

Stretching and exercise can strengthen the bones and ligaments surrounding the affected areas and can greatly improve the range of motion and overall strength. The most helpful exercises are swimming, walking, and biking.

Water exercises using floats, buoyancy vests, kickboards, resistance gloves, and other devices can be beneficial to those patients who do not swim or find swimming too strenuous.

*Gilliland, B., "Arthritis and Periarthritic Disorders," *The Management of Pain*, vol. 2, ed. Bonica, J. (Philadelphia: Lea & Febiger, 1990), 329.

Hydrotherapy warms the joints and improves circulation. In older patients this should be supervised.

Affected joints should not be overused, and high-impact sports should be avoided.

Canes, special shoes, lifts, crutches, etc., can be helpful.

Some patients find that keeping the joint warm helps to reduce the pain. Others find that alternating cold and warm therapies works best.

Surgical replacement of the joint may be necessary for patients whose ability to function is impaired and who experience serious discomfort or disability. Total hip and knee replacements are the most common.

Rheumatoid Arthritis

This is an autoimmune disorder in which the antibodies from the patient's immune system attack the tissues in the joints of the body. *If rheumatoid arthritis is suspected, it is important to seek medical treatment as early as possible.*

Indications

- Morning stiffness in and around the joints lasting at least one hour before improvement is noted.
- Warm and swollen (known as inflamed) joints.
- The wrists and knuckles are almost always involved.
- Lumps may form under the skin.
- Hand grip may be reduced.
- Sometimes there is deformity of the hand.
- Sometimes the knees and joints of the ball of the foot can be involved.
- Any joint may be affected.
- Signs have been present for at least six weeks.

Other Signs

- Fatigue and muscle aches and pains.
- Patients sometimes say they feel as if they have the flu or a virus.
- Fluid buildup around the ankles.
- Anemia.
- Sudden pain and inflammation in a single joint.

Diagnosis

- *Blood tests:* A high sedimentation rate may suggest active rheumatoid arthritis. Rheumatoid factor is most commonly used. Joint fluid is sometimes examined to look for inflammatory cells and/or infection.
- *X-rays:* X-ray evidence of erosion in joints of the hand, wrist, or both. Sometimes x-rays don't show any effects of rheumatoid arthritis in the early stages.

  Baseline x-rays are suggested to compare with future ones to check for changes in bone or joints.

Assessment

The use of the *Arthritis Self-Efficacy Scale* can help health care professionals understand the level of impairment suffered by a patient.

Arthritis Self-Efficacy Scale

SELF-EFFICACY PAIN SUBSCALE

In the following questions, we'd like to know how your arthritis pain affects you. For each of the following questions, please circle the number which corresponds to your certainty that you can *now* perform the following tasks.

1. How certain are you that you can decrease your pain *quite a bit?*
2. How certain are you that you can continue most of your daily activities?
3. How certain are you that you can keep arthritis pain from interfering with your sleep?
4. How certain are you that you can make a *small-to-moderate* reduction in your arthritis pain by using methods other than taking extra medication?
5. How certain are you that you can make a *large* reduction in your arthritis pain by using methods other than taking extra medication?

SELF-EFFICACY FUNCTION SUBSCALE

We would like to know how confident you are in performing certain daily activities. For each of the following questions, please circle the number which corresponds to your certainty that you can perform the tasks as of *now, without* assistive devices or help from another person.

Please consider what you *routinely* can do, not what would require a single extraordinary effort.

AS OF NOW, HOW CERTAIN ARE YOU THAT YOU CAN:

1. Walk 100 feet on flat ground in 20 seconds?
2. Walk 10 steps downstairs in 7 seconds?
3. Get out of an armless chair quickly, without using your hands for support?
4. Button and unbutton 3 medium-size buttons in a row in 12 seconds?
5. Cut 2 bite-size pieces of meat with a knife and fork in 8 seconds?
6. Turn an outdoor faucet all the way on and all the way off?
7. Scratch your upper back with both your right and left hands?
8. Get in and out of the passenger side of a car without assistance from another person and without physical aids?
9. Put on a long-sleeve front-opening shirt or blouse (without buttoning) in 8 seconds?

SELF-EFFICACY OTHER SYMPTOMS SUBSCALE

In the following questions, we'd like to know how you feel about your ability to control your arthritis. For each of the following questions, please circle the number which corresponds to the certainty that you can *now* perform the following activities or tasks.

1. *How certain* are you that you can control your fatigue?
2. *How certain* are you that you can regulate your activity so as to be active without aggravating your arthritis?
3. *How certain* are you that you can do something to help yourself feel better if you are feeling blue?
4. As compared with other people with arthritis like yours, *how certain* are you that you can manage arthritis pain during your daily activities?
5. *How certain* are you that you can manage your arthritis symptoms so that you can do the things you enjoy doing?
6. *How certain* are you that you can deal with the frustration of arthritis?

Note. Each question is followed by the scale:

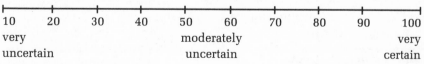

| 10 | 20 | 30 | 40 | 50 | 60 | 70 | 80 | 90 | 100 |
| very uncertain | | | | moderately uncertain | | | | | very certain |

The course of the disease is highly variable. Some patients experience remission; others continue on with active disease. Most patients fall between the two groups. Rheumatoid arthritis has a tendency to flare up and wane into remission.

The cause is unknown.

Treatment

Treatment is often complicated. The goals are to reduce swelling and pain, preserve joint function, and allow the patient to continue daily activities.

Because the inflammation of the joint membrane causes damage to the joint itself, anti-inflammatory drugs are used to reduce the inflammation. Pain medications do not reduce the inflammation.

Be instructed by your doctor in ways to protect joints, sustain muscle strength and tone, cope with stress, modify diet, and learn self-management techniques.

The drugs used include:

Anti-inflammatory Drugs:
- Aspirin
- Ibuprofen (Motrin, Advil, Nuprin)
- Fenoprofen (Fenoprofen Calcium capsules, tablets, Nalfon pulvules)
- Ketoprofen (Orudis capsules)
- Diclofenac (Voltaren tablets)
- Naproxen (Naprosyn)
- Sulindac (Clinoril tablets, Sulindac tablets)
- Indomethacin (Indocin IV, capsule, oral suspension, suppositories)
- Tolmetin (Tolectin)
- Mecolfenamate sodium (Meclomen)
- Piroxicam (Feldene capsules)
- Diflunisal (Dolobid tablets)
- Phenylbutazone (Butazolidin capsules and tablets)
- Choline salicylate (Arthropan)
- Choline magnesium salicylate (Trilisate)
- Etodolac (Lodine)

Anti-rheumatic Drugs:
- Methotrexate (in small doses)
- Gold (Myochrysine, Solganal)
- Penicillamine (Cuprimine, Depen)

- Hydroxychloroquine (Plaquenil)
- Azathioprine (Imuran)

   These may be effective in moderating the course of the disease process. In the past they were used after other measures failed. They may be effective in the early stages of rheumatoid arthritis.

Glucocorticoids:

- Prednisone (Deltasone tablets, Prednisone tablets, Sterapred)
- Dexamethasone (Decadron tablets and elixir)

   Patients should be monitored carefully.

Topical Analgesic Cream:

- Capsaicin (Zostrix) may provide temporary relief of pain. It appears that capsaicin renders the skin and joints insensitive to pain. It can also be used for osteoarthritis.

Some patients who cannot achieve pain control through the use of anti-inflammatory drugs may benefit from weak opioids. A case-by-case evaluation should be made for the use of stronger opioids.

The AngioLaz company makes use of biomagnetics to treat arthritis. The Biomagnetic Treatment Center in Melville, New York, claims their treatment reduces pain and may increase bone growth.

An indication for surgery would be the failure of drugs or therapy to affect the course of rheumatoid arthritis. Patients with severe loss of function may benefit from joint replacement. Removal of joint membrane is sometimes performed.

Self-management

Relaxation techniques, biofeedback, and individual and group therapy may help. Contact the resources listed at the end of this chapter.

Occupational therapy is suggested to learn how to best use impaired joints to improve function, conserve strength, and reduce fatigue and pain. For example, patients learn how to open jars, use spray cans, close containers, sit, stand, walk, climb stairs, and sleep.

Learn about special products that allow easier manipulation of objects by using less force. Some special products are:

- *Extenders* for: Door knob which allow opening of a door with the palm of the hand rather than fingers. Car doors for opening with palm of hand. Key holder devices to allow palm opening.
- *Convenience items:* Enlarged knobs to place on lamps, stoves, etc. Lightweight dishes, pots and pans, luggage, etc.
- *Other:* Foam-wrapped pens, electric toothbrushes. Raised toilet

seats, grab bars in bathroom, stools in showers, shower hoses, long-handled combs and brushes. Velcro closing on clothes and shoes, large rings on zippers. Special beds, joint warmers, home Jacuzzis, heating pad, etc.

• Other tools that can be employed are pain diaries and goal diaries.

It is important to seek the help of a rheumatologist as soon as rheumatoid arthritis is suspected. He or she is the most familiar with early management and treatment options. The Arthritis Foundation or Arthritis Society can be contacted to locate a specialist. The goal is to control the disease, relieve pain, and help the patient to maintain function and activity.

Lorig and Fries note, "People who become good arthritis self-managers have less pain and are more active than those people who feel there is nothing they can do for themselves. The bottom line is that arthritis self-managers feel better."[69]

SUMMARY

No one truly understands why two individuals can suffer the same injury and have such different outcomes. When patients suffer from chronic pain, there often is no easy answer as to why the pain continues unabated. This is especially true when there appears to be no medical reason for the pain. Many doctors treat all pain in the acute pain model, an approach that does not take into account the complex physical and psychological profiles of the chronic pain sufferer.

There is no question that chronic pain affects millions of Americans and costs hundreds of billions in health care and loss-of-job dollars. In addition, the patient may restrict activity, exercise, hobbies, friends, intimacy, and family interaction. Patients who suffer intermittent or continuous chronic pain are often isolated and depressed. There is evidence that psychological factors may contribute to the patient's pain and acceptance of impairment.

A thorough medical history and medical and psychological evaluation must be carried out by the various health care specialties in order to individualize treatment programs for patients.

Patients need to learn how to actively participate in getting well by relinquishing a passive approach to their pain management and regaining interest in exercise, hobbies, family, job, and self-determination.

The following chronic pain resources may be of help.

CHRONIC PAIN RESOURCES

NATIONAL ASSOCIATIONS

American Council for Headache
  Education
875 Kings Highway, Suite 200
West Deptford, NJ 08096
(800) 255-ACHE

American Chronic Pain Association
P.O. Box 850
Rocklin, CA 95677
(916) 632-0922

Arthritis Foundation
1314 Spring Street, N.W.
Atlanta, GA 30309
(404) 872-7100

Arthritis Society of Canada
National Office
250 Bloor Street East, Suite 401
Toronto, Ontario M4W 3P2
(416) 967-1414

Commission on Accreditation of
  Rehabilitation Facilities
2500 N. Pantano Road, Suite 226
Tucson, AZ 85715
(602) 748-1212

National Chronic Pain Outreach
  Association
7979 Old Georgetown Road, Suite 100
Bethesda, MD 20814
(301) 652-4948

National Headache Foundation
5252 North Western Avenue
Chicago, IL 60625
(800) 523-8858 in Illinois
(800) 843-2256 all other states

National Chronic Pain Outreach Association—Local Chapters, U.S.A.

CALIFORNIA
Ann Bradley
16699 Sequoia
Fountain Valley, CA 92708

CONNECTICUT
Rita Fiero
P.O. Box 388
Hartford, CT 06141-0388

ILLINOIS
Rose Kaplan
400 E. Randolph, #2601
Chicago, IL 60601

Becky Heiman
28 Bay Shore Drive
Lacon, IL 61540

IOWA
Joanne Hansen
5706 Fillmore
Davenport, IA 52806

MARYLAND
Janet Hayes
2907 Virginia Avenue
Baltimore, MD 21227

Martha Heinrich
24129 Pecan Grove Lane
Gaithersburg, MD 20879

MASSACHUSETTS
Mary Ellen Davis
14 Robert Dyer Circle
Springfield, MA 01109

Sheryl A. Homer
190 Walnut Street
Stoughton, MA 02072

Alice Zalucki
P.O. Box 1096
Westfield, MA 01086

MICHIGAN
Carl Ebach
46171 Village Green Drive
Belleville, MI 48111

MISSOURI
Lona Polk
P.O. Box 786
Manchester, MO 63011

NEW JERSEY
Dr. Kenneth Leight
Betty Bachrach Rehabilitation Hospital
Pomona, NJ 08240

NEW YORK
Marcelle Simon
44 E. 67th Street
New York, NY 10021

Clare Trautman
37 Beechwood Drive
Glen Head, NY 11545

NORTH CAROLINA
JoAnn Wood
2719 W. Polo Road
Winston-Salem, NC 27106

OHIO
Joann Lovejoy
1855 Doral Drive
Fairfield, OH 45014

Stephanie Smith
4534 Queens Avenue
Dayton, OH 45406

OKLAHOMA
Kathy Rinehart
P.O. Box 55372
Tulsa, OK 74155

SOUTH CAROLINA
June Minske
15 Turret Shell Lane
Hilton Head, SC 29928

TEXAS
Pat Church
5850 Beltline Road, #407
Dallas, TX 75240

VIRGINIA
Joel Friedman
Rehabilitation Medical Center of
  Northern Virginia
5201 Leesburg Pike
Falls Church, VA 22041

Evelyn Purcell
510 Heather Circle
Highland Spring, VA 23075

Arthritis Society of Canada—Local Chapters

ALBERTA
301, 1301—8th Street S.W.
Calgary, Alberta T2R 1B7
(403) 228-2571/2572

BRITISH COLUMBIA and YUKON
895 West Tenth Avenue
Vancouver, British Columbia V5Z 1L7
(604) 879-7511

MANITOBA
386 Broadway Avenue, Suite 105
Winnipeg, Manitoba R3C 3R6
(204) 942-4892

NEW BRUNSWICK
65 Brunswick Street
Fredericton, New Brunswick E3B 1G5
(506) 454-6114

NEWFOUNDLAND
Box 522, Station C
St. John's, Newfoundland A1C 5K4

NOVA SCOTIA
5516 Spring Garden Road
Halifax, Nova Scotia B3J 1G6
(902) 429-7025

ONTARIO
250 Bloor Street East, Suite 401
Toronto, Ontario M4W 3P2
(416) 967-1414

PRINCE EDWARD ISLAND
P.O. Box 1537
Charlottetown, P.E.I. C1A 7N3

QUEBEC
2075 University Street, Suite 1206
Montreal, Quebec H3A 2L1
(514) 842-4026/4848

SASKATCHEWAN
864 Victoria Avenue East
Regina, Saskatchewan S4N 0P2
(306) 352-3312

PUBLICATIONS

Advantage: A Magazine for People with Chronic Health Conditions. 119 N. Fourth Street, #513, Minneapolis, MN 55401.

The Arthritis Handbook by Dr. Theodore W. Rooney and Patty Ryan Rooney. Ballantine Books, 1985.

The Arthritis Helpbook by Kate Lorig and James F. Fries. Addison-Wesley Publishing Co., 1990.

Awareness: Exploring, Experimenting, Experiencing by J. O. Stevens. Real People Press, 1971.

Chronic Pain Control Work Book, Ellen M. Catalano, editor. New Harbinger Publications, 1987.

Chronic Pain Letter. Box 1303, Old Chelsea Station, New York, NY 10011. Bimonthly information for those with chronic pain. Cost: $20/year.

Conquering Back Pain by Judylaine Fine. Prentice-Hall Press, 1987.

Coping with Stress by Donald Meichenbaum. John Wiley & Sons, 1982.

Evaluation and Treatment of Chronic Pain, second edition, by Gerald M. Aronoff. Williams & Wilkins, 1992.

The Fight Against Pain by Charles B. Stacy, Andrew S. Kaplan, Gray Williams, Jr., and by the editors of Consumer Reports Books. Consumer Reports Books, 1992.

Freedom from Headaches by the American Medical Association. Simon & Schuster, 1981.

The Headache Book by Seymour Solomon and Steven Fraccaro. Consumers Union, 1991.

Healing Back Pain by John Sarno. Warner Books, 1991.

Help for Headaches by Joel R. Saper. Warner Books, 1987.

National Directory of Pain Treatment Centers. Oryx Press, 2214 N. Central, Suite 103, Phoenix, AZ 85004, (602) 254-6156.

New Harbinger Publications, 5674 Shattuck Avenue, Oakland, CA 94609, (800) 621-0851, ext. 287. Sells publications on chronic pain.

The Nuprin Pain Report by H. Taylor and N. M. Curran. Louis Harris & Associates, 1985.

Pain and Behavioral Medicine: A Cognitive-Behavioral Perspective by D. C. Turk, D. Meichenbaum, and M. Genest. Guilford Press, 1983.

Pain Resources, 1940 S. Greely Street, #202, Stillwater, MN 55082, (612) 430-3892.

Patient or Person—Living with Chronic Pain by Penney Cowan. Gardner Press, 1992.

"Program Evaluation in Chronic Pain Management Programs." Commission on Accreditation of Rehabilitation Facilities, 2500 Pantano Road, Tucson, AZ 85715, (602) 886-8575.

The Relaxation and Stress Workbook by Marsha Davis, Elizabeth Eshelman, and Matthew McKay. New Harbinger Publications, 1988.

The Relaxed Body by Daniel Goleman and Tara Bennett-Goleman. Doubleday, 1986.

Relief from Chronic Arthritis Pain by Helene MacLean. Dell, 1990.

We Are Not Alone: Learning to Live with Chronic Illness by Sefra Kobrin Pitzele. Workman Publishing, 1985.

NOTES

[1]Bonica, J., *Evaluation and Treatment of Chronic Pain*, second edition, ed. G. Aronoff (Baltimore: Williams & Wilkins, 1992), xx.

[2]Sullivan, L., letter, *American Journal of Pain Management*, vol. 2, no. 4 (October 1992), 223.

[3]American Pain Society, *Principles of Analgesic Use in the Treatment of Acute Pain and Chronic Cancer Pain: A Concise Guide to Medical Practice* (1987), 1.

[4]Bond, M. B., Kosterlitz, H. W., Terenius, L. Y., *Pain and Society*, Dahlem Konferenzen 1980 (Weinheim: Verlag Chemie GmbH), 53–62.

[5]Loeser, J. D., "What Is Chronic Pain?," *Theoretical Medicine* 12 (1991), 213–25.

[6]Bennett, G., "Experimental Models of Painful Peripheral Neuropathies," *NIPS*, vol. 5 (June 1990), 128–33.

[7]Loeser, J. D., "What Is Chronic Pain?," *Theoretical Medicine* 12 (1991), 213–25.

[8]Bonica, J., *Evaluation and Treatment of Chronic Pain*, second edition, ed. G. Aronoff (Baltimore: Williams & Wilkins, 1992), xxiii.

[9]Aronoff, G., *Evaluation and Treatment of Chronic Pain*, second edition (Baltimore: Williams & Wilkins, 1992), Preface.

[10]McCaffery, M., Beebe, R. N., *Pain: Clinical Manual for Nursing Practice* (St. Louis: C. V. Mosby, 1989), 235.

[11]McCaffery, M., Beebe, R. N., *Pain: Clinical Manual for Nursing Practice* (St. Louis: C. V. Mosby, 1989), 235.

[12]McCaffery, M., Beebe, R. N., *Pain: Clinical Manual for Nursing Practice* (St. Louis: C. V. Mosby, 1989), 235.

[13]International Pain Foundation, "About Living with Chronic Pain" (Seattle: Channing Bete Company, 1987).

[14]Wall, P., *Textbook of Pain*, ed. Wall, P., Melzack, R. (Churchill Livingstone, 1984), 1.

[15]Price, D. D., Harkins, S. W., "The Affective-Motivational Dimension of Pain: A Two-Stage Model," *Journal American Pain Society*, vol. 1, no. 4 (Winter 1992), 229–39.

[16]Turk, D., Nash, J., "Chronic Pain: The Interface of Mind and Body, Mind/Body Medicine," ed. Goleman and Gurin. In press.

[17]Turk, D., Nash, J., "Chronic Pain: The Interface of Mind and Body, Mind/Body Medicine," ed. Goleman and Gurin. In press.

[18]Evans, W., "Chronic Pain Syndrome: Evaluation and Treatment," *Indiana Medicine*, May 1984, 370.

[19]Turk, D., personal communication, 1993.

[20]Philips, C., *The Psychological Management of Chronic Pain: A Treatment Manual* (New York: Springer Publishing Co., 1988), 4.

[21]Turk, D., Nash, J., "Chronic Pain: The Interface of Mind and Body, Mind/Body Medicine," ed. Goleman and Gurin. In press.

[22]Turk, D., Nash, J., "Chronic Pain: The Interface of Mind and Body, Mind/Body Medicine," ed. Goleman and Gurin. In press.

[23]Loeser, J. D., "What Is Chronic Pain?," *Theoretical Medicine,* 12 (1991), 213–25.

[24]McCaffery, M., Beebe, R. N., *Pain: Clinical Manual for Nursing Practice* (St. Louis: C. V. Mosby, 1989), 235.

[25]Edwards, L., Pearce, S., Turner-Stokes, L., Jones, A., "The Pain Beliefs Questionnaire: An Investigation of Beliefs in the Causes and Consequences of Pain," *Pain,* 51 (1992), 267–72.

[26]Brown, G. K., Nicassio, P. M., "Development of a Questionnaire for the Assessment of Active and Passive Coping Strategies in Chronic Pain Patients, *Pain,* 31 (1987), 53–64.

[27]Roy, R., "Impact of Chronic Pain on Marital Partners: Systems Perspective," *Proceedings of the Fifth World Congress on Pain,* 1988, ed. Dubner, Gebhart, and Bond (Elsevier Science Publishers BV), 286.

[28]Rustad, L., "Family Adjustment to Chronic Illness and Disability in Mid-life," *Chronic Illness and Disability Through the Life Span: Effects on Self and Family,* ed. Eisenberg, M., Sutkin, L., Jansen, M. (New York: Springer Publishing Co., 1984), 222–42.

[29]Rustad, L., "Family Adjustment to Chronic Illness and Disability in Mid-life," *Chronic Illness and Disability Through the Life Span: Effects on Self and Family,* ed. Eisenberg, M., Sutkin, L., Jansen, M. (New York: Springer Publishing Co., 1984), 222–42.

[30]Turk, D., Melzack, R., "Trends and Future Directions in Human Pain Assessment," *Handbook of Pain Assessment,* ed. Turk and Melzack (New York: Guilford Press, 1992), 473–79.

[31]Kinney, W. W., Brin, E. D., "Diagnostic Evaluation and Management of the Patient with Chronic Pain," *Evaluation and Treatment of Chronic Pain,* second edition, ed. Aronoff, G. (Baltimore: Williams & Wilkins, 1992), 26–55.

[32]Loeser, J. D., "Disability, Pain and Suffering," *Clinical Neurosurgery,* 1989, vol. 35, 398–408.

[33]Chapman, C. R., Syrjala, K. L., "Measurement of Pain," *The Management of Pain,* second edition, ed. Bonica, J. (Philadelphia: Lea & Febiger, 1990), 580.

[34]Adapted from Kinney, W. W., Brin, E. D., "Diagnostic Evaluation and Management of the Patient with Chronic Pain," *Evaluation and Treatment of Chronic Pain,* second edition, ed. Aronoff, G. (Baltimore: Williams & Wilkins, 1992).

[35]Reeves, J., personal communication, 1993.

[36]Chapman, C. R., Syrjala, K. L., "Measurement of Pain," *The Management of Pain,* second edition, ed. Bonica, J. (Philadelphia: Lea & Febiger, 1990), 580.

[37]Bradley, L., McDonald Haile, J., Jaworski, T., "Assessment of Psychological Status Using Interviews and Self-Report Instruments," *Handbook of Pain Assessment,* ed. Turk, D., Melzack, R. (New York: Guilford Press, 1992), 203–204.

[38]Turk, D., Rudy, R., "A Cognitive-Behavioral Perspective on Chronic Pain: Beyond the Scalpel and Syringe." In press.

[39]Kerns, R. D., personal communication, 1993.

[40]Kerns, R. D., Jacob, M. C., "Assessment of the Psychosocial Context of the Experience of Chronic Pain," *Handbook of Pain Assessment,* ed. Turk, D., Melzack, R. (New York: Guilford Press, 1992), 235–53.

[41]Kerns, R. D., personal communication, 1993.

[42]Wilensky, J., "Physiatric Approach to Chronic Pain," *Evaluation and Treatment of Chronic Pain,* second edition, ed. Aronoff, G. (Baltimore: Williams & Wilkins, 1992), 176–201.

[43]Dalessio, D. J., "A Clinical Classification of Headache," *Wolff's Headache and Other Head Pain,* fifth edition, ed. Dalessio (Oxford University Press, 1987), 3.

[44]F. Andrasik, "Assessment of Patients with Headaches," *Handbook of Pain Assessment,* ed. Turk, D., Melzack, R. (New York: Guilford Press, 1992), 344.

[45]Dalessio, D. J., "A Clinical Classification of Headache," *Wolff's Headache and Other Head Pain,* fifth edition, ed. Dalessio (Oxford University Press, 1987), 3.

[46]Dalessio, D. J., "A Clinical Classification of Headache," *Wolff's Headache and Other Head Pain,* fifth edition, ed. Dalessio (Oxford University Press, 1987), 3.

[47]Bonica, J., *Evaluation and Treatment of Chronic Pain,* second edition, ed. Aronoff, G. (Baltimore: Williams & Wilkins, 1992), xx.

[48]Bonica, J., *The Management of Pain* (Philadelphia: Lea & Febiger, 1990).

[49]Phillips and Jahanshahi, from *Evaluation and Treatment of Chronic Pain,* second edition, ed. Aronoff, G. (Baltimore: Williams and Wilkins, 1992).

[50]Andrasik, F., "Assessment of Patients with Headaches," *Handbook of Pain Assessment,* ed. Turk, D., Melzack, R. (New York: Guilford Press, 1992), 344.

[51]Andrasik, F., Burke, E. J., in *Applications in Behavioral Medicine and Health Psychology: A Clinician's Source Book,* ed. Blumenthal, J. A., McKee, D. C. (Sarasota, Fla.: Professional Resource Exchange, 1987).

[52]Solomon, S., Fraccaro, S., *The Headache Book: Effective Treatments to Prevent Headaches and Relieve Pain* (Consumer Reports Books, Sarabande Press, 1991), 44.

[53]Friedman, M., personal communication, 1993.

[54]Definitions and treatments of headaches adapted from Graham, J. R., Bana, D. S., "Headache," *Evaluation and Treatment of Chronic Pain,* second edition, ed. Aronoff, G. (Baltimore: Williams & Wilkins, 1992).

[55]Graff-Radford, S. B., "The Differential Diagnosis of Facial Pain," "Clarks Clinical Dentistry." In press.

[56]Graff-Radford, S. B., Reeves, J., Jaeger, B., "Management of Chronic Head and Neck Pain: Effectiveness of Altering Factors Perpetuating Myofascial Pain," *Headache Journal,* vol. 27, no. 4 (April 1987), 186.

[57]Frymoyer, J. W., Cats-Baril, W. L., "An Overview of the Incidence and Costs of Low Back Pain," *Causes and Cure of Low Back Pain and Sciatica, Orthopedic Clinics of North America,* vol. 22, no. 2 (April 1991), 263–71.

[58]Loeser, J., Bigos, S., Fordyce, W., Volinn, E., "Low Back Pain," *The Management of Pain,* vol. 2, ed. Bonica, J. (Philadelphia: Lea & Febiger, 1990), 1449.

[59]Polatin, P. B., Mayer, T. G., "Quantification of Function in Chronic Low Back Pain," *Handbook of Pain Assessment,* ed. Turk, D., Melzack, R. (New York: Guilford Press, 1992), 37.

[60]Polatin, P. B., Mayer, T. G., "Quantification of Function in Chronic Low Back Pain," *Handbook of Pain Assessment,* ed. Turk, D., Melzack, R. (New York: Guilford Press, 1992), 37.

[61]Loeser, J., Bigos, S., Fordyce, W., Volinn, E., "Low Back Pain," *The Management of Pain*, vol. 2, ed. Bonica, J. (Philadelphia: Lea & Febiger, 1990), 1449.

[62]Sarno, J., *Mind Over Back Pain* (New York: William Morrow, Berkley Edition, 1986), 11.

[63]Sarno, J., *Mind Over Back Pain* (New York: William Morrow, Berkley Edition, 1986), 11.

[64]Adapted from Loeser, J., Bigos, S., Fordyce, W., Volinn, E., "Low Back Pain," *The Management of Pain*, vol. 2, ed. Bonica, J. (Philadelphia: Lea & Febiger, 1990).

[65]Frymoyer, J. W., Cats-Baril, W. L., "An Overview of the Incidence and Costs of Low Back Pain," *Causes and Cure of Low Back Pain and Sciatica, Orthopedic Clinics of North America*, vol. 22, no. 2 (April 1991), 263–71.

[66]Saberski, L., personal communication, 1993.

[67]Lorig, K., Fries, J., *The Arthritis Helpbook*, third edition (New York: Addison-Wesley Publishing Co., 1990), xiii.

[68]Gilliland, B., "Arthritis and Periarthritic Disorders," *The Management of Pain*, vol. 2, ed. Bonica, J. (Philadelphia: Lea & Febiger, 1990), 329.

[69]Lorig, K., Fries, J., *The Arthritis Helpbook*, third edition (New York: Addison-Wesley Publishing Co., 1990), xiii.

3

INFANTS AND CHILDREN

Not to adequately treat pain in infants and childrens caused by diagnostic, medical, or surgical procedures or disease is "now known to be medically unsound as well as barbaric," writes Neil Schechter, M.D.,[1] Director of Development Pediatrics at St. Francis Hospital in Hartford, Connecticut.

Infants and children feel pain. Treatment for the relief of pain is a basic human right, regardless of age.

In 1987 a survey of the ten most used textbooks on pediatrics contained only one page on pain out of twelve thousand clinical pages. This appalling lack of interest in the subject results in millions of infants and children suffering horrible unrelieved pain.[2]

A myth still exists that infants don't feel the same level of pain at birth because their nervous systems are not completely formed. Dr. Clifford Woolf, a neurobiologist at University College in London, published findings that infants have the same fully developed pain pathways as adults. In fact, he said, pain pathways are in full operation before birth.[3]

Infants show the physical stress of pain just as adults do. There is an increase in heart rate, and they will often scream and recoil when they are in pain. Recently a four-day-old baby was taken back to the hospital because of fever. After being in the hospital only one day, the baby screamed in anticipation of the needle stick to come every time the nurse swabbed his skin with alcohol.

Lack of pain control can be dangerous to infants. Agitation and physiologic stress for some infants can lead to excessive crying, which can affect oxygen levels. Margo McCaffery, R.N., writes, "Pain can be life-threatening. Continuous crying decreases oxygenation, which may result in intraventricular hemorrhaging, a major cause of death in premature infants."[4] Other infants may respond differently to pain. Some may withdraw. Nancy Hester, Ph.D., R.N., notes that "some infants may not cry if they find out crying means they will be hurt more."[5]

Myron Yaster, M.D., of the Johns Hopkins Children's Center, is a crusader for children in pain. In a recent interview he said, "It's really scandalous. It's appalling. The situation now exists that getting pain relief is the exception rather than the rule. I think ten years from now people are going to look back and say, 'You won't believe what we used to do,' because that is how absurd it will seem."[6]

Circumcision in newborns is almost always performed without anesthesia or analgesia. There is usually pain, crying, distress, and physiologic changes. A 1987 study compared twenty newborns who had a penile nerve block for circumcision with ten who had no anesthesia. The results were dramatic. The heart rate and blood pressure rose in infants who had no anesthesia and were unchanged in infants receiving the nerve block. Oxygen saturation declined 10% in the unanesthetized infants and was unchanged in those who had the nerve block.[7]

Recently, at a major medical center, a mother asked her doctor if her newborn would feel any pain when he was circumcised. The doctor said, "It doesn't make any difference anyway. He'll never remember it." The doctor's comment on a newborn's memory is out of date. Several studies show evidence that infants do have a capacity for memory.[8] When the mother asked for a penile nerve block, the doctor refused. Finally the mother was able to get the doctor to agree to use a topical anesthetic before the circumcision. Since circumcision is an elective procedure, the mother could have waited to find a doctor who used penile nerve blocks. A recent study demonstrated that using a topical anesthetic gel before a nerve block and for several days afterward on the wound significantly decreased the infant's crying and agitation.[9]

Until the late 1980s it was common practice to perform surgery on young infants with no anesthesia. Infants may now receive anesthesia, but often it is used sparingly. "Unfortunately, in its extremes this policy has resulted in children being pharmacologically paralyzed with muscle relaxants without the concomitant use of analgesics, hypnotics, or amnesics. This occurs despite the fact that muscle relaxants have absolutely no sedative or analgesic properties. What can be more chilling and cruel than to be paralyzed while awake? Is a scream silenced because there is no sound?" writes Yaster.[10]

Yet studies have shown that anesthesia can reduce complications after surgery. Dr. K. J. Anand studied week-old infants who were scheduled for heart surgery. Thirty received deep anesthesia for surgery followed by twenty-four hours of sedation with opioids (morphine-like drugs). Fifteen infants received only anesthesia. The infants who had both anesthesia and sedation had fewer postoperative complications. In another study, of premature infants undergoing surgery with "minimal" anesthesia, Dr. Anand noted that there was a high stress response to the surgery, which resulted in postoperative complications and a higher death rate.[11]

As mentioned in Chapter 1, regional anesthesia is a choice for infants and children. Epidural anesthesia can be used for this age group for urologic, orthopedic, and general surgical procedures below the diaphragm. Complications are rare.[12]

Epidurals combined with or without light general anesthesia reduce pain during surgery and postoperatively.

At the Hospital for Special Surgery, in New York City, 90% of the children who have nonspinal orthopedic surgery "benefit from regional anesthesia," says Dr. Victor Zayas, who is both a pediatrician and an anesthesiologist. "We try to minimize the trauma of hospitalization and anesthesia for all children."[13]

WHY ARE INFANTS AND CHILDREN NOT GIVEN ENOUGH PAIN MEDICATION?

Dr. Nancy Hester, of the University of Colorado Health Sciences Center, a researcher who is dedicated to alleviating pain in children, notes that there is a paucity of research on assessing pain in infants.

A 1986 study found that 59% of the surgeons surveyed thought children could not feel pain at two years of age. Forty percent thought that newborns did not require pain medication following surgery.[14]

Many doctors and nurses are reluctant to administer opioids to infants and children because they are fearful of depressing respiration. However, respiration can be monitored by a machine called an Oximeter. Dr. Schechter writes, "For children over 1 month old, there is no evidence of increased respiratory suppression, nor is there support for decreasing frequency of morphine administration."[15]

Philip A. Pizzo, M.D., Chief of Pediatrics at the National Cancer Institute, notes that "assessment of airway and respiratory rate by an experienced observer is a critical component of management of patients receiving morphine-like drugs, especially intravenous medications."

Another reason for hesitancy to use opioids is the incorrect assumption by doctors, nurses, and families that children may easily become addicted. In fact, studies show that addiction is extremely rare. As mentioned earlier, a study showed that only four adult patients out of eleven thousand who received opioids became addicted. There is no reason to suspect that children would be different. "To withhold adequate pain relief from a suffering patient on the theoretic ground of addiction potential is not only inhumane, but incorrect."[16]

It is difficult to assess pain in infants because they can't tell anyone what hurts or where they are hurting. Although crying is one indicator, not all infants cry. Some are withdrawn or too sick to react.

Hospitalized infants often have to endure endless needle sticks or be subjected to invasive procedures that cause pain. In fact, studies have shown that repeated lancing of an infant's heel over days and weeks results in skin hypersensitivity. It has been proposed that the use of topical and local anesthetics can greatly reduce infants' and children's pain in procedures that must be repeated.[17]

POSTOPERATIVE PAIN IS UNDERTREATED

In Schechter's 1974 study of twenty-five children age four to eight years revealed that "only 12 received any analgesics throughout their hospital stay. In total this group received only 24 doses of analgesics, of which half were narcotics. Thirteen children received no pain medications despite diagnoses such as traumatic amputation of the foot, excision of neck mass, and atrial defect repair."[18]

A 1983 study by Mather and Mackie of postoperative pain in 170 children found:

. . . up to 40% of the children reported moderate to severe pain during the operative and first postoperative day. The medical staff had variable prescribing habits, and the doses for pain relief were too small and/or infrequent. The majority of orders were written PRN [as needed], which was often interpreted by the nursing staff as "as little as possible." The nursing staff preferred not to give narcotic medications and substituted non-narcotic analgesics, even soon after surgery. Up to 45% of the children continued to report moderate to severe pain even after receiving pain medications. Many of the children became withdrawn, which was interpreted as coping with pain. Other children expressed a dread of "the needle" as a way of administering analgesics and preferred to suffer pain to an injection.[19]

The undertreatment of pain in children is considered such a national health care concern that the Agency for Health Care Policy and Research recently published a guide for clinicians: "Acute Pain Management in Infants, Children, and Adolescents: Operative or Medical Procedures and Trauma." According to the guide:

Infants and children vary greatly in their cognitive and emotional development, medical conditions and operations, responses to pain and interventions and personal preferences. Therefore, rigid prescriptions for pain management are inappropriate. Children who may have difficulty communicating their pain require particular attention. Postoperative pain should be assessed frequently. For example, assessment after major surgery should occur every 2 hours for the first 24 hours and every 4 hours thereafter. More frequent assessment is necessary if pain is poorly controlled.[20]

The American Academy of Pediatrics is also formulating guidelines on children's pain management. It can't happen fast enough. Parents need to become informed, educated, and involved.

EVALUATING PAIN IN CHILDREN

McCaffery and Beebe note that "when the patient is an infant or child, the rights to which a patient is entitled are essentially transferred to the parents. As guardians of those rights, the parents need information that will enable them to make decisions about the care of their child. Further, the child's family can be a great asset in the assessment and relief of the child's pain."[21]

Charles Berde, M.D., and Dr. Carol Warfield, both of Harvard University, write, "For children, the response to acute pain and illness is intimately associated with fear and anxiety."

Parents must act as advocates for their infants and children. Dr.

Nancy Hester and Carol Barcus, P.N.P., write that doctors and nurses need to conduct a *Pain Experience History.* Accordingly,

> The parent and child (if verbal) discuss the child's experience with previous pain. This history should be completed prior to antici- pated potentially painful experiences (such as a well child visit or at the time of admission to the hospital). The first question should be to find out if the child understands what pain is. Most school-age children do not know what *pain* is, but they know what *hurt* is. Children under 7, however, may not know what the word "hurt" means, but do relate to the word "owie!" Therefore, it is important for the doctor or nurse to use a variety of words for pain when talking with a child.[22]

Following are examples of the *Pain Experience History* for both parent and child.

Pain Experience History: Parent

Name of child:_____

Age:_____Parent_____

Date:_____

What word(s) does your child use in regard to pain?_____
_____

Describe the pain experiences your child has had before._____
_____

Does your child tell you or others when he or she is hurting?____
_____

How do you know when your child is in pain?_____
_____

What do you do for your child when he/she is hurting?_____
_____

What does your child do for him/herself when he/she is hurting?
_____

What works best to decrease or take away your child's pain?____
_____

Is there anything special that you would like me to know about your child and pain? (If yes, have parent[s] describe.)_____
_____

Pain Experience History: Child Informant

Name of child:_____

Age_____Parent_____

Date_____

Tell me what pain is._____

_____

Tell me about the hurt you have had before._____

_____

What do you do when you hurt?_____

_____

Do you tell others when you hurt? If yes, who?_____

_____

What do you want others to do for you when you are hurting?__

_____

What don't you want others to do for you when you hurt?_____

_____

What helps the most to take away your hurt?_____

_____

Is there anything special that you want me to know about you when
you hurt? (If yes, have child describe.)_____

_____

© Hester and Barcus. Reprinted with permission, 1993.

It is important to know how a child reacts to pain. Each child is different and has his or her own method of coping with pain. Some may lie still; others want to be held by a parent, to have their "blankie" or favorite toy, or the light on or off. Schechter, Berde, and Yaster write, "We do not know the true impact of children's sex, age and cognitive level on their 'hurting'—specifically, the manner in which these characteristics may modify children's understanding of pain, their actual perception of pain, the type of tissue damage sustained and their behavioral responses to pain."[23]

Parents and other family members should be informed and involved with the child's medical treatment. The parents should be familiar with every aspect of diagnostic, medical, or surgical treatment. They should know what to expect so they can prepare the child and allay his or her fears. If a procedure will hurt, it is best to let the child know that it will hurt and for how long. Saying that something won't hurt when it will is not only dishonest, it can damage child's future relationships with adults and even cause the child to conceal illness for fear of being hurt again.

PAIN PLAN

A parent has a right to develop a Pain Plan with the doctor. Never should any diagnostic, medical, or surgical procedure be initiated without a detailed discussion about pain. A parent needs to be involved in the decision-making process of what pain medications will be given, in what form, how often, who will give them, who will assess the pain, and who will be responsible if the pain is inadequately controlled.

Dr. Nancy Hester says, "The parent should enter into a contract with the physician as to what the Pain Plan will be. If pain management is not addressed and agreed upon, the parent should either get a second opinion or look for another hospital. Sometimes this is difficult, but no child should suffer from poor pain management."[24]

The parent should always be with the child before, during, and after any diagnostic or nonsurgical procedure.

If surgery is to be performed, the parent should be with the child up until surgery. The ideal choice is for the parent to be with the child in the operating room until the child is sedated or asleep. Dr. Myron Yaster reports that at the John Hopkins Children's Center it is routine to allow a parent into the operating room during that process. He notes, "There is nothing detrimental about this practice. It is helpful to the child and it is of equal importance to the parent. It allays the parents' fears that they are deserting the child."[25] At the Hospital for Special Surgery, in New York City, oral premedication is used instead of injections. A parent holds the child until he or she is asleep. The parent leaves the operating room after the child is asleep.

The parent should be with the child immediately following the surgery—preferably as the child wakes up in the recovery room. Margo McCaffery, R.N., notes, "There is no general medical reason a parent cannot be with a child in the recovery room."[26] At the Hospital for Special Surgery and John Hopkins the parents are brought to the recovery room after surgery to further eliminate the child's separation anxiety.

After a procedure, parents should be asked frequently by the staff about their child's level of pain and whether the pain is being relieved. The parent knows how the child reacts to pain and can communicate that information for overall assessment.

The coping and control methods that work in a child's home as he or she experiences the usual cuts, scrapes, and bruises are usually inadequate in the medical arena of severe pain. A goal must be to provide the child with some level of control in the medical setting. Attaining that goal depends on the doctor or nurse's gaining the child's trust.

McCaffery and Beebe write about how a child should be approached in the health care setting:

- Allow the child time to feel comfortable with the nurse (or doctor).
- Avoid sudden or rapid advances.
- Talk to the parent initially if the child is shy.
- Try talking through objects such as dolls or puppets before directly questioning a young child.
- Give the older child an opportunity to talk without parents or friends being present. [Author's note: It is generally accepted that parents should stay with the young child.]
- Assume a position that allows for eye contact but do not force eye contact or maintain it for long periods.
- Speak in a quiet, unhurried voice.
- Use simple word and sentences, but avoid upsetting terms such as "shot" instead of injection or "deaden" instead of numb.
- Offer physical contact. Once an infant or toddler makes eye contact and shows no fear, hand her a toy and gradually increase physical contact, eventually holding her. A similar approach can be used with an older child, beginning with handing her a toy or touching her arm or shoulder, eventually offering physical comfort such as an arm around the shoulder or holding her hand.
- *Be honest,* especially about the possibility of pain occurring.
- Give the child an opportunity to express his concerns and ask questions. Ask open-ended questions, wait for answers, and do not interrupt. Avoid "putting words in his mouth."
- Use actual equipment or pictures in explanations. Demonstrate on self or doll, or use figure drawings. Be sensitive to the older child's desire not to be treated childishly.[27]

No child should be rushed through a process that will cause pain. A recent study of surgical patients aged three to twelve showed that systematic preparation, rehearsal, and supportive care conducted prior to each stressful procedure resulted in less anxiety and upset and more cooperation.[28]

If the child is in the hospital, any painful procedure should be performed "outside the child's room," so the child will "feel safe in their bed" and hurts take place somewhere else.[29]

Children so hate the pain associated with needles that they will sometimes deny pain or illness, as previously noted. Recently a five-year-old girl sliced open the palm of her hand with a knife. Even though she sustained a painful, gaping, bleeding wound, she did not want to go to the hospital, because she didn't want the doctor to hurt her with a needle.

Parents taking their child to an emergency room should be prepared to "insist that they stay with their child and insist that their child's pain be adequately managed consistently, and not at the convenience of the staff," notes Margo McCaffery.[30]

A recent study by Steven Selbst, M.D., Director of the Emergency Department at Children's Hospital of Philadelphia, found that "children usually do not get the same treatment as adults with similar painful conditions who present to the emergency department. Children with second degree burns and lower extremity fractures rarely received analgesics. . . . Children, especially those under 2 years old, were less likely to receive prescriptions for analgesics than were the adults."[31]

Selbst and Henretig have noted the paucity of data about the practice of pediatrics in emergency departments. However, they write about the importance of including the help of parents as much as possible. Doctors should approach the child slowly, avoid condescension, and speak at age-appropriate levels.[32]

Dr. Yaster points out that "sedation techniques are underused for children who are hurt and/or have overwhelming anxiety."[33] Liquids, tablets, suckers, or nasal forms of medication can be used for sedation and pain relief. For children under two, a rectal route can be used. If intermittent or continuous pain medication infusions are needed, it is preferable to start an IV line, so that the child will have to suffer through only one needle stick. An intramuscular injection is the *least* desirable, because of the pain from the injection and delayed absorption time (see Chapter 1).

Procedure-Related Pain

The parent should ask for topical or local anesthetics to be used before needle sticks, sutures, or other invasive procedures commence. It takes a little more time, but the result is a less painful procedure.

There are two topical anesthetics that can be applied to skin to diminish the pain of needles from sticks, injections, punctures, or sutures:[34]

- *EMLA:* Can be placed on the skin under a gauze pad dressing one hour prior to the procedure. (It is suggested that two sites be chosen for the application of EMLA if the procedure's purpose is to take blood; if one site does not work, another will already be prepared.)
- *TAC:* A solution that can be dripped into open wounds to numb the area to be sutured. It takes effect in five to nineteen minutes. It must be mixed by the pharmacy at the hospital. Note: It should not be used on mucous membranes, the penis, fingers, or ears, because of its tissue-constricting qualities.

When these are not available, ice or a chilling spray called Frigiderm can be used at the site to help offset the pain of needle sticks.

For invasive wounds, spinal taps, placing chest tubes, or other invasive procedures, a local anesthetic—one that is injected under the skin—is used. The most common, Lidocaine, can burn and sting as it is injected. It is suggested that the burning can be eliminated by using a buffer of sodium bicarbonate, warming the solution, using small needles, and injecting it slowly.[35] It is reported that Marcaine stings only for two or three seconds and can produce numbness for up to ten hours.[36]

If the child is extremely anxious, an antianxiety drug should be used. In addition, nitrous oxide provides analgesia for short procedures that are very painful. It requires the child's cooperation because a mask is used over the nose and mouth. The child should be over five.

For bone marrow aspirations, the use of general anesthesia or an opioid mixed with relaxants should be used.[37]

When children must endure ongoing procedure-related pain from chronic illness or cancer, it is essential that the child be prepared for the procedure slowly and premedicated adequately. *Children do not get used to pain from repeated procedures. They need sensitive and compassionate care to ensure that they do not suffer needlessly as well as having to cope with illness.*

Acute Pain Control

As discussed in other chapters, during the acute pain experience the central nervous system can be imprinted with the pain message. In order to prevent the immediate and long-term results of pain, analgesia must be used. Administration of opioids in concert with anesthesia before and during surgery decreases postoperative pain.

For acute postoperative pain in children, the goal is the same as it is for adults: prevention and control of pain. Pain relief should allow for deep breathing and mobility (if appropriate), to reduce pain-related respiratory, cardiac, blood, and gastrointestinal complications which can become life-threatening.

As with adults, PRN ("as needed") pain medication is the least desirable method. "As needed" means that when pain is felt, medication is requested. This leads to unsatisfactory fluctuations of the drug dose in the blood. A continuous twenty-four-hour schedule of drugs, either orally or intravenously, provides ongoing pain control and avoids runaway pain. The parent should ask about "rescue doses" of pain medication, in case the child experiences a pain breakthrough (see Chapter 1).

If the doctor refuses twenty-four-hour pain coverage, parents should be told that *they or the child must ask for pain medication.* Often parents or children do not know what medication has been ordered and how often it is to be given. It is important for a parent to write down the name of the drug, in what form it is given, and how often. (The parent can use the Parent's Daily Pain Chart for Young Children, page 152.)

PCA

By age five or six, a child is capable of using PCA (patient-controlled analgesia), which offers intravenous pain medication via a programmed bedside pump.

If the child feels pain, he or she can press a button for a measured dose of medication. The computer in the pump allows a set dose to be delivered within a timed interval. *This method adds the element of control for a child.*[38] Children need to be taught how to use PCA. If the

Parent's Daily Pain Chart for Young Children

Name_____Date_____

Doctor_____

Medication(s)?_____Dose?_____

How given? (IV, Oral, other)_____

How often?_____

0 = No pain   4 = Worst pain

0	1	2	3	4
no		moderate		worst
pain		pain		pain

Time A.M./P.M.	Pain Score 0–4	Dose Received	Pain Score 30 min. IV or 60 min. oral 0–4	Comments

Describe your child's pain_____

_____

_____

© 1992, Jane Cowles, Ph.D.

child cannot press the dose button, a parent or nurse can do it. The child should be monitored hourly if on PCA.

PCA-plus provides twenty-four-hour continuous infusion as well as the availability of a measured dose. Dr. Myron Yaster notes, "If children can play Nintendo they can operate PCA." He adds, "Although PCA is usually thought of as 'patient controlled,' we use it with children younger than five years of age. The parent or nurse can push the button. This is common in my practice for children with cancer and/or children with decreased mental capacity."[39]

Even with PCA, constant assessment is needed to make certain that analgesia is taking place. As the recovery period progresses, a combination of oral analgesic and PCA can be given until the pain begins to abate; then the intravenous line is removed, and oral administration is continued.

Extra Doses of Pain Medication

If a child is required to do anything that causes pain, such as walking, doing breathing exercises or physical therapy, or undergoing dressing changes or tests, an extra dose of pain medication should be ordered. The timing of the extra dose should be tailored to the method of administration. For example, if an intravenous route is used, the extra dose will take effect in minutes, whereas the absorption time of oral drugs can be up to sixty minutes. The ideal time for the child to make a painful effort is when the drug used for pain relief is at its peak level.[40]

Side Effects

Side effects from drugs should be anticipated for children, just as they should be for adults. Older children may be able to verbalize such side effects as itching, nausea, or feelings of disorientation, but younger children cannot tell an adult what is wrong. Extra care and assessment are needed to make certain that pain is being relieved and side effects are not occurring.

Regional Analgesia

Regional analgesia such as an epidural can be used with local anesthetic, opioids, or both. An epidural combined with light general anesthesia can be used preoperatively and postoperatively for a child undergoing orthopedic, abdominal, chest, or urinary procedures. As noted in Chapter 1, the use of an epidural can reduce pain during surgery and reduce the need for postoperative pain medications. PCA or PCA-plus can also be used with an epidural line left in place as a method of postoperative pain treatment. However, some children don't like the feeling of numbness associated with an epidural.

Nerve Blocks

Various forms of nerve blocks, as discussed in Chapter 1, can be employed for single, intermittent, and continuous analgesia. Nerve block techniques can interrupt the pain transmission in nerves targeting the head and neck, upper extremities, chest, upper abdomen, lower abdomen, pelvis, or lower extremities. As discussed previously, only those familiar with these procedures should make use of them.

As cautioned in Chapter 1, parents should request that a board-certified anesthesiologist treat their child. To repeat, discussions about analgesia should take place well before any procedure is begun. *If parents feel that their concerns and questions are not being addressed, they should seek a second opinion.*

Since children may not be able to describe their pain, side effects, or other discomforts, it is critical for both the health care team and the parents to be ever vigilant. Each child's pain is unique and cannot be treated on the average.

It is worthwhile to note again that the fear of addiction to morphine-like drugs is unfounded. It is not an excuse for adults or health care providers to cut or withhold pain medications from infants or children who are experiencing pain. Undertreatment of pain in children has been termed by Dr. Schechter "medically unsound and barbaric." In addition, there is no evidence that children who have been given opioids for pain relief are at greater risk for abusing drugs at a later age.[41]

Analgesics

Nonopioid analgesics also play a role in pain management. As reported in Chapter 1, the use of these analgesics along with opioids can enhance their effect. When pain subsides, these drugs can be used alone.

Mild Pain:
- Acetaminophen (Tylenol).
- Can be used orally and rectally (rectal is not the preferred route for children over two).
- Thirty to sixty minutes or longer to take effect.

Mild to Moderate Pain:

- NSAIDs (nonsteroidal anti-inflammatory drugs).
- These are used to reduce the severity of postoperative pain.
- Thirty to sixty minutes or longer to take effect.

The above drugs have a ceiling effect. This means after a certain point there is no further pain relief achieved.

Moderate Pain:

- Acetaminophen with codeine can be taken orally.
- Thirty minutes or longer to take effect.
- Should be given round-the-clock.
- Can be combined with NSAIDs for pain relief.

Severe Pain:

- Morphine is considered the first line of defense.
- Can be given in oral form, which takes thirty minutes or longer to take effect.
- Can be combined with NSAIDs for added pain relief.
- Intravenous takes effect in ten to fifteen minutes.
- Should be given round-the-clock.

See Chapter 1 for more information on side effects and drugs that can enhance pain relief.

Distraction

Forms of distraction such as a pop-up book, mirrors, storytelling, music tapes, toys, story books, coloring books, watching TV, or playing games can help a child through a painful period. Holding, stroking, rocking, swinging, or swaying rhythmically can make a child feel better. Even blowing soap bubbles can divert attention. Relaxation techniques such as counting, breathing, and recalling a special place where the child had no pain (the beach, the circus, etc.) may be of help.

The parent should be involved as much as possible in helping to distract, hold, rock, or use whatever techniques work in comforting the child. It is important to note that a playing or sleeping child can be experiencing pain.

It is helpful for parents to keep a *Pain Diary* to note periods of pain, relief, methods of comfort that do or do not work, and eating or sleeping habits.

PAIN ASSESSMENT

Using the *Young Child's Pain Assessment Scale* of 0 = no pain to 4 = worst pain, parents can note the assessment of pain on a regular basis and discuss it with doctors and nurses.[42] The 0–4 scale seems to be about what a young child can grasp. Using crying as a sole measure of pain is unreliable. A sleeping or playing child can still be in pain.

The following is a *Pain Assessment Scale* for children, which can be copied and taken to the hospital or used at home by the parent.

A parent can track a child's pain levels, what medication they receive, how often, and with what result. Other pain-relieving methods that work for the child may also be noted, along with side effects and comments.

Young Child's Pain Assessment Scale

0	1	2	3	4
no pain		moderate pain		worst pain

Dr. Hester makes use of the *Pain Interview* when pain is occurring or may be occurring. The questions are open-ended, and the interview requires the child to give the information in any way he or she chooses. These types of questions facilitate the child's participation in her/his pain.

If the child is young or in extreme pain, a supplied question format can be substituted. This type of question requires that the child only agree or disagree. For example, instead of asking, "What would you like me to do?" the nurse might ask the child, "Do you want medication? Do you want me to hold you? Do you want the light on?" The supplied question still allows the child to participate, but the freedom of choice is limited to the options supplied by the nurse.[43]

In addition, the nurse might ask the child to choose reasonable alternatives, such as "Do you want me to use heat or cold?" on a site when an IV is being pulled out.

The parent form of *Pain Interview* is also important in providing knowledge about the child's pain.

Tell me about the hurt you're having now.
Elicit descriptor, location and cause.
What would you like me to do for you?

Tell me about the pain your child is having now.
Elicit descriptors, location, and cause.
What would you like me to do for your child?

Interviews by permission of N. O. Hester, © 1992.

The Poker Chip Tool of Pain Assessment

This tool consists of four red poker chips—four pieces of "hurt." Each poker chip represents a different pain level, one being the least and four being the worst hurt.

If poker chips are not available, parents or health care professionals can make their own out of cardboard or paper circles.

The Wong-Baker Faces Pain Rating Scale

Another pain assessment tool which notes a child's "distress" is the *Wong-Baker Faces Pain Rating Scale.*

A parent can easily use these methods of assessing pain in the home setting, so that a child can become familiar with them.

It is important to note that many children assume that someone will magically know if they are having pain and do something to relieve it. *It is safe to suppose that if the child has sustained an injury or had a procedure that would hurt an adult, it will also hurt the child.*

It has also been documented that poorly treated acute pain may lead to imprinting of pain into the pain pathways of the central nervous system, resulting in chronic pain (see Chapter 1).

Parents and health care staff need to understand that pain relief is a vital part of a child's overall medical care, equal in importance to other parts of the treatment program.

Poker Chip Tool Instructions

English Instructions
1. Use four red poker chips.
2. Align the chips horizontally in front of the child on the bedside table, a clipboard or other firm surface.
3. Tell the child, *"These are pieces of hurt."* Beginning at the chip nearest the child's left side and ending at the one nearest the right side, point to the chips and say, *"This* (the first chip) *is a little bit of hurt and this* (the fourth chip) *is the most hurt you could ever have."*

   For a young child or for any child who does not comprehend the instructions, clarify by saying, *"That means this* (the first chip) *is just a little hurt; this* (the second chip) *is a little more hurt; this* (the third chip) *is more hurt; and this* (the fourth chip) *is the most hurt you could ever have."*
4. Ask the child, *"How many pieces of hurt do you have right now?"* Children without pain will say they don't have any.
5. Clarify the child's answer by words such as "Oh, you have a little hurt? Tell me about the hurt." (Use the Pain Interview.)
6. Record the number of chips selected on the bedside flowsheet.

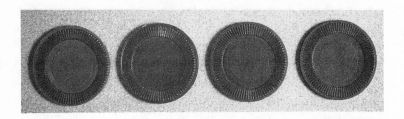

Spanish Instructions
1. Follow the English instructions, substituting the following words.
2. Tell the parent, if present: *"Estas fichas son una manera de medir dolor. Usamos cuatro fichas."*
3. Say to the child: *"Estas son pedazos de dolor: una es un poquito de dolor y cuatro son el dolor maximo que tu puedes sentir. Cuantos pedazos de dolor tienes?"*

Wong-Baker Faces Pain Rating Scale

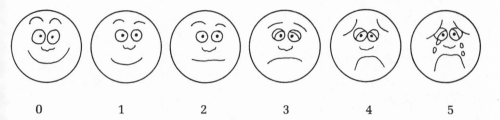

| 0 | 1 | 2 | 3 | 4 | 5 |

Explain to the person that each face is for a person who feels happy because he has no pain (hurt) or sad because he has some or a lot of pain. Face 0 is very happy because he doesn't hurt at all. Face 1 hurts just a little bit. Face 2 hurts a little more. Face 3 hurts even more. Face 4 hurts a whole lot. Face 5 hurts as much as you can imagine, although you don't have to be crying to feel this bad. Ask the person to choose the face that best describes how he is feeling. *Recommended for persons age 3 years and older.*

© D. Wong, 1993. Reprinted by permission.[44]

CONTROL-COPING MEASURES

Children should be given as much control over what is happening to their bodies as possible. Some control-coping measures are:

- If a child must have an injection, let him/her choose the site.
- If painful dressing changes must be made, let him/her help.
- Let the child participate in picking a time for a painful procedure, within the framework of reality.
- Always be honest as to what is about to happen to the child so he/she can be prepared and be part of the process rather than having the process "done" to him/her.

In addition to drug intervention, distraction, imagery, and comforting measures to relieve pain, other therapies may also be of help. These include:

- Self-hypnosis or guided imagery
- Psychotherapy

- Life changes such as diet, exercise, stretching
- Physical therapy
- Heat and cold therapy
- TENS (transcutaneous electrical nerve stimulation)
- Acupuncture
- Massage (for older children)

CHRONIC PAIN

It is not uncommon for children to experience chronic pain. Berde writes that "recurrent headaches and abdominal and limb pains each occur repeatedly for perhaps 5% to 10% of school children."[45] Pain can result in serious disruption of a child's family and social interaction and school attendance. "With increasing frequency, pediatricians encounter patients with chronic disease, either of a genetic, congenital or acquired origin, and many of these chronic diseases—cancer, cystic fibrosis, sickle cell anemia, migraine, Crohn's disease and AIDS— severely impact lives."[46]

It is estimated that roughly ten million children in the United States have a chronic illness; about two million are severely impaired. For many, hospital confinement is the norm rather than the exception. For these children, home care is an option that should be explored. It is now possible to bring medical technology to the home. Children can receive infusions of antibiotics, pain-relieving drugs, chemotherapy, and parenteral nutrition at home. Some children can be sent home on ventilators that do their breathing for them.

It is important that every effort be made not only to treat the medical problem but to make certain that chronic pain is managed, making use of all available pain-relieving techniques, so that these chronically ill children can enjoy their lives to the fullest of their capacity.

CHILDREN'S CANCER PAIN

The acknowledgment of pain and the necessity to treat pain in infants, children, and adolescents has been discussed. However, for cancer pain there are some special considerations. (See children's cancer resources in Chapter 5.)

Drs. Neil Schechter, Arnold Altman, and Steven Weisman, editors

Children's Pain Bill of Rights

As a parent, you have a right to:
- Act on behalf of your child
- Have your child's pain prevented or controlled adequately
- Discuss your child's pain history and pain behavior
- Tell what special name for hurt your child uses (such as "boo-boo" or "owie" or other)
- What comforts your child when he/she is in pain
- Know what kind of pain can be expected and for how long
- Know how pain will be controlled before, during, and after any procedure
- Know the risks, benefits, and side effects of pain medications
- Sign a statement of informed consent about a pain plan
- Be with your child before, during, and after a medical procedure
- Be with your child up to and immediately after surgery
- Have a commitment from doctors and nurses to assess pain on a regular basis
- Know who is accountable for your child's pain relief
- Have doctors and nurses use topical and/or local anesthetics before any injections, needle sticks, or invasive procedures
- Have postoperative pain managed aggressively
- Request painless methods of administering medications (oral or intravenous line, instead of injection). Avoid rectal administration in children over two whenever possible.
- Have doctors and nurses listen to your assessment of how much pain your child is experiencing
- Remind those who care for your child that pain management is an important part of any diagnostic, medical, or surgical procedure
- Request a second opinion if you feel your child's pain is being poorly managed or if doctors and nurses do not share your concerns about preventing and controlling your child's pain
- Act as an aggressive advocate for your child

REMINDERS

Remember: You can never assume that your child's pain will be taken care of automatically. You should always ask about pain control.

Do not assume that if your child has received medication for pain, the pain has been adequately and appropriately treated. Assessment should continue.

of the *Report of the Consensus Committee on Pain in Childhood Cancer,* write:

> Inadequate management of pain is a significant problem in all aspects of pediatric care. In every clinical situation which has been studied, children's pain receives far less attention than that of adults. Nowhere is this situation more unfortunate, however, than in the management of pain associated with childhood cancer. Poor controlled cancer pain validates the worst fears of parents and children that cancer is accompanied by inevitable and excruciating pain. Inadequate control of the pain associated with diagnostic procedures creates an anticipatory dread in the child of the next procedure and colors his or her attitudes toward the hospital and the staff providing care.[47]

How children are treated for their pain can have long-term results, in relation not only to their physical pain but to their perception of the world in general. Children need to have their pain treated aggressively and with compassion.

Following is a list of resources for infants and children.

INFANTS' AND CHILDREN'S RESOURCES

PUBLICATIONS

Acute Pain Management in Infants, Children and Adolescents: Operative and Medical Procedures. Clinical Practice Guideline, Quick Reference Guide for Physicians. U.S. Department of Health and Human Services, AHCPR Pub. #92-0020.

Pain in Infants, Children and Adolescents by Neil L. Schechter, Charles B. Berde, and Myron Yaster. Williams & Wilkins, 1993.

CHILDREN'S PAIN PROFESSIONALS

Jane Allen, P.T.
Department of Physical Therapy and
Occupational Therapy Services
Consultant, Pain Treatment Service
Children's Hospital
Boston, Massachusetts

K. J. S. Anand, M.D.
Clinical Fellow in Pediatric Intensive
Care
Harvard Medical School
Massachusetts General Hospital
Boston, Massachusetts

Corrie T. M. Anderson, M.D.
Assistant Professor of Anesthesiology
and Pediatrics
Co-Director, Pediatric Pain Program
Chief, Division of Pediatric
Anesthesiology
Departments of Anesthesiology and
Pediatrics
University of California at Los Angeles
Los Angeles, California

Paul A. Aubuchon, Ph.D.
Clinical Psychologist
Diplomate in Acupuncture
Landmark Medical Center
Milford-Whitinsville Regional Hospital
Woonsocket, Rhode Island

Ronald G. Barr, M.A., M.D.C.M.,
F.R.C.P.(C)
Associate Professor of Pediatrics
McGill University
Director, Child Development Programme
Montreal Children's Hospital
Montreal, Quebec, Canada

Carlene Bartolotta, R.N., B.S.N.
Nursing Manager, Pediatrics
Department of Nursing
John Dempsey Hospital
University of Connecticut Health Center
Farmington, Connecticut

Charles B. Berde, M.D., Ph.D.
Associate Professor of Anaesthesia
(Pediatrics)
Department of Anaesthesia
Harvard Medical School
Director, Pain Treatment Service
Children's Hospital
Boston, Massachusetts

Bruce A. Bernstein, Ph.D.
Director of Research
Department of Pediatrics
Saint Francis Hospital and Medical
Center
Assistant Professor
Department of Pediatrics
University of Connecticut Health Center
Hartford, Connecticut

Daniel B. Carr, M.D.
Associate Professor
Department of Anaesthesia
Harvard Medical School
Director, Division of Pain Management
Department of Anesthesia
Massachusetts General Hospital
Shriners Burns Institute
Boston, Massachusetts

Charles S. Cleeland, Ph.D.
Director, Pain Research Group
University of Wisconsin Medical School
Madison, Wisconsin

David E. Cohen, M.D.
Director, Pain Management Program
Assistant Anesthesiologist
The Children's Hospital of Philadelphia
Assistant Professor of Anesthesia and
Pediatrics
The University of Pennsylvania School
of Medicine
Philadelphia, Pennsylvania

Maria Dietrich, R.N., B.S.
Madison, Wisconsin

Joëlle F. Desparmet, M.D.
Visiting Professor
Montreal Children's Hospital
Montreal, Quebec, Canada

Jo Eland, Ph.D., R.N., F.A.A.N., N.A.P.
Associate Professor of Nursing
College of Nursing
University of Iowa
Iowa City, Iowa

Debra Fanurik
Assistant Research Psychologist
Pediatric Pain Program
Department of Pediatrics
University of California at Los Angeles
Los Angeles, California

Judy Feret, R.N., M.S.
Clinical Nurse Specialist, Pediatrics
Department of Nursing
John Dempsey Hospital
University of Connecticut Health Center
Farmington, Connecticut

Nalton F. Ferraro, D.M.D., M.D.
Instructor
Harvard School of Dental Medicine
Associate in Surgery
Children's Hospital
Boston, Massachusetts

Betty R. Ferrell, Ph.D., R.N., F.A.A.N
Research Scientist, Nursing Research
City of Hope Medical Center
Durate, California

Linda S. Franck, M.S., R.N.
Director, Critical Care Nursing
Children's Hospital
Oakland, California

M. Alex Geertsma, M.D., F.A.A.P.
Associate Professor of Pediatrics
University of Connecticut Health Center
Director, Early Childhood Development
  Program
Hartford Hospital
Hartford, Connecticut

Sharon Gerrity, R.N., B.S.
Department of Psychiatry
Dean Medical Center
Madison, Wisconsin

George A. Gregory, M.D.
Professor of Anesthesia and Pediatrics
University of California, San Francisco
San Francisco, California

Eric Heiligenstein, M.D.
Psychiatrist
Department of Psychiatry
Dean Medical Center
Madison, Wisconsin

Nancy K. Hester, R.N., Ph.D.
Assistant Director, Center for Nursing
  Research
Associate Professor, School of Nursing
University of Colorado Health Sciences
  Center
Golden, Colorado

Sheila Jacobsen, M.D.
Department of Pharmacology and
  Toxicology
The Hospital for Sick Children
University of Toronto
Toronto, Ontario, Canada

Beverly Pray Jedlinsky, P.T.
Department of Physical Therapy and
  Occupational Therapy Services
Consultant, Pain Treatment Service
Children's Hospital
Boston, Massachusetts

Celeste Johnston, R.N., D.Ed.
Department of Nursing
McGill University and Montreal
  Children's Hospital
Montreal, Quebec, Canada

Stephen R. King, Ph.D.
Instructor, Department of Pediatrics
University of Connecticut School of
  Medicine
Director, Pediatric Psychology
Saint Francis Hospital and Medical
  Center
Hartford, Connecticut

Gideon Koren, M.D.
Department of Pharmacology and
  Toxicology
The Hospital for Sick Children
University of Toronto
Toronto, Ontario, Canada

Leora Kuttner, M.D.
Clinical Psychologist
B.C. Children's Hospital
Department of Pediatrics
University of British Columbia
Vancouver, British Columbia, Canada

Alan M. Leichtner, M.D.
Clinical Director
Combined Program in Gastroenterology
  and Nutrition
Children's Hospital
Assistant Professor
Harvard Medical School
Boston, Massachusetts

Yuan-Chi Lin, M.D., M.P.H.
Assistant Professor
Department of Anesthesia
Stanford University School of Medicine
Stanford, California

Joseph R. Madsen, M.D.
Assistant Professor
Department of Neurosurgery
Children's Hospital
Boston, Massachusetts

Bruce J. Masek, Ph.D.
Assistant Professor of Psychology
Department of Psychiatry
Harvard Medical School
Director, Behavioral Medicine
Department of Psychiatry
Children's Hospital
Boston, Massachusetts

Judith R. Mathews, Ph.D.
Assistant Professor
Department of Psychology
West Virginia University
Morgantown, West Virginia

Eeva-Liisa Maunuksela, M.D., Ph.D.
Helsinki University Eye Hospital
Helsinki, Finland
Associate Professor in Anesthesiology
University of Kuopio
Kuopio, Finland
Visiting Professor in Anesthesiology
Texas Tech University
Health Sciences Center
Lubbock, Texas

Lynne G. Maxwell, M.D.
Assistant Professor
Departments of Anesthesiology/Critical
  Care Medicine and Pediatrics
The Johns Hopkins Medical Institutions
Baltimore, Maryland

Margo McCaffery, R.N., M.S., F.A.A.N.
Consultant in the Nursing Care of
  Patients with Pain
Los Angeles, California

Claire F. McCarthy, P.T., M.S.
Director
Department of Physical Therapy and
  Occupational Therapy Services
Children's Hospital
Boston, Massachusetts

Melanie L. McGrath, Ph.D.
Instructor in Psychology
Department of Psychiatry
Harvard Medical School
Children's Hospital
Boston, Massachusetts

Patricia A. McGrath, Ph.D.
Director, Child Health Research
  Institute
Associate Professor
Department of Paediatrics
University of Western Ontario
London, Ontario, Canada

Patrick J. McGrath, Ph.D.
Professor of Psychology, Paediatrics,
  Psychiatry, and Occupational
  Therapy
Co-ordinator of Clinical Psychology
Dalhousie University
Halifax, Nova Scotia, Canada

Angela W. Miser, M.B.B.S.
Associate Professor
Department of Anesthesiology and
  Pediatrics
University of Washington
Seattle, Washington

Kathleen Nolan, M.D., M.S.L.
Medical Ethicist
Mount Tremper, New York

Tim F. Oberlander, M.D., F.R.C.P.(C)
Clinical Fellow in Medicine
Pain Treatment Service
Children's Hospital
Boston, Massachusetts

Patricia F. Osgood, Ph.D.
Assistant Professor
Department of Anaesthesia
Harvard Medical School
Massachusetts General Hospital
Shriners Burns Institute
Boston, Massachusetts

Lee M. Pachter, D.O.
Associate Director
Pediatric Inpatient Unit
St. Francis Hospital and Medical Center
Assistant Professor
Department of Pediatrics
University of Connecticut Health Center
Hartford, Connecticut

Heléne Pigeon, Ph.D.
Clinician, Child Study Centre
University of Ottawa
Ottawa, Canada

Philip Pizzo, M.D.
Chief of Pediatrics
Head, Infectious Disease Section
National Cancer Institute
National Institutes of Health
Bethesda, Maryland

Fran Porter, Ph.D.
Assistant Professor
Department of Pediatrics
Washington University School of
    Medicine
St. Louis, Missouri

Leonard A. Rappaport, M.D.
Associate Chief, General Pediatrics
Children's Hospital
Assistant Professor
Harvard Medical School
Boston, Massachusetts

Eugene Rossitch, Jr., M.D.
Chief Resident
Division of Neurosurgery
Duke University Medical Center
Durham, North Carolina

A. David Rothner, M.D.
Head, Section of Pediatric Neurology
Cleveland Clinic Foundation
Cleveland, Ohio

Marilyn Savedra
School of Nursing
University of California, San Francisco
San Francisco, California

Neil L. Schechter, M.D.
Professor of Pediatrics
Head, Division of Developmental and
    Behavioral Pediatrics
University of Connecticut School of
    Medicine
Co-Director, Children's Pain Service
University of Connecticut Health Center
Director, Section of Developmental and
    Behavioral Pediatrics
Saint Francis Hospital and Medical
    Center
Hartford, Connecticut

Steven M. Selbst, M.D.
Director, Emergency Department
Children's Hospital of Philadelphia
Associate Professor of Pediatrics
University of Pennsylvania School of
    Medicine
Philadelphia, Pennsylvania

Navil Sethna, M.D.
Associate in Anesthesia
Associate Director
Pain Treatment Service
Children's Hospital
Instructor in Anaesthesia
Harvard Medical School
Boston, Massachusetts

Barbara S. Shapiro, M.D.
Assistant Professor of Pediatrics
University of Pennsylvania School of
    Medicine
Associate Director
Pain Management Service
Children's Hospital of Philadelphia
Philadelphia, Pennsylvania

Maureen Strafford, M.D.
Assistant Professor of Anaesthesia
    (Pediatrics)
Harvard Medical School
Associate in Anesthesia
Children's Hospital
Boston, Massachusetts

Stanislaw K. Szyfelbein, M.D.
Associate Professor of Anaesthesia
Harvard Medical School
Anesthetist
Massachusetts General Hospital
Director of Anesthesia
Shriners Burns Institute
Boston, Massachusetts

Joseph R. Tobin, M.D.
Assistant Professor
Department of Anesthesiology/Critical
    Care Medicine
The Johns Hopkins Medical Institutions
Baltimore, Maryland

Anita M. Unruh, B.Sc.(O.T.), M.S.W.
Lecturer in Occupational Therapy
Dalhousie University
Halifax, Nova Scotia, Canada

Gary A. Walco, Ph.D.
Chief of Behavioral Medicine
Tomorrow's Children's Institute
Hackensack Medical Center
Hackensack, New Jersey

Steven J. Weisman, M.D.
Associate Professor of Pediatrics
Division of Hematology/Oncology
Co-Director, Children's Pain Service
University of Connecticut Health Center
Farmington, Connecticut

Robert T. Wilder, M.D., Ph.D.
Instructor in Anaesthesia
Harvard Medical School
Assistant in Anesthesia
Pain Treatment Service
Children's Hospital
Boston, Massachusetts

Tara Lee Wilson, P.T.
Department of Physical Therapy and
 Occupational Therapy Services
Consultant, Pain Treatment Service
Children's Hospital
Boston, Massachusetts

Donna L. Wong, R.N., M.N., P.N.P.,
 C.P.N.
Nurse Consultant
Saint Francis Hospital Children's Center
Tulsa, Oklahoma
Arkansas Children's Hospital
Little Rock, Arkansas
Children's Medical Center of Dallas
Dallas, Texas

Myron Yaster, M.D.
Associate Professor
Departments of Anesthesiology/Critical
 Care Medicine and Pediatrics
Director, Multidisciplinary Pain Service
The Children's Medical and Surgical
 Center
The Johns Hopkins Medical Institutions
Baltimore, Maryland

John D. Yee, M.D.
Resident in Pediatrics
Children's Hospital
Clinical Fellow in Pediatrics
Harvard Medical School
Boston, Massachusetts

Lonnie K. Zeltzer, M.D.
Professor of Pediatrics
Director, Pediatric Pain Program
Department of Pediatrics
University of California at Los Angeles
Los Angeles, California

NATIONAL ASSOCIATION OF CHILDREN'S HOSPITALS AND RELATED INSTITUTIONS, INC.

Freestanding Hospitals

ALABAMA

BIRMINGHAM

Children's Hospital of Alabama
1600 Seventh Avenue South, 35233
(205) 939-9100
Jim Dearth, M.D.
Chief Executive Officer and Medical
 Director

ALASKA

ANCHORAGE

North Star Hospital
1650 South Bragaw, 99508
(907) 277-1522
Steve Berkshire

ARIZONA

PHOENIX

Phoenix Children's Hospital
1111 East McDowell Road, 85006
(602) 239-2400
Leland Clabots
President and Chief Executive Officer

Westbridge
1830 E. Roosevelt, P.O. Box 5750,
 85006
(602) 254-0884
John F. Capurso
President and Chief Executive Officer

Westbridge Center for Children
720 East Montebello, 85014
(602) 277-5437
Sheri Capurso
Chief Executive Officer

TUCSON

Desert Hills Center for Youth
2797 North Introspect Drive, 85745
(602) 622-5437
Karen F. Wiese
Administrator

ARKANSAS

BENTON

Rivendell Psychiatric Center
100 Rivendell Drive, 72015
(501) 794-1255
Chalres E. West
Executive Director

LITTLE ROCK

Arkansas Children's Hospital
800 Marshall Street, 72202
(501) 320-1100
Randall L. O'Donnell, Ph.D.
Chief Executive Officer

CALIFORNIA

EL CAJON

Rancho Park Hospital
109 E. Chase Avenue, 92020
(619) 579-1666
Izabela Vaught, R.N.
Administrator

FRESNO

Valley Children's Hospital
3151 North Millbrook Avenue, 93703
(209) 225-3000
James D. Northway, M.D.
President and Chief Executive Officer

LOS ANGELES

Childrens Hospital of Los Angeles
4650 Sunset Boulevard, P.O. Box 54700,
    Mail Stop 1, 90027
(213) 660-2450
Terry Bonecutter
COO and Vice President, Ambulatory
    Services

Crossroads Hospital
6323 Woodman Avenue, 91401
(818) 782-2470
Jeanne Prichard
Administrator

Shriners Hospital for Crippled Children
3160 Geneva Street, 90020
(213) 388-3151
Paul D. Hargis
Administrator

NEWPORT BEACH

Newport Harbor Hospital and Child
    Adolescent Mental Health Center
1501 East 16th Street, 92663
(714) 650-9752
Edward C. Morton, Jr.
Chief Executive Officer

OAKLAND

Children's Hospital Oakland
747 52d Street, 94609
(510) 428-3000
Antonie H. Paap
President and Chief Executive Officer

ORANGE

Children's Hospital of Orange County
455 South Main Street, 92668
(714) 997-3000
Thomas Penn Jones
President and Chief Executive Officer

PALO ALTO

Lucile Salter Packard Children's
    Hospital at Stanford
725 Welch Road, 94304
(415) 497-8000
Lorraine Zippiroli
President and Chief Executive Officer

SAN DIEGO

Children's Hospital and Health Center
8001 Frost Street, 92123
(619) 576-1700
Blair L. Sadler
President and Chief Executive Officer

San Diego County Loma Portal Mental
    Health Facility
3485 Kenyon Street, 92110
(619) 692-5501
Eric Eliason
Chief Executive Officer

SAN FRANCISCO

Shriners Hospital for Crippled Children
1701 19th Avenue, 94122
(415) 665-1100
Margaret Williams
Administrator

COLORADO

DENVER

The Children's Hospital
1056 East 19th Avenue, Box 020, 80218
(303) 861-8888
Lua R. Blankenship, Jr.
President and Chief Executive Officer

WESTMINSTER

Cleo Wallace Center Hospital
8405 West 100th, 80021
(303) 466-7391
James Cole
President and Chief Executive Officer

CONNECTICUT

MERIDEN

Henry D. Altobello Children and Youth
   Center
Undercliff Road, 06450
(203) 238-6054
Margery S. Stahl
Superintendent

MIDDLETOWN

Riverview Hospital for Children
River Road, Box 621, 06457
(203) 344-2700
Richard J. Wiseman, Ph.D.
Superintendent

NEWINGTON

Newington Children's Hospital
181 East Cedar Street, 06111
(203) 667-5437
A. John Menichetti
President and Chief Executive Officer

NEWTOWN

Housatonic Adolescent Hospital
Box 5525, 06470
(203) 270-2700
Brenda McGavran
Superintendent

DELAWARE

NEW CASTLE

Meadow Wood Hospital for Children
   and Adolescents
575 South Dupont Highway, 19720
(302) 328-3330
Scott C. Stamm
Administrator and Chief Executive
   Officer

WILMINGTON

Alfred I. DuPont Institute
1600 Rockland Road, P.O. Box 269,
   19899
(302) 651-4000
Thomas P. Ferry
Administrator

DISTRICT OF COLUMBIA

WASHINGTON

Children's National Medical Center
111 Michigan Avenue, N.W., 20010
(202) 745-5000
Donald L. Brown
President and Chief Executive Officer

Hospital for Sick Children
1731 Bunker Hill Road, N.E., 20017
(202) 832-4400
Constance U. Battle, M.D.
Chief Executive Officer and Medical
   Director

FLORIDA

FORT WALTON BEACH

Harbor Oaks Hospital
1015 Mar Walt Drive, 32547
(904) 863-4160
J. F. Gallagher III
Administrator

LAND O'LAKES

Florida Camelot
P.O. Box 1101, 33549
(813) 949-7491
James E. Spicer, Ph.D.
Executive Director

MELBOURNE

Devereux Hospital and Children's
Center of Florida
8000 Devereux Drive, 32940
(407) 242-9100
Nancy Dion
Acting Executive Director

MIAMI

Miami Children's Hospital
6125 S.W. 31st Street, 33155
(305) 666-6511
Thomas F. Jones
President and Chief Executive Officer

ST. PETERSBURG

All Children's Hospital
801 Sixth Street, S., 33701
(813) 898-7451
J. Dennis Sexton
President and Chief Executive Officer

TAMPA

Shriners Hospital for Crippled Children,
Tampa Unit
12502 North Pine Drive, 33612
(813) 972-2250
Donna Durden
Administrator

WEST PALM BEACH

Charter Hospital
1950 Benoist Farms Road, 33411
(407) 687-1511
Martin Schappell
Administrator

GEORGIA

ATLANTA

Charter Brook Hospital
3913 North Peachtree Road, 30341
(404) 457-8315
Randall Schlichting
Chief Executive Officer

Egleston Children's Hospital at Emory
University
1405 Clifton Road, N.E., 30322
(404) 325-6000
Alan J. Gayer
President, CEO

Hillside Hospital
690 Courtney Drive, N.E., 30306
(404) 875-4551
Thomas Corbett
Executive Director

Scottish Rite Children's Medical Center
1001 Johnson Ferry Road, N.E.,
30363-3101
(404) 256-5252
James E. Tally, Ph.D.
President and Chief Executive Officer

DOUGLASVILLE

Inner Harbour Hospitals
4685 Dorsett Shoals Road, 30135
(404) 942-2391
Tony Mobley
Chief Executive Officer

KENNESAW

Devereux Center—Georgia
1291 Stanley Road, 30144
(404) 427-0147
Ralph L. Comerford
Director

HAWAII

HONOLULU

Shriner's Hospitals for Crippled
Children
1310 Punahou Street, 96826
(808) 941-4466
James B. Brasel
Administrator

ILLINOIS

CHICAGO

LaRabida Children's Hospital and
Research Center
East 65th Street at Lake Michigan,
60649
(312) 363-6700
Arthur F. Kohrman, M.D.
Director

Shriners Hospitals for Crippled
Children
2211 North Oak Park Avenue, 60635
(312) 622-5400
A. James Spang
Administrator

Children's Memorial Hospital
2300 Children's Plaza, 60614
(312) 880-4000
Earl J. Frederick
President and Chief Executive Officer

INDIANA

INDIANAPOLIS

Lifelines Children's Rehabilitation
  Hospital
1707 West 86th Street, P.O. Box 40407,
  46240-0407
(317) 872-0555
William A. Schmidt
Administrator

KANSAS

ELLSWORTH

St. Francis at Ellsworth
P.O. Box 127, 67439
(913) 472-4453
Rev. Phillip Rapp
President

SALINA

St. Francis at Salina
5097 Cloud Street, 67401
(913) 825-0563
Rev. Phillip Rapp
President

TOPEKA

Children's Division of Menninger Clinic
P.O. Box 829, 66601
(913) 273-7500
Leland Koon
Administrator

KENTUCKY

COVINGTON

Children's Psychiatric Hospital of
  Northern Kentucky
502 Farrell Drive, Box 2680, 41012
(606) 331-1900
William Poll
Administrator

LEXINGTON

Shriners Hospitals for Crippled
  Children, Lexington Unit
1900 Richmond Road, 40502
(606) 266-2101
Jeffrey T. Mitchell
Administrator

OWENSBORO

Valley Institute of Psychiatry
1000 Industrial Drive, P.O. Box 4010,
  42302
(502) 686-8477
Alvin Freedman, Ph.D.
Administrator

LOUISIANA

GREENWELL SPRINGS

Greenwell Springs Hospital
23260 Greenwell Springs Road, 70739
(504) 261-2730
Donna K. Bourque, M.D.
Chief Executive Officer

NEW ORLEANS

Children's Hospital
200 Henry Clay Avenue, 70118
(504) 899-9511
Steve Worley
Executive Director

New Orleans Adolescent Hospital
210 State Street, 70118
(504) 987-3400
Robert Varnado
Acting Chief Executive Officer

SHREVEPORT

Shriners Hospital for Crippled Children,
  Shreveport Unit
3100 Samfort Avenue, 71103
(318) 222-5704
Thomas R. Schneider
Administrator

MARYLAND

BALTIMORE

Mt. Washington Pediatric Hospital, Inc.
1708 West Rogers Avenue, 21209-4597
(410) 578-8600
Francis A. Pommett, Jr.
President

Kennedy Krieger Institute
707 North Broadway, 21205
(410) 550-9000
Gary W. Goldstein, M.D.
President and Chief Executive Officer

MASSACHUSETTS

BOSTON

Children's Hospital
300 Longwood Avenue, 02115
(617) 735-6000
David S. Weiner
President

Franciscan Children's Hospital and
    Rehabilitation Center
30 Warren Street, 02135
(617) 254-3800
Kevin W. Ryan
President and Chief Executive Officer

Shriners Hospitals for Crippled
    Children, Boston Unit
51 Blossom Street, 02114
(617) 722-3000
Salvatore P. Russo, Ph.D.
Administrator

CANTON

Massachusetts Hospital School
3 Randolph Street, 02021
(617) 828-2440
John H. Britt
Chief Executive Officer

SPRINGFIELD

Shriners Hospital for Crippled Children,
    Springfield Unit
516 Carew Street, 01104
(413) 787-2000
Edwin C. Thorn
Administrator

MICHIGAN

DETROIT

Children's Hospital of Michigan
3901 Beaubien Boulevard, 48201
(313) 745-5437
Thomas M. Rozek
President

NORTHVILLE

Hawthorn Center
18471 Haggerty Road, 48167
(313) 349-3000
Harold J. Lockett, M.D.
Director

MINNESOTA

FARIBAULT

Wilson Center for Adolescent
    Psychiatry
Box 917, 55021
(507) 334-5561
Kevin J. Mahoney
President and Chief Executive Officer

MINNEAPOLIS

Minneapolis Children's Medical Center
2525 Chicago Avenue, S., 55404
(612) 863-6100
Lawrence J. Whalen
Chief Executive Officer

Shriners Hospital for Crippled
    Children—Twin Cities Unit
2025 East River Road, 55414
(612) 335-5300
Laurence E. Johnson
Administrator

ST. PAUL

Gillette Children's Hospital
200 East University Avenue, 55101
(612) 291-2848
Margaret Perryman
President and Chief Executive Officer

NEW HAMPSHIRE

SPOFFORD

Spofford Hall Hospital
Route 9A, Box 225, 03462
(603) 363-4545
Tom Murphy
Executive Director

NEW JERSEY

MOUNTAINSIDE

Children's Specialized Hospital
150 New Providence Road, 07092
(908) 233-3720
Richard B. Ahlfeld
President

PEAPACK

Matheny School
Main Street, 07977
(908) 234-0011
Robert Schonhorn
President

VOORHEES

Voorhees Pediatric Facility
1304 Laurel Oak Road, 08043-4392
(609) 346-3300
Carl W. Underland
Administrator

NEW MEXICO

ALBUQUERQUE

Carrie Tingley Hospital
1127 University, N.E., 87102-1701
(505) 272-5200
James C. Drennan, M.D.
Medical Director and Chief Executive
  Officer

University of New Mexico
Children's Psychiatric Hospital
1001 Yale Boulevard, N.E., 87131
(505) 843-2945
Christiana B. Gunn
Administrator

NEW YORK

BAYSIDE

St. Mary's Hospital for Children, Inc.
29-01 216th Street, 11360
(718) 281-8800
Burton Grebin, M.D.
President

BELLEROSE

Queens Children's Psychiatric Center
74-03 Commonwealth Boulevard, 11426
(212) 464-2900
Gloria Faretra, M.D.
Director

BRONX

Bronx Children's Psychiatric Center
1000 Waters Place, 10461
(718) 892-0808
E. Richard Feinberg, M.D.
Executive Director

BUFFALO

Children's Hospital of Buffalo
219 Bryant Street, 14222
(716) 878-7000
John P. Davanzo
President and Chief Executive Officer

DIX HILLS

Sagamore Children's Psychiatric Center
197 Half Hallow Road, 11747
(516) 673-7700
Robert Schweitzer, Ed.D.
Executive Director

ORANGEBURG

Rockland Children's Psychiatric Center
Convent Road, 10962
(914) 359-7400
Oleh Riznyk
Deputy Director Administration

VALHALLA

Blythedale Children's Hospital
Bradhurst Avenue, 10595
(914) 592-7555
Robert Stone
President

WEST SENECA

Western New York Child's Psychiatric
  Center
1010 East and West Road, 14224
(716) 674-9730
Allen R. Morganstein, M.D.
Clinical Director

NORTH CAROLINA

WINSTON-SALEM

Amos Cottage Rehabilitation Hospital
3325 Silas Creek Parkway, 27103
(919) 765-9916
Douglass M. Cody
Administrator

OHIO

AKRON

Children's Hospital Medical Center of
    Akron
281 Locust Street, 44308
(216) 379-8200
William H. Considine
President and Chief Executive Officer

CINCINNATI

Children's Hospital Medical Center
Elland and Bethesda Avenues,
    45229-2899
(513) 559-4200
William K. Schubert, M.D.
President and Chief Executive Officer

Shriners Burns Institute
3229 Burnet Avenue, 45229
(513) 872-6000
Ronald R. Hitzler
Administrator

CLEVELAND

Health Hill Hospital for Children
2801 Martin Luther King, Jr., Drive,
    44104
(216) 721-5400
Thomas A. Rathbone
President and Chief Executive Officer

COLUMBUS

Children's Hospital
700 Children's Drive, 43205
(614) 461-2000
Stuart Williams
Executive Director

DAYTON

Children's Medical Center
One Children's Plaza, 45404
(513) 226-8300
Laurence P. Harkness
President and Chief Executive Officer

NORTHFIELD

Sagamore Hills Children's Psychiatric
    Hospital
11910 Dunham Road, 44067
(216) 467-7955
D. W. Thernes, Jr.
Chief Executive Officer

YOUNGSTOWN

Belmont Pines Hospital
615 Churchill Hubbard Road, 44505
(216) 759-2700
Richard I. Feldman
Administrator

Western Reserve Care System—Tod
    Children's Hospital
500 Gypsy Lane, 44501
(216) 740-3898
Kris Hoce
Administrator

OKLAHOMA

NORMAN

J. D. McCarty Center for Children with
    Developmental Disabilities
1125 East Alameda, 73071
(405) 321-4830
Curtis A. Peters
Administrator

TULSA

Children's Medical Center
5300 East Skelly Drive, P.O. Box 35648,
    74153-0648
(918) 664-6600
Gerard J. Rothlein, Jr.
President and Chief Executive Officer

Shadow Mountain Institute
6262 South Sheridan, 74133
(918) 492-8200
Harold M. Katz
Chief Executive Officer

OREGON

PORTLAND

Shriners Hospital for Crippled Children
3101 S.W. Sam Jackson Park Road,
    97201
(503) 241-5090
Patricia J. Sadowski
Administrator

PENNSYLVANIA

DEVON

Devereux Foundation—French Center
119 Old Lancaster Road, P.O. Box 400,
  19333
(215) 964-3214
Gery Sasko
Executive Director

ERIE

Shriners Hospitals for Crippled
  Children
1645 West Eighth Street, 16505
(814) 452-4164
Richard W. Brzuz
Administrator

MALVERN

Devereux Foundation—Mapleton
  Psychiatric Institute—Earl D. Bond
  Center
655 Sugartown Road, P.O. Box 400,
  19355
(215) 296-6923
Kenneth Tenley
Director

PHILADELPHIA

Children's Rehabilitation Hospital
3905 Ford Road, 19131
(215) 581-3100
Robert Moylan
Administrator

Children's Seashore House
Philadelphia Center for Health Care
  Sciences
3405 Civic Center Boulevard, 19104
(215) 895-3600
Richard W. Shepherd
President and Chief Executive Officer

Shriner's Hospital for Crippled
  Children, Philadelphia Unit
8400 Roosevelt Boulevard, 19152
(215) 332-4500
Sharon J. Rajnic
Administrator

St. Christopher's Hospital for Children
Erie Avenue at Front Street, 19134-1095
(215) 427-5000
Calvin Bland
President and Chief Executive Officer

Children's Hospital of Philadelphia
34th Street and Civic Center Boulevard,
  19104
(215) 590-1000
Edmond F. Notebaert
President and Chief Executive Officer

PITTSBURGH

Children's Hospital of Pittsburgh
One Children's Place,
3705 Fifth Avenue at DeSoto Street,
  15213-2583
(412) 692-5325
Edwin K. Zechman, Jr.
President

Southwood Psychiatric Hospital
2575 Boyce Plaza Road, 15241
(412) 257-2290
Alan A. Axelson, M.D.
Medical Director and Chief Executive
  Officer

Children's Home of Pittsburgh
5618 Kentucky Avenue, 15232-2696
(412) 441-4884
B. Marlene West
Executive Director

TREVOSE

Eastern State School and Hospital
3740 Lincoln Highway, 19047
(215) 671-3141
Robert E. Switzer, M.D.
Superintendent

RHODE ISLAND

RIVERSIDE

Emma Pendleton Bradley Hospital
1011 Veterans Memorial Parkway,
  02915
(401) 434-3400
Ellen R. Nelson, Ph.D.
President and Chief Executive Officer

SOUTH CAROLINA

GREENVILLE

Shriners Hospital for Crippled Children,
  Greenville Unit
950 West Faris Road, 29605
(803) 271-3444
Gary Fraley
Administrator

SOUTH DAKOTA

SIOUX FALLS

Crippled Children's Hospital and
  School
2501 West 26th Street, 57105
(605) 336-1840
Charisse S. Oland
President and Chief Executive Officer

TENNESSEE

KNOXVILLE

East Tennessee Children's Hospital
2018 West Clinch Avenue, P.O. Box
  15010, 37916
(615) 541-8000
Robert F. Koppel
President

MEMPHIS

Le Bonheur Children's Medical Center
One Children's Plaza, 848 Adams
  Avenue, 38103
(901) 522-3000
Eugene K. Cashman, Jr.
President and Chief Executive Officer

St. Jude Children's Research Hospital
332 North Lauderdale Street, Box 318,
  38101
(901) 522-0300
Frederick F. Nowak
Chief Operating Officer

NASHVILLE

Vanderbilt Child and Adolescent
  Psychiatric Hospital
1601 23d Avenue, S., 37212
(615) 320-7770
William Nolan
Administrator

TEXAS

AUSTIN

Meridell Achievement Center
P.O. Box 203638, 78720
(512) 259-0774
Michele Toth, M.D.
Managing Director

Oaks Treatment Center
1407 West Stassney Lane, 78745
(512) 444-9561
Diane G. Stewart
Director

CORPUS CHRISTI

Ada Wilson Children Center for
  Rehabilitation
3511 South Alameda Street, 78411
(512) 853-9977
Teresa Barron
Administrator

Driscoll Children's Hospital
3533 South Alameda, 78411
(512) 850-5000
Joel T. Allison, F.A.C.H.E.
Chief Executive Officer

DALLAS

Children's Medical Center of Dallas
1935 Motor Street, 75235
(214) 640-2000
George D. Farr
President and Chief Executive Officer

Texas Scottish Rite Hospital for
  Children
2222 Welborn, P.O. Box 19567, 75219
(214) 521-3168
J. C. Montgomery, Jr.
President

FORT WORTH

Cook–Fort Worth Children's Medical
  Center
801 Seventh Avenue, 76104
(817) 885-4000
Russell K. Tolman
President

GALVESTON

Shriners Hospital for Crippled Children,
  Burn Institute
815 Market Street, 77550
(409) 770-6600
John A. Swartwout
Administrator

HOUSTON

Shriners Hospitals for Crippled
  Children, Houston Unit
1402 North MacGregor Drive, 77030
(713) 797-1616
Steven B. Reiter
Administrator

Texas Children's Hospital
6621 Fannin Street, Mail Code 1-4460,
  77030
(713) 770-1000
Mark A. Wallace
Executive Director and Chief Executive
  Officer

SAN ANTONIO

Monte Vista Hospital
210 West Ashby Place, 78212
(512) 736-2211
Anne G. Anthony
Executive Director

Southwest Neuropsychiatric Institute—
  Woodlawn
2939 West Woodlawn, 78228
(512) 736-4273
Carl M. Pfeifer, M.D.
Executive Director

VICTORIA

Devereux Foundation—Texas Center
120 David Wade Drive, 77902
(512) 575-8271
Gail Atkinson
Executive Director

UTAH

SALT LAKE CITY

Primary Children's Medical Center
100 North Medical Drive, 84113
(801) 588-2000
Donald R. Poulter
Chief Executive Officer

Shriners Hospital for Crippled
  Children—Intermountain Unit
Fairfax Avenue and Virginia Street,
  84103
(801) 532-5307
Marie N. Holm
Administrator

WEST JORDAN

Rivendell Psychiatric Center
5899 West Rivendell Drive, 84084
(801) 561-3377
Jared U. Balmer
Executive Director

VIRGINIA

LEESBURG

Graydon Manor
301 Children's Center Road, 22075
(703) 777-3485
Bernard Haberlein
Executive Director

NEW KENT

Cumberland Hospital for Children
P.O. Box 150, 23124
(804) 966-2242
Leslie Wyatt
Administrator

NORFOLK

Children's Hospital of the King's
  Daughters
601 Children's Lane, 23507
(804) 628-7000
Stephen S. Perry, Jr.
President

RICHMOND

Children's Hospital
2924 Brook Road, 23220
(804) 321-7474
George Comstock
Hospital Administrator

STAUNTON

De Jarnette Center
Richmond Road, Drawer 2309, P.O. Box
  2309, 24401
(703) 332-8800
Andrea C. Newsome
Director

WASHINGTON

SEATTLE

Children's Hospital and Medical Center
P.O. Box 5371
4800 Sand Point Way, N.E., 98105
(206) 526-2000
Treuman Katz
President and Chief Executive Officer

SPOKANE

Shriners Hospitals for Crippled
  Children
911 West Fifth Avenue, 99204
(509) 455-7844
Howard L. Parrett
Administrator

TACOMA

Mary Bridge Children's Hospital and
  Health Center
317 South K Street, P.O. Box 5299,
  98405-0987
(206) 594-1000
Karen Lynch, R.N.
Associate Administrator for Patient
  Services

WISCONSIN

MILWAUKEE

Children's Hospital of Wisconsin
9000 West Wisconsin Avenue, P.O. Box
  1997, 53201
(414) 266-2000
Jon E. Vice
President

Nonfreestanding Hospitals in the United States

ARIZONA

PHOENIX

Children's Health Center
St. Joseph's Hospital
350 West Thomas Road, 85013
(602) 285-3160
Joseph DeSilva
President

TUCSON

University Medical Center Children's
  Hospital
1501 North Campbell Avenue, 85724
(602) 694-0111
Martha Enriquez, R.N., M.S.N.
Director, Women and Children's
  Services

CALIFORNIA

LOMA LINDA

Loma Linda University Children's
  Hospital
11234 Anderson Street, 92350
(714) 824-4223
David B. Hinshaw, Sr., M.D.
President of Loma Linda University
  Medical Center

LONG BEACH

Memorial Miller Children's Hospital
2801 Atlantic Avenue, P.O. Box 1428,
  90801-1428
(310) 933-2000
Jonathan R. Bates, M.D.
Senior Vice President/Administrator

SACRAMENTO

University Children's Hospital
University of California–Davis, Medical
  Center
2315 Stockton Boulevard, 95817
(916) 734-2011
Frank J. Loge
Director

FLORIDA

HOLLYWOOD

Memorial Hospital Children's Center
3501 Johnson Street, 33021
(305) 987-2000
Frank V. Sacco
Administrator and Chief Executive
  Officer

JACKSONVILLE

Wolfson Children's Hospital
800 Prudential Drive, 32207
(904) 393-2000
Larry J. Freeman
Administrator

MIAMI

Baptist Hospital of Miami
8900 North Kendall Drive, 33176-2197
(305) 596-1960
Brian E. Keeley
President

ORLANDO

Arnold Palmer Hospital for Children
and Women
Orlando Regional Healthcare System
1414 Kuhl Avenue, 32806
(407) 649-9111
J. Gary Strack
President and Chief Executive Officer

PENSACOLA

Children's Hospital at Sacred Heart
Hospital
5151 North Ninth Avenue, 32504
(904) 474-7000
Sr. Virginia Cotter
President and Chief Executive Officer

TAMPA

St. Joseph's Children's Hospital
3001 West Martin Luther King
Boulevard, P.O. Box 4227, 33677
(813) 870-4662
Michael D. Aubin
Chief Executive Officer

GEORGIA

AUGUSTA

Children's Medical Center, Medical
College of Georgia
1120 15th Street, 30912-6001
(706) 721-0211
R. Edward Howell
Executive Director, MCG Hospital and
Clinics

MACON CITY

Children's Hospital at the Medical
Center of Central Georgia
777 Hemlock Street, P.O. Box 6000,
31201
(912) 744-1104
Damon D. King, F.A.C.H.E.
President

SAVANNAH

Children's Hospital at Memorial
Medical Center
4700 Waters Avenue, P.O. Box 23039,
31403-3089
(912) 350-8000
John E. Ives
President, Chief Executive Officer

IDAHO

BOISE

St. Luke's Regional Medical Center
190 East Bannock, 83712
(208) 386-2113
Vera M. Fink
Divisional Director Woman/Children
Services

ILLINOIS

CHICAGO

Sylvain and Arma Wyler Children's
Hospital
University of Chicago Hospitals
5841 South Maryland, MC 1051, 60637
(312) 702-6239
Susanne Banz
Associate Director, Wyler Children's
Hospital and Pediatrics

MOLINE

Trinity Medical Center—East Campus
P.O. Box 934, 61265
(309) 757-2968
Barry J. Halm
President and Chief Executive Officer

PARK RIDGE

Lutheran General Children's Medical
Center
1775 Dempster Street, 60068
(708) 696-2210
Kevin S. Wardell
President and Chief Executive Officer

PEORIA

Children's Hospital of Illinois at Saint
Francis Medical Center
530 N.E. Glen Oak Avenue, 61637
(309) 655-7171
Sr. M. Canisia, O.S.F.
Administrator

ROCKFORD

Rockford Memorial Hospital—
Children's Center
2400 North Rockton Avenue, 61103
(815) 968-6861
Thomas Defauw
President

INDIANA

INDIANAPOLIS

James Whitcomb Riley Hospital for
Children
Indiana University Hospitals
1100 West Michigan Street, 46202
(317) 274-5000
David J. Handel
Director

KENTUCKY

LOUISVILLE

Kosair Children's Hospital, Alliant
Health System
200 East Chestnut, P.O. Box 35070,
40232-5070
(502) 629-6000
G. Rodney Wolford
President and Chief Executive Officer of
Alliant Health System

MARYLAND

BALTIMORE

Johns Hopkins Children's Center
600 North Wolfe Street, CMSC 2-121,
21205
(410) 955-5000
Ted Chambers
Administrator

MASSACHUSETTS

BOSTON

Floating Hospital for Infants and
Children
New England Medical Center
750 Washington Street, 02111
(617) 956-5000
Jerome H. Grossman, M.D.
President

SPRINGFIELD

Baystate Medical Center's Children's
Hospital
759 Chestnut Street, 01199
(413) 784-0000
Mark Tolosky
Chief Executive Officer and President

NEVADA

LAS VEGAS

Humana Children's Hospital—Las
Vegas
3186 Maryland Parkway, P.O. Box
98530, 89193
(702) 731-8000
Allan Stipe
Executive Director

NEW HAMPSHIRE

LEBANON

Dartmouth-Hitchcock Medical Center
Children's Hospital at Dartmouth
One Medical Center Drive, 03756
(603) 650-5000
James W. Varnum
President

NEW JERSEY

NEWARK

Children's Hospital of New Jersey
United Hospital Medical Center
15 South Ninth Street, 07107
(201) 268-8760
Richard H. Rapkin, M.D.
Medical Director

NEW YORK

NEW HYDE PARK

Schneider Children's Hospital
Long Island Jewish Medical Center
269-01 76th Avenue, 11042
(718) 470-3000
Martin Fink
Administrator

NORTH CAROLINA

CHAPEL HILL

North Carolina Children's Hospital
University of North Carolina Hospitals
101 Manning Drive, 27514
(919) 966-4131
Thomas D. Kmetz
Assistant Director of Operations

CHARLOTTE

Carolinas Medical Center
1000 Blythe Boulevard, P.O. Box 32861,
    28232-2861
(704) 355-2000
Harry A. Nurkin, Ph.D.
President

FAYETTEVILLE

Cape Fear Valley Medical Center
Cumberland County Hospital System
1638 Owen Drive,
P.O. Box 2000, 28302
(919) 323-6151
John T. Carlisle
Administrator

NORTH DAKOTA

BISMARCK

Medcenter One
300 North Seventh Street, 58501
(701) 224-6000
Terrance G. Brosseau
President

Children's Center
St. Alexius Medical Center
900 East Broadway, Box 5510, 58502
(701) 224-7600
Richard A. Tschider
Administrator, Chief Executive Officer

FARGO

Children's Hospital—Meritcare
720 4th Street North, 58122
(701) 234-6000
Lloyd Smith
President, St. Luke's Hospitals

OHIO

CLEVELAND

Cleveland Clinic Children's Hospital
9500 Euclid Avenue, A 120, 44195-5045
(216) 444-2200
Douglas S. Moodie, M.D.
Chairman, Center for Children and
    Youth

Rainbow Babies and Children's Hospital
2074 Abington Road, 44106
(216) 844-3762
Richard R. Evens
Acting Senior Vice President and
    General Manager

OKLAHOMA

OKLAHOMA CITY

Children's Hospital of Oklahoma
Oklahoma Medical Center
940 N.E. 13th Street, P.O. Box 26307,
    73126
(405) 271-6165
Mike Noel
Administrator

TULSA

Children's Center
Saint Francis Hospital
6161 South Yale, 74136
(918) 494-2200
Sr. Mary Blandine Fleming
Administrator

OREGON

PORTLAND

Children's Healthcare Center at
   Emanuel Hospital and Health Center
2801 N. Gantebein Avenue, 97227
(503) 280-3500
James May
President and Chief Executive Officer

Doernbecher Children's Hospital at the
   Oregon Health Sciences University
3181 S.W. Sam Jackson Park Road,
   97201-3098
(503) 494-8811
Timothy M. Goldfarb
Hospital Director

PENNSYLVANIA

DANVILLE

Geisinger Medical Center
North Academy Avenue, 17822-0150
(717) 271-6211
F. Kenneth Ackerman, Jr.
President

PITTSBURGH

Rehabilitation Institute of Pittsburgh
6301 Northumberland Street, 15217
(412) 521-9000
John A. Wilson
President and Chief Executive Officer

RHODE ISLAND

PROVIDENCE

Rhode Island Hospital
593 Eddy Street, Potter Building, 02903
(401) 444-4000
Eleanor Elbaum
Director, Pediatric Patient Services

SOUTH CAROLINA

CHARLESTON

Children's Hospital, Medical University
   of South Carolina
171 Ashley Avenue, 29425
(803) 792-3522
Stuart Smith
Executive Director, MUSC

GREENVILLE

Children's Hospital of the Greenville
   Hospital System
701 Grove Road, 29605
(803) 455-8860
William F. Schmidt, M.D., Ph.D.
Medical Director

TENNESSEE

JOHNSON CITY

Children's Hospital at Johnson City
   Medical Center
400 State of Franklin Road, 37604-6094
(615) 461-6111
Dennis Vonderfecht
Administrator/Chief Executive Officer

NASHVILLE

Children's Hospital of Vanderbilt
   University
1211 22d Avenue South, 37232
(615) 322-3377
Norman B. Urmy
Executive Director

TEXAS

GALVESTON

Children's Hospital at the University of
   Texas Medical Branch Hospitals
301 University Boulevard, 77555-0518
(409) 772-3460
James F. Arens, M.D.
Chief Executive Officer

HOUSTON

Hermann Children's Hospital
6411 Fannin Street, 77030-1501
(713) 797-2170
Lynn M. Walts
Vice President of Operations

SAN ANTONIO

Santa Rosa Children's Hospital
Santa Rosa Health Care Corp.
519 West Houston Street, 78207-3108
(512) 228-2011
Sharon Smith
Interim Chief Executive Officer

VERMONT

BURLINGTON

Medical Center Hospital of Vermont,
    Women's and Children's Services
111 Colchester Avenue, 05401
(802) 656-2345
James H. Taylor
President

WEST VIRGINIA

MORGANTOWN

Children's Hospital of West Virginia
    University Hospitals
Medical Center Drive, 26506-8111
(304) 293-7086
Bernard G. Westfall
President

MAIL ORDER

Kids At Home Mail Order USA
P.O. Box 19083
Washington, DC 20036
    Write for a $3 catalog of listings for
children with special needs.

NOTES

[1]Schechter, N., Berde, C., Yaster, M., *Pain in Infants, Children and Adolescents* (Baltimore: Williams and Wilkins, 1993), 2.

[2]Rana, S., "Pain: A Subject Ignored" (letter), *Pediatrics,* 79 (1987), 309.

[3]Woolf, C. J., "Central Mechanisms of Acute Pain," *Proceedings of the Sixth World Congress on Pain, Pain RES and Clinical Management,* vol. 4, ed. Bond, M. R., et al. (Amsterdam: Elsevier, 1991), 25–34.

[4]McCaffery, M., Beebe, A., "About Pain in Children," *Nursing,* vol. 20, no. 7 (July 1990), 81.

[5]Hester, N., personal communication, 1992.

[6]Yaster, M., "When Pain Strikes," *20/20* interview, August 18, 1989.

[7]Maxwell, L. G., Yaster, M., Wetzel, R. C., Niebyl, J. R., "Penile Nerve Block for Newborn Circumcision," *Obstetrics and Gynecology,* vol. 70, no. 9 (September 1987), 415.

[8]Kolata, G., "Research News: Early Signs of School Age IQ," *Science,* 236 (1987), 774–75.

[9]Tree Trakatn, T., Pirayavaraporn, W., Lertakyamanee, J., "Topical Analgesia for Relief of Post-Circumcision Pain," *Anesthesiology,* vol. 67, no. 3 (September 1987), 395–99.

[10]Yaster, M., Bean, J., Tremlett, M., et al., "Pain, Sedation, and Postoperative Anesthetic Management in the Pediatric Intensive Care Unit," *Surgical and Anesthetic Considerations,* section 9, chapter 45, 1519.

[11]Anand, K. J., Aynsley-Green, A., "Measuring the Severity of Surgical Stress in Newborn Infants," *Journal of Pediatric Surgery,* 23 (1988), 297–305.

Anand, K. J., Brown, M. J., Causon, R. C., et al., "Can the Human Neonate Mount an Endocrine and Metabolic Response to Surgery?" *Journal of Pediatric Surgery,* 20 (1985), 41–48.

[12]Yaster, M., Maxwell, L. G., "Pediatric Regional Anesthesia," *Anesthesiology* (February 1989), 324–38.

[13]Zayas, V., "Pioneering Changes in Anesthesia Practice at Hospital for Special Surgery," *Horizon,* 1992, 17–18.

[14]Schechter, N., "The Undertreatment of Pain in Children," *Pediatric Clinics of North America,* vol. 36, no. 4 (August 1989), 788.

[15]Schechter, N., "The Undertreatment of Pain in Children," *Pediatric Clinics of North America,* vol. 36, no. 4 (August 1989), 787.

[16]Pizzo, P., personal communication, 1993.

[17]Fitzgerald, M., Shaw, A., McIntosh, N., "Postnatal Development of the Cutaneous Flexor Reflex: Comparative Study of Preterm Infants and Newborn Rat Pups," *Dev.-Med.Child.Neuro.,* 30 (1988), 520–26.

Fitzgerald, M., Millard, C., McIntosh, N., "Cutaneous Hypersensitivity Following Peripheral Tissue Damage in Newborn Infants and Its Reversal with Topical Anesthesia," *Pain,* 39 (1989), 31–36.

[18]Schechter, N., "Acute Pain in Children," *Pediatric Clinics of North America,* vol. 36, no. 4 (August 1989), 782.

[19]Mather, L., Mackie, J., "The Incidence of Postoperative Pain in Children," *Pain,* 15 (1983), 211–82.

[20]Agency for Health Care Policy and Research, "Acute Pain Management in Infants, Children, and Adolescents: Operative or Medical Procedures and Trauma," February 1992, 2.

[21]McCaffery, M., Beebe, A., *Pain: Clinical Manual for Nursing Practice,* St. Louis: C. V. Mosby, 1989), 271.

[22]Hester, N., Barcus, C., "Assessment and Management of Pain in Children," *Pediatrics: Nursing Update,* vol. 1, lesson 14 (1986), 2–8.

[23]Schechter, N., Berde, C., Yaster, M., *Pain in Infants, Children, and Adolescents* (Baltimore: Williams & Wilkins, 1993), 42.

[24]Hester, N., personal communication, 1992.

[25]Yaster, M., personal communication, 1992.

[26]McCaffery, M., personal communication, 1992.

[27]McCaffery, M., Beebe, A., *Pain: Clinical Manual for Nursing Practice* (St. Louis: C. V. Mosby, 1989), 271.

[28]Visintainer, M., Wolfer, J., "Psychological Preparation for Surgery on Pediatric Patients: The Effects on Children's and Parents' Stress Responses and Adjustment," *Journal Pediatrics,* vol. 50, no. 2 (August 1975), 107.

[29]Schechter, N., Berde, C., Yaster, M., *Pain in Infants, Children, and Adolescents* (Baltimore: Williams & Wilkins, 1993), 310.

[30]McCaffery, M., personal communication, 1992.

[31]Selbst, S., "Pain Management in the Emergency Department," *Pain in Infants, Children, and Adolescents* (Baltimore: Williams and Wilkins, 1993), 505–18.

[32]Selbst, S., Henretig, F., "The Treatment of Pain in the Emergency Department," *Pediatric Clinics of North America,* vol. 36, no. 4 (August 1989), 967.

[33]Yaster, M., personal communication, 1992.

[34]Schechter, N., "Acute Pain in Children," *Pediatric Clinics of North America,* vol. 36, no. 4 (August 1989), 310.
  McCaffery, M., Beebe, A., *Pain: Clinical Manual for Nursing Practice,* St. Louis: C. V. Mosby, 1989), 283.

[35]McKay, W., Morris, R., Mushlin, P., "Sodium Bicarbonate Attenuates Pain on Skin Infiltration with Lidocaine, with or without Epinephrine," *Anestha.Analg.,* 86 (1987), 856–57.
  Yaster, M., personal communication, 1992.

[36]McCaffery, M., Beebe, A., *Pain: Clinical Manual for Nursing Practice,* St. Louis: C. V. Mosby, 1989), 284.

[37]Schechter, N., "Why Do We Care?" Memorial-Sloan Kettering Cancer Center and European School of Oncology, April 2–4, 1992, New York.

[38]Berde, B., Lehn, B. M., Yee, J. D., et al., "Patient Controlled Analgesia in Children and Adolescents: A Randomized, Prospective Comparison with Intramuscular Administration of Morphine for Postoperative Analgesia," *Journal of Pediatrics,* 118 (1991), 460–66.

[39]Yaster, M., personal communication, 1993.

[40]Hester, N., personal communication, 1992.

[41]Hester, N., personal communication, 1992.

[42]Hester, N., personal communication, 1992.

[43]Hester, N., personal communication, 1992.
  Hester, N., Barcus, C., "Assessment and Management of Pain in Children," *Pediatrics: Nursing Update,* vol. 1, lesson 14 (1986), 4–5.

[44]From Whaley, L., Wong, D., *Nursing Care of Infants and Children,* third edition (St. Louis: C. V. Mosby, 1987), 1070.

[45]Berde, C., "Chronic Pain in Pediatrics," *Evaluation and Treatment of Chronic Pain,* second edition, ed. Aronoff, G. (Baltimore: Williams & Wilkins, 1992), 349.

[46]Foundation for Hospice and Homecare, "The Crisis of Chronically Ill Children in America: Triumph of Technology—Failure of Public Policy," report by the Caring Institute, congressional hearings, Washington, D.C., March 23, 1987.

[47]American Academy of Pediatrics, *Report of the Consensus Conference on the Management of Pain in Childhood Cancer,* vol. 86, no. 5 (November 1990), part 2.

4

ADOLESCENTS

The treatment of pain in adolescents must be combined with an understanding that the various stages of adolescence are fraught with extremely complex physical, emotional, and psychological struggles. Not to consider these highly charged adolescent stressors usually leads to inadequate pain control.

The study of pain in adolescents is almost as scarce as the study of pain in infants. Adolescents are often treated as either children or adults, resulting in poor pain management.

As mentioned in other chapters, pain is an "unpleasant sensory and emotional experience associated with actual or potential tissue damage, or described in terms of such damage."[1] Pain is a very complex physical, cultural, behavioral, and neurophysiological experience. It is as individual in the human as a fingerprint. No two persons experience pain in the same way, making it is impossible to know or even to guess how much pain someone is experiencing. Only the patient knows how much pain he or she is having or not having. It is of critical importance for doctors, nurses, and family members to take the time to assess pain and to make certain that pain relief is taking place. All persons, regardless of age, have a right to adequate pain control.

Within the general backdrop of the individuality of pain, the adolescent adds to the task of assessing pain by bringing his or her own complex emotional and physical stressors to the evaluation. The authors of the *Textbook of Adolescent Medicine* write, "The experience of pain associated with injury, disease or repeated invasive diagnostic and treatment procedures can threaten the adolescent's physical, emotional and psychological adjustment during an already vulnerable period. Untreated or untreated pain not only may have a significant emotional impact but also may result in poor medical outcome and maladaptive behavior."[2]

THE STAGES OF ADOLESCENCE

To understand the adolescent patient first requires the understanding of the different stages of adolescence. *The Hospitalized Adolescent: A Guide to Managing the Ill and Injured Youth* notes the following:[3]*

Puberty:
- Begins in the United States at about *11¾ years for boys and 11¼ for girls.*
- On the average, this is when the physical changes of adolescence begin to manifest themselves. There can be a variation in the pace of development. Consequently, there is a variation in emotional maturity.

As adolescence progresses, the youth also tries out new behaviors to match his or her physical and emotional growth. Part of the trying out of behaviors results in adolescents putting distance between themselves and their parents. On the way to becoming an adult, the adolescent travels a road full of what Erikson calls "the tasks of adolescence." Some of those tasks are:

- *Emancipation:* The youth trying to achieve autonomy
- *Role definition:* Trying to find out who he or she is through intellectual, sexual, and functional development. Part of this search is learning abstract thinking.

At various stages of adolescence, illness may mean different things at different ages to each youth.

Early Adolescence:
- This extends from *twelve to fifteen in females and thirteen to sixteen in males.*
- During this period both males and females possess fully developed hormone levels. Body image is of critical importance to this age group. Early adolescents of both sexes are preoccupied with how

*Adapted from Hofmann, A., Becker, R., Gabriel, H., *The Hospitalized Adolescent: A Guide to Managing the Ill and Injured Youth* (New York: Free Press, 1976), 121.

they look and feel. Acceptance can often revolve around interaction with friends. This period is generally not fraught with parent-teen tension and confrontation.

Marilyn Savedra, D.N.S., R.N., of the Department of Family Health Care Nursing, University of California–San Francisco, says, "The normal adolescent is so caught up with all the physical and emotional changes that the major question they have is 'Am I normal?' "[4]

If illness occurs at this age, the parents usually act on the adolescent's behalf. At this stage there are few issues about being dependent on parents', doctors', and nurses' decisions.

Midadolescence:

- This period ranges from approximately *fourteen to seventeen or eighteen.*
- Physical growth is usually completed. During this time there can be great conflict between the parent and the adolescent, generated by such issues as independence, dating, and control. Physical image is extremely important, since it directly relates to the success or failure to attract the opposite sex. This age represents a time when the adolescent has achieved a sense of self-worth and is capable of making most of his or her own decisions.

    If illness comes at this age, it is not tolerated well. Any change in the body can be devastating, since body image is of such importance. Dependence and the inability to make one's own decisions during the course of illness can add to a downward spiral in self-image, due to the loss of hard-won control and sense of self-worth.

Late Adolescence:

- This extends from approximately *seventeen to twenty-two years.*
- Typically, men and women of this age group are concerned with functional roles such as education, career, possible marriage, and the choice of how they are going to conduct their lives. Family relationships have quieted down, and interaction is on an adult level. Romantic relationships are calmer and less physically oriented and more adult, with emphasis on caring and sharing.

    Illness for this age can mean a serious interruption or deprivation of such fundamental lifetime goals as school, job, career, love, marriage, and life-style choices.

No two teenagers grow physically or mature emotionally at the same age or in the same way. Consequently, no two teens will respond to illness and pain in the same way. Among the many variables are:

- *The nature of illness:* What it is, how long it will last, what it will do to change the body, and what it will do to affect the youth's autonomy.
- *The age:* The age of onset can be psychologically critical when all the things that should be going right physically and emotionally are blocked by the limitations of illness or disability.
- *Chronic illness:* If chronic illness or disability occurs, the youth must face the long-term effects of possible alteration of the physical, social, school, work, and family structures. Feelings of wanting to be independent opposed to the reality of dependence make finding his or her own self-defining image emotionally depleting. Peer group interaction can be impossible, leading to confusion and isolation and further inhibiting the growth cycles that would normally take place. The normal exploration of independence within the family structure is also obstructed.
- *The course of the illness:* When an illness turns unstable and symptoms begin to affect such things as mobility, function, and interaction at school or with peers, causing isolation, maladaptive behavior may result. Hyperanxiety, depression, anger, panic, withdrawal, and acting out are but a few of the possible behaviors that can be exhibited.

  Illness itself may be the only focus, with either intense preoccupation with every aspect of the illness or, at the other extreme, intense denial of the illness. Mourning the loss of normal life, or a body part, or the possible loss of life itself, is common.

In the face of illness, it is entirely possible for an older adolescent to act grown up one day and regress suddenly another day. This can lead to confusion on the part of parents, doctors, and nurses as to how to interact with the adolescent. It is generally a poor idea to leave the adolescent to cope alone, as such behavior can be construed as abandonment and lack of caring.

Because adolescents are so involved with body image, it is important for family, doctors, nurses, and staff to be sensitive to these patients' right to privacy. Adolescents may find examinations and tests performed by strangers to be excruciatingly embarrassing and stressful.

An adolescent is not a child. He or she should be told, as simply as possible, what is wrong and what the proposed treatment plan might be. Honesty must prevail. Each patient should be prepared well ahead of time for any tests, invasive or not. Surprise can cause panic or evoke a combative attitude.

"We again iterate the imperative need to be tuned in to the teenager's specific fears about forced dependence, diminished mastery and control, bodily invasions, loss of privacy, humiliation and embarrassment, rejection by his peers, physical mutilation, and possible forced alteration of career and life-style hopes and dreams."[5]*

The stage of adolescent development can greatly influence how pain is perceived and how it is handled. As opposed to children, who may scream or cry, adolescents are usually more controlled in their behavior. Because adolescents without illness are attempting to achieve control and autonomy in their lives, it is important to allow them to participate in their pain management. "Asking adolescents about their pain, allowing them to individualize their experience and play a role in the control of their pain becomes an increasingly important aspect of pain assessment during this developmental period," write Hofmann et al.[6]

Savedra notes that there is a paucity of literature which provides baseline data on adolescents' experience with pain. A study of 156 adolescents thirteen to seventeen years of age in two schools and four hospitals focused on how adolescents describe pain. Questions were asked about how adolescents feel when they are in pain, how they describe pain, how they cope with pain, and what measures to relieve it were helpful. The adolescents reported having felt pain as the result of a wide range of experiences. Although pain was largely associated with physical pain, some equated pain with mental distress, such as the death of a parent or friend, divorce, or breaking up a relationship. The color red was most often associated with pain, but 40% did not mention color.

Sensory words were used most often to describe pain. Almost all were able to list one strategy they used to manage pain, such as not looking at the area of pain, listening to music, thinking about something else, getting into an altered state of consciousness, and turning to God. Sixty-five percent thought there was nothing good about pain.

*Adapted from Hofmann, A., Becker, R., Gabriel, H., *The Hospitalized Adolescent: A Guide to Managing the Ill and Injured Youth* (New York: Free Press, 1976), 121.

Hospitalized adolescents indicated that they had experienced pain in relation to surgery, treatment, or a specific disease. They also indicated that they most often felt scared and that they had no control when they were in pain. Medication was most frequently listed by hospitalized adolescents as a strategy for relieving pain.

In addition, the researchers found that adolescents were explicitly descriptive about how they felt when they were in pain. Descriptions of pain varied from a one-word answer ("terrible," "awful") to a vivid characterization ("like an earthquake with waves of vibrations pounding to your brain").[7]

As mentioned in Chapter 1, Melzack writes that there are "many words in the English language to describe the varieties of pain experience. To describe pain solely in terms of intensity, however, is like specifying the visual world in terms of light flux only, without regard to pattern, color, texture and the many other dimensions of visual experience."[8] Based on this information, it is critical to use assessment tools to describe and locate pain and to determine whether pain is impacting on the adolescent's quality of life.

ASSESSMENT

The *Adolescent Pediatric Pain Tool* (pages 192–93) can help the adolescent indicate the presence of pain and describe his or her pain so that family, doctors, and nurses can assess and treat it.[9]

The third part of the *Adolescent Pediatric Pain Tool* is a word descriptor. The words are selected from three categories to measure the "quality" of the pain, i.e.:

Sensory:
- Aching
- Pounding

- Biting
- Cutting, etc.

Evaluative:
- Bad
- Horrible

- Uncontrollable
- Never goes away, etc.

Affective:
- Crying
- Screaming

- Terrifying
- Frightening

Beyer and Wells write, "It is important to note that adolescents who are ill may regress to earlier stages of development. Thus, simpler

Adolescent Pediatric Pain Tool (Appt)

Instructions:

1. Color in the areas on these drawings to show where you have pain. Make the marks as big or small as the place where the pain is.

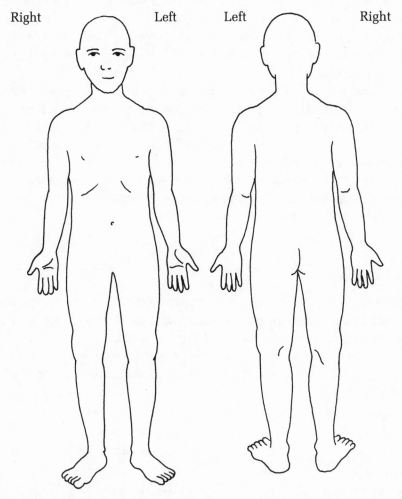

Right   Left   Left   Right

2. Place a straight, up and down mark on this line to show how much pain you have.

No	Little	Medium	Large	Worst
Pain	Pain	Pain	Pain	Possible
				Pain

3. Point to or circle as many of these words that describe your pain.

1	4	8	13
annoying	biting	shocking	never goes away
bad	cutting	shooting	uncontrollable
horrible	like a sharp knife	splitting	14
miserable	pin like	9	always
terrible	sharp	numb	comes and goes
uncomfortable	stabbing	stiff	comes on all of a
2	5	swollen	sudden
aching	blistering	tight	constant
hurting	burning	10	continuous
like an ache	hot	awful	forever
like a hurt	6	deadly	15
like a hurt	cramping	dying	off and on
sore	crushing	killing	once in a while
3	like a pinch	11	sneaks up
beating	pinching	crying	sometimes
hitting	pressure	frightening	steady
pounding	7	screaming	
punching	itching	terrifying	If you like, you
throbbing	like a scratch	12	may add other
	like a sting	dizzy	words:
	scratching	sickening	_____
	stinging	suffocating	_____
			_____

Reprint permission granted by M. C. Savedra, 1992.[10]

scales may be necessary during acute illness episodes." They add, "Pain assessment is most useful and accurate when frequent and systematic measurements are obtained. Pain assessment should be as systematic and more frequent than the monitoring of vital signs."[11]

In addition, adolescents are capable of using the *0–10 Numeric Pain Intensity Scale:* 0 = no pain, 10 = worst pain.

It can be used visually and/or verbally. Some patients may be too ill or too immobilized to use the scale visually. All the adolescent has to remember is "0 = no pain, 10 = worst pain."

Involving the adolescent in assessing his or her own pain allows the adolescent to participate in his or her own pain management. This active participation goes to the core of the adolescent's need for control and mastery.

Adolescents can also make use of the *Adolescent Daily Pain Chart.* They can chart their pain scores, the type of medication, dose, timing, and relief score. This chart can be particularly helpful when communication between staff and patient is limited.

PAIN CONTROL

Acute pain that results from diagnostic procedures can provide the adolescent with a high level of anxiety that must be coped with. "For example," writes McAnarney, "past successes or failures contribute to the adolescent's perceived self-effectiveness in coping with the expected pain, and to real or exaggerated memories of the pain itself. For some adolescents, the anxiety related to an anticipated pain event may become so overwhelming that he or she attempts to avoid the experience. Arguments with parents about pain may become a serious problem for adolescents with chronic illness."[12]

As with children, some adolescents may dislike pain control measures. Blanket orders do not work, hence each adolescent must be treated individually. Some may not be bothered by sedation before a procedure, and others may perceive sedation as a further loss of control. The caregiver must take the time to talk to the adolescent patient, prepare the patient, and investigate the adolescent's preferences for pain relief.

Since control is an important factor for adolescents, PCA (patient-controlled analgesia) and PCA-plus are good choices for *most* patients in the age group (see Chapter 1). As Dr. Myron Yaster mentioned earlier, PCA may be used unless the patient cannot understand how to use it, does not want to assume the responsibility for his or her own care, or is too sick or weak to push the button.

When oral medication is indicated, it has been suggested that adolescents be given the opportunity to self-administer oral medication, which is known as oral bedside PCA.[13]

As has been pointed out throughout this book, there is little chance of addiction. Remember the study of twelve thousand hospitalized adults? Only four patients in the study became addicted. The goal should be prevention and control of pain, not the preoccupation of restricting pain-relieving drugs based on misinformation. An adolescent receiving opioids for pain is totally different from a teen on the

Adolescent Daily Pain Chart

Name_____Date_____

Doctor_____

Medication(s)?_____

How often?_____What form? (Oral, IV, etc.)_____

What dose?_____

$$0 = \text{no pain} \qquad 10 = \text{worst pain}$$

```
 ├──┼──┼──┼──┼──┼──┼──┼──┼──┼──┤
 0   1   2   3   4   5   6   7   8   9   10
No                      Moderate              Worst
pain                      pain                possible
                                               pain
```

Time A.M./P.M.	Pain Score 0–10	Dose Received	Pain Score 30 min. IV or 60 min. oral	Comments

Describe pain in your own words_____

_____

_____

street corner seeking out drugs to get high. Failure to relieve acute pain may cause medical complications and lead to excessive emotional and psychological stress. In fact, adolescents need to be reminded that opioids prescribed for pain are safe to take. The war on drugs has even frightened some adolescents into enduring horrible pain out of fear of addiction.

The authors of *The Textbook of Adolescent Medicine* write, "The most effective approach to adolescent pain management is often a combination of pharmacological agents and psychological intervention. However, the approach taken depends on the type of pain and the adolescent's needs. In general, pain management methods should be implemented within the background of the individual adolescent and his or her family, assessing individual needs, capitalizing on personal resources, establishing predictability and control as appropriate, and fostering feelings of self-control and self-efficacy."[14]

Dr. Savedra urges "doctors, nurses and parents to elicit from the adolescent how they personally manage their pain. Some teens may retreat, some may really want to talk or some may want to listen to music. It is very important to listen to the techniques that they have developed over time, especially for repeated painful procedures."[15]

Medications

As mentioned in Chapter 1, a variety of drugs are available for pain control. With rigorous assessment and the direct involvement of the adolescent, they should be used to prevent and control pain. The goal is to ease the pain with the fewest side effects in order to return the youth to as normal a life as possible.

The drugs that are most commonly used are:

Mild Pain:
- Aspirin, nonacetylated salicylates (Trilisate)
- Acetaminophen (Tylenol)
- NSAIDs (ibuprofens: Nuprin, Advil, Motrin)

Moderate Pain:
- NSAIDs
- Codeine
- Dihydrocodeine

Severe Pain:
- Morphine. See Chapter 1 for other, morphine-like drugs.

Anxiety:
- Miadazolam (known as Versed) is commonly used, producing relaxation, amnesia, sedation, and muscle relaxation. This drug is used prior to medical procedures and when a patient's anxiety is overwhelming.[16]
- Diazepam (Valium) is an alternative.

Other Methods of Pain Relief

As with children and adults, nonpharmacological psychological methods of relieving pain would be:

- *Distraction:* Focusing attention on something other than the pain. Teens can play video games, watch TV, have conversations, etc.
- *Self-hypnosis or guided imagery:* Getting deeply involved with the fantasy of going into another setting, away from the painful event. Parents and nurses can help the adolescent find special places they like to go to, either a happy memory or a setting they make up.
- *Relaxation techniques:* Deep breathing, counting, etc. (For the basic relaxation exercise, see page 55.)

SUMMARY

Adolescents must have attention and understanding that relates to their complex physical and emotional development. Doctors, nurses, and family members must assess the adolescent's pain frequently, using as many tools as possible. Each youth should be prepared for any treatment well in advance, and be involved as a partner in planning his or her pain care.

See Chapter 2 for chronic pain and Chapter 5 for cancer pain.

NOTES

[1]International Association for the Study of Pain.

[2]McAnarney, E., Kreipe, R., Orr, D., Comerci, G., *Textbook of Adolescent Medicine* (Philadelphia: W. B. Saunders, 1992), 140.

[3]Adapted from Hofmann, A., Becker, R., Gabriel, H., *The Hospitalized Adolescent: A Guide to Managing the Ill and Injured Youth* (New York: Free Press, 1976), 3–89.

[4]M. Savedra, personal communication, 1992.

[5]Hofmann, A., Becker, R., Gabriel, H., *The Hospitalized Adolescent: A Guide to Managing the Ill and Injured Youth* (New York: Free Press, 1976), 121.

[6]Adapted from Hofmann, A., Becker, R., Gabriel, H., *The Hospitalized Adolescent: A Guide to Managing the Ill and Injured Youth* (New York: Free Press, 1976), 121.

[7]Savedra, M., Tesler, M., Ward, J., Wegner, C., "How Adolescents Describe Pain," *Journal of Adolescent Health Care,* 9 (1988) 315–20.

[8]Melzack, R., Torgerson, W. S., "On the Language of Pain" (1971).

[9]Tesler, M., Savedra, M., Holzemer, W., et al., "The Word-Graphic Rating Scale as a Measure of Children's and Adolescents' Pain Intensity," *Research in Nursing and Health,* 14 (1991), 361–71.

[10]Savedra, M. C., Tesler, M. D., Holzemer, W. L., Ward, J. A., University of California, San Francisco, School of Nursing (1989).

[11]Schechter, N., "Acute Pain in Children," *Pediatric Clinics of North America,* vol. 36, no. 4 (August 1989), 849.

[12]McAnarney, E., Kreipe, R., Orr, D., Comerci, G., *Textbook of Adolescent Medicine,* (Philadelphia: W. B. Saunders, 1992), 141–42.

[13]Litman, R., Shapiro, B., "Oral Patient-Controlled Analgesia in Adolescents," *Journal of Pain and Symptom Management,* vol. 7, no. 2 (February 1992), 78–81.

[14]McAnarney, E., Kreipe, R., Orr, D., Comerci, G., *Textbook of Adolescent Medicine* (Philadelphia: W. B. Saunders, 1992), 142.

[15]Savedra, M., personal communication, 1993.

[16]Yaster, M., personal communication, 1992.

CANCER PAIN

"Fear is an inherent feature of cancer, and one which, unfortunately, cannot be excised with a scalpel," writes John Stehlin, M.D., of the Stehlin Foundation for Cancer Research.[1]

More than 1,000,000 new cancer patients are diagnosed each year in the United States. It is estimated that there are 6,000,000 patients living with cancer, of whom 520,000 will die of the disease this year.[2]

Up to 60% to 90% of patients with advanced *cancer will experience significant pain, and up to 25% will die in pain.*[3] *The World Health Organization states that 80% to 90% of all cancer pain could be controlled or eliminated.*[4]

Pain is one of the most feared consequences of cancer, notes Kathleen Foley, M.D., Chief of the Pain Service at Memorial Sloan-Kettering Cancer Center in New York.[5]

Carol Moinpour, Ph.D., and C. Richard Chapman, Ph.D., write:

> Because of advances in early diagnosis and treatment, more patients are surviving cancer, and many who ultimately succumb do so only after a period of significantly extended life. Unfortunately, many patients pay a high price for effective treatment. Both the neoplasm [cancer] and the cytodestructive [cell destruction] interventions directed at it degrade the well-being of a cancer patient. Some patients who survive cancer suffer reduced functional capability, chronic symptom problems and/or persisting pain.
>
> Consequently, patient comfort and function during extended life and survival are emerging as pressing concerns in cancer care. Pain control is a critical element in the comprehensive care of many cancer patients. Multiple painful diagnostic and therapeutic events

and pain problems occur in the long interval between disease diagnosis and termination of treatment. . . . Unremitting pain over-shadows every other aspect of human existence, destroys hope and courage, and brings the family as well as the patient to the brink of desperation.[6]

Dr. John Bonica writes:

Many people regard cancer as being associated with pain, destruc-tion, loss and often with death. Individuals are concerned not only about the eventual outcome of their illness but also with the possi-bility of further suffering, especially severe pain, before their lives end. Thus, the diagnosis of disease brings with it a sense of help-lessness and provokes significant anxiety and fear. Cancer patients develop anxiety and fear of separation from family and friends, of loss of work and of life's goals, and of the consequences of the illness for others. They are also anxious and fearful in regard to increasing dependency and to loss of self-esteem, personal control and of their faculties, and mutilation by surgery.[7]

PAIN UNDERTREATED

Despite the profound anxiety, pain, and suffering that cancer produces, the undertreatment of cancer pain cruelly continues.

"Undertreatment of pain and other symptoms of cancer is a serious and neglected public health problem. Every patient with cancer should have the expectation that pain control will be an integral aspect of care throughout the course of the the disease," writes James Mason, M.D., head of the Public Health Service's Agency for Health Care Policy and Research. Pain management is so often ignored by doctors and health care professionals that the agency has formed a panel of fourteen private-sector health care experts and consumers to develop clinical practice guidelines for managing cancer pain.[8]

Dr. Bonica writes, "Inadequate or total lack of interest or concern by oncologists about the problem of pain is attested to by the fact that very little, if any, information on proper management of the pain problem is found in the oncologic [cancer] literature, voluminous as it is."[9]

Margo McCaffery, R.N., and Betty Ferrell, Ph.D., F.A.A.N., note, "A recent survey of pain content in the curriculum of 305 baccalaureate nursing programs accredited by the National League for Nursing re-vealed that 48% spend 4 hours or less on the subject of pain." They reviewed fourteen textbooks, which contained 10,000 pages of text. Only 133 pages, or 1.6% of the textbook pages, contained sections on pain and comfort. In addition, much of the information was misleading, inaccurate, or confusing when discussing the likelihood of addiction.

They also reported on 1,781 practicing nurses' specific knowledge deficits regarding opioid (morphine-like) analgesics. They found that *"Many nurses have exaggerated concerns about the rare consequence of addiction from the use of opioids for pain relief. This can result in reluctance to administer an opioid, causing needless suffering."*[10]

In 1990 David Weissman, M.D., and June Dahl, Ph.D., provided a brief questionnaire to 317 first-year medical students to assess their attitudes about cancer pain. The researchers discovered that students greatly exaggerated the incidence of psychological dependence (addiction) in patients treated with opioid analgesics, and believed that increasing pain was invariably related to the development of drug tolerance rather than to the progression of the disease.[11]

Marilee Donovan, R.N., Ph.D., and Paula Dillon, R.N., M.S., of St. Luke's Medical Center in Chicago, interviewed ninety-six randomly selected cancer patients regarding their experiences with pain during hospitalization. *"More than 50% had suffered from pain that was horrible or excruciating, yet only 43% of the patients could recall a nurse having discussed anything about their pain with them."*[12]

The most frequently noted reasons for undertreatment of cancer pain are:

- *Lack of knowledge:* Not enough emphasis on the cancer process. Cancer pain management not taught in school or in hospital programs.
- *Fear of addiction:* Unreasonable and unfounded fears based on myth and misinformation.
- *Underuse of drugs:* Lack of understanding of pharmacology of drugs, how quickly and how long drugs provide relief, and fear of not being able to deal with side effects.
- *Failure of assessment:* Patient self-report of pain levels doubted by staff; little attempt made to assess pain using pain assessment measures.
- *Pain not a priority:* No hospital dedication or national dedication to pain management; lack of accountability.

- *Patient barriers:* Lack of education, fear of addiction, loss of control, desire to be a "good patient," equating pain with the progression of cancer.

The Wisconsin Cancer Pain Initiative noted other reasons for poor pain management:

- *Lack of coordination of care:* Patients are moved from one setting to another—for example, from a hospital to a nursing home.
- *Fragmentation of care:* Cancer patients often consult with three to fifteen specialists.
- *Unwillingness of pharmacies:* Pharmacies in large cities don't stock opioids because of theft. In less urban areas, resources for pain-relieving neurosurgical and other procedures are not available.[13]

A study by the Eastern Cooperative Oncology Group (ECOG) of 1,177 cancer specialists who had treated 70,000 cancer patients in the six months prior to the survey showed that almost 60% of the doctors reported poor pain assessment as a major barrier to good pain control.

Other results showed that doctors who faced state regulations which required triplicate prescription forms were reluctant to prescribe drugs as often as they were needed. Hypothetical patient cases were presented. Up to 86% of the doctors thought that cancer patients were undermedicated. The majority doctors thought that medical school cancer pain training was poor, and 73% reported that their hospital residency training in cancer pain management was poor or fair.[14]

Cancer pain is extremely complex. A patient must face not only the diagnosis of cancer, the invasion and alteration of the body, but the possible progression of the cancer as well. There can also be an erosion in the quality of life enjoyed, change in or loss of job, and increasing dependence on the family. There may be an overlay of psychological suffering, such as anxiety, depression, anger, fear of abandonment, sadness, helplessness, or hopelessness. Pain is "often experienced not only as an immediate threat to body, comfort or activity, but also to well-being and life in general," write Drs. Donald Price and Stephen Harkins, of the Medical College of Virginia.[15] Finally, the worst fear is that any pain may signal a hastening of death.

Judith Spross, a professor of Nursing at Massachusetts General Hospital in Boston, refers to unrelieved cancer pain as "an emergency for the patient, regardless of the underlying pathology." She states that "professionals must apply the science and art of pain relief as if a life depended on it; certainly the quality of life does."[16]

Stuart Grossman, M.D., of the Johns Hopkins Pain Center, says, "At a cancer center, we discovered that M.D.s and nurses didn't have any idea of how much pain cancer patients have. If they don't know how much pain patients have, how can they treat the pain?"[17]

Dr. Grossman gave a lecture to eighty-eight medical students and medical residents. He presented them with typical pain management questions, like this one: "Mrs. C has been taking 60 milligrams of codeine and 60 milligrams of methadone every six hours. What hourly rate of intravenous morphine will you choose to keep Mrs. C's cancer pain well controlled?" The students were given textbooks, handbooks, and permission to discuss the problem among themselves. Only seven students got the right answer. After the results were in, Dr. Grossman asked the students if these were fair questions. All agreed that "these were things they had to do every day and were embarrassed to admit that they just had never been taught how to do them."[18]

Mitchell Max, M.D., of the National Institutes of Health, writes, "The quality of care would benefit, no doubt, if clinicians deepened their knowledge of the finer points of analgesic pharmacology . . . 'inadequate education,' however, does not account for the commonest lapse: very often, when a patient gets little relief from an initial analgesic dose, no increase is made in the dose."[19]

Russell Portenoy, M.D., Director of Analgesic Studies at Memorial Sloan-Kettering Cancer Center, says:

> With cancer patients, the M.D. is often more preoccupied with how the cancer is doing than how the patient is doing. M.D.s are woefully trained in medical school. They lack the skills in the assessment of pain and lack a pharmacological background to treat pain in a state-of-the-art manner. Undertreatment originates with the M.D. and is directly related to fears of toxicity and addiction. Those fears are often wildly overestimated. Toxicity is usually treatable and addiction occurs in less than 1% of the population. Nurses compound the problem with the same lack of education as M.D.s. They too are not taught to assess pain. Often the patient complaining of pain never gets past the nurse to the M.D.[20]

TYPES OF CANCER PAIN

In order to understand cancer pain, it is important to know about the different types of pain and how they occur. Kathleen Foley, M.D., writes:

> Patients with cancer have two types of pain: Acute and Chronic.
> Group I comprises patients with acute cancer-related pain.
> The first subgroup of this category includes patients in whom pain is the major symptom leading to the diagnosis of cancer. For this group, pain has a special meaning as the harbinger of their illness. The occurrence of pain during the course of the illness, or after successful therapy, has the immediate implication of recurrent disease.[21]

Although it is widely believed that cancer is not painful early in its course, Randall Daut, Ph.D., and Charles Cleeland, Ph.D., found that pain is an early symptom of cancer in 40% to 50% of patients with cancer of the breast, ovary, prostate, colon, and rectum and in about 20% of patients with cancer of the uterus and cervix.[22]

Foley continues:

> The second subgroup includes patients who have acute pain associated with cancer therapy—e.g. pain after surgery or secondary to the acute effects of chemotherapy. The cause of the pain is readily identified, and its course is predictable and self-limited. Such patients endure pain for the promise of a successful outcome.[23]

Bonica adds that acute pain can "occur during and after certain diagnostic procedures and various anticancer therapies, particularly postoperative pain, pain during chemotherapy and radiation therapy and in the acute [pain] secondary to steroid withdrawal."[24]

In the textbook The Management of Pain, the following chart notes types of acute pain:[25]

> Group II consists of patients with chronic cancer-related pain, and represents difficult diagnostic and therapeutic problems. This group can be subdivided into patients with chronic pain from tumor progression and those with chronic pain related to cancer treatment.
> Group III includes patients with a history of chronic, nonmalignant pain who have cancer and associated pain. Psychological

Acute Pain Associated with Cancer Management

Diagnostic Procedures

Blood samples
Lumbar puncture
Angiography
Endoscopy
Biopsy
Lymphangiogram

*Radiotherapy**

Skin burns
Mucositis
Pharyngitis
Esophagitis
GI distress
Proctitis
Itching
Painful fractures

*Can cause delayed onset and chronic pain.

*Treatment-Related Infections**

Bacterial
Fungal
Viral
Herpes—oral. So painful it is impossible to eat or speak.
Herpes zoster. Excruciatingly painful; can result in postherpetic neuralgia.

*Substantial pain problems for cancer patients who undergo surgical biopsy, exploratory surgery, or therapeutic surgery that produces postoperative pain.

Chemotherapy

Mucositis
Myalgia
Arthralgia
Pancreatitis
GI distress
Nausea/Vomiting
Cardiomyopathy
Extravasation of drug into tissues

*Surgical Therapy**

Postoperative pain
Ileus, colic
Urinary retention distress

*Chemotherapy and radiation weaken and may destroy the patient's immune system, leaving the patient vulnerable to infections.

Adapted from Bonica, J., *The Management of Pain*, second edition (Philadelphia: Lea & Febiger, 1990).

factors play an important part in these patients, whose psychological and functional status is already compromised. They are at high risk for further functional incapacity and escalating chronic pain.[26]

(Group IV and Group V patients who are dying with pain are discussed in Chapter 10.)

Single or multiple areas of pain can be the result of the cancer itself, the effects of radiation and chemotherapy, other noncancer disorders, or a combination of several causes. The pain can involve tissue, nerves, bones, and skin.

Chronic Cancer-Related Pain Syndromes

Up to 78% of persons in an inpatient cancer population and 62% of persons in an outpatient cancer population will have pain.[27]

Those chronic cancer-related pain syndromes are:

Invasion of the bone:
   Spine, base of skull, pelvis, long bones, ribs, shoulders, etc.
Tumor compression or infiltration of peripheral nerves or plexus:
   Peripheral, cranial, spine, etc.
Tumor involvement of viscera:
   Abdominal area—all internal organs
Other types of tumor involvement:
   Blood vessels—infiltration or obstruction; mucous membranes
Postsurgical pain
Postchemotherapy pain
Postradiation therapy pain
Pain unrelated to cancer:
   Other chronic pain from arthritis, osteoporosis, migraine, etc.[28]

INDIVIDUAL RESPONSE TO PAIN

Along with the physical pain, and of equal impact, is the complex individual response to pain. As mentioned earlier, pain is as individual as the human fingerprint. *There is no way to know how much pain a person is experiencing. Only the person who has the pain knows.*

No two cancer patients experience pain in the same way. Each patient brings along the uniqueness of his or her cancer and his or her coping skills, as well as attitudes about pain and what it means to the individual. Gary Donaldson, Ph.D., a specialist in Pain and Toxicity

Research at the Fred Hutchinson Cancer Research Center in Seattle, says, "In research there is no average response. Patients have individual traits and predispositions. When treating a patient, whatever makes people different will account for differences in outcome . . . personality, life events, family. There is no such thing as a typical patient."[29]

Relieving pain allows patients the energy to live their lives to the fullest of their capacity. Not to relieve pain is to condemn the patient to a life darkened by pain. Pain can reduce one's life to stress, fatigue, sleeplessness, helplessness, dependence, depression, and hopelessness. Continuous pain is a "constant unremitting sensation, often of such intensity that it dominates an individual's entire existence, disturbing sleep, thought, and everyday activity," notes Mehta.[30]

In addition, there is mounting evidence that poor cancer pain management might impair the immune system. John Liebeskind, Ph.D., professor of Psychology at UCLA, studies pain stress and immunity. He states, "Pain can kill. If you look at the killer cells—the body's first line of defense against virus and cancer—you'll see a reduced killing of the cells in animals who are pain stressed. Opiates [morphine-like drugs] can block this effect."[31]

The very simple things in life that we take for granted—eating, sleeping, dressing, laughing, walking, independence, choices, socialization, job and family interaction—can all be lost for the cancer patient in pain.

THE VICIOUS CIRCLE OF POOR PAIN CONTROL

It is important to look at the vicious circle of poor pain control that makes thousands of patients in thousands of hospitals victims every day.

In the classic scenario, the doctor prescribes an opioid shot to be given intramuscularly every four hours. We already know that many doctors do not acknowledge the level of pain the patient is experiencing. Since he is fearful of addiction and side effects, and often does not understand the pharmacology of drugs, he will underprescribe the amount of drug, as well as the timing of the dosage.

His prescription is ordered "PRN" (as needed). That means patients must ask for a shot when they feel pain. When the patient complains of pain, he must first find a nurse who has the time to check the patient.

As reported in Chapter 1, there is clear evidence from research that the majority of nurses will cut the dose prescribed by the doctor. By the time the nurse looks at the patient, the key to the drug cabinet is obtained, and the dose drawn and administered, up to an hour may have passed. When the patient gets an intramuscular shot—a shot that hurts—it sometimes takes more than ninety minutes for it to be absorbed into the bloodstream. The patient suffers. Because the pain level was too high to begin with and the dose too low, the patient complains of pain and begs the nurse for more medication. She refuses, on "doctor's orders." The nurse can often be as biased as the doctor. Her concern is not to addict the patient.

When the patient is reduced to desperate, demanding pleas for more medication, McCaffery points out, many nurses *incorrectly* assume that the patient is "overstating the pain" and "preoccupied with desire for more drug." The patient is tagged by the nursing staff as "only wanting drugs," "exhibiting addictive drug behavior," or, the worst misconception, "a drug addict."[32]

If only the medical staff would put aside their misconceptions and become educated about pain and the pharmacology of drugs, they would find that a cancer patient who is adequately managed for pain will very likely not be preoccupied with drugs.

THE ETHICS OF PAIN RELIEF

There have been reports of doctors and nurses who "turn off the patient's suffering" and become immune to it. This brings up the human, medical, and legal ethics of allowing patients to suffer needless pain. A very basic tenet of our humanity is that we are capable of compassion. As the Reverend Robert Smith, Ph.L., notes, *"The treatment of pain is a moral imperative. Professional health care providers and patients have a shared human-ness with the patients and there is a need to humanize the medical experience. Health care providers have a clear moral duty to alleviate pain and it is simply not enough to just 'treat the pain'; there must be a clear developed strategy."*[33]

He writes, *"Pain consequent upon disease, or related to therapy, which can be but is not controlled is an instance of ethical failure on the part of the care giver. It is a violation of the principle of benevolence which grounds all health care. It violates the covenant of mutual trust implicit in the relationship between care giver and patient, because fear of being abandoned to overwhelming pain is constantly mentioned as the principal cause of dread in cancer patients. Lastly, it is a straightforward failure to live by the codes of both nurses' and physicians' professional organizations."* [34]

You read in the Introduction about a man who had cancer which had spread to his bones. He was in crushing pain. His doctor had ordered morphine to be administered every four hours. However, the nurse in charge decided the dose was too high. She gave him an over-the-counter drug. He finally stopped eating and sitting up. He just lay in bed suffering. After he died, the family filed suit against the nurse and the institution for failure to adequately treat the man's pain. The court awarded his family $7.5 million in punitive damages and $7.5 million dollars for suffering. The federal government and the state testified against the nurse and the institution, stating that both had violated the legal standards of care.

One must ask how any health care professional can allow incapacitating cancer pain to exist, either based on ignorance of pain management or because of underdosing or cutting patients' pain medications.

THE EFFECTS OF UNRELIEVED PAIN

Acute

As you have read, unrelieved acute pain can lead to pain-related physical complications, such as:

- Increased heart rate and blood pressure
- Negative emotions, such as anxiety, depression, fear, helplessness, etc.

At the very least, these unnecessary side effects of unrelieved acute pain can extend a stay in the hospital, which adds to the expense.

The worst effect may be serious, life-threatening complications such as pneumonia or blood clots. For the elderly and those who are already weak, it is possible for these complications to lead to death.

Chronic

Some of the effects of unrelieved chronic pain are sleeplessness and loss of appetite.

Emotional side effects include fear, anger, depression, hopelessness, and suicidal feelings. These are just some of the side effects of un-relieved chronic cancer pain.

Up to 90% of all cancer pain can be controlled, and almost all patients can enjoy some level of relief.

ASSESSMENT

The cornerstone of cancer pain management is assessment, assessment, and assessment.

Your doctor should first obtain a detailed medical and pain history and a review of your past medical or surgical records, treatments, or any other therapies (your pain can be related to treatments and/or progression of the disease).

Bonica writes, *"A careful examination of the painful region and general physical, neurologic and orthopedic examinations are also essential to acquire objective data and to substantiate the clinical history."* [35]

Radiologic and laboratory diagnostic tests need to be performed "to confirm the clinical diagnosis and to define, in those patients with metastatic disease, the site and extent of tumor infiltration," writes Bonica. These tests can include x-rays, CT scans, bone scans, liver scans, and blood workups, to name a few. In some patients, biopsy or surgical exploration may be necessary.

"It deserves re-emphasis that, early in the evaluation course, it is important to provide the patient with effective pain relief. In addition to the obvious humanitarian reason, partial relief will markedly improve the patient's ability to participate in the various diagnostic procedures," adds Bonica. [36]

The Pain Service, Department of Neurology, at Memorial Sloan-Kettering Cancer Center evaluated 276 patients with cancer pain. The researchers noted how important a comprehensive evaluation is in the management of patients with cancer pain. During the pain consultation they "identified a previously undiagnosed etiology for the pain in 64% of the patients." Spread of the cancer was the most common finding, along with the discovery that 36% of the patients had neurologic diagnoses and 4% had unsuspected infections. [37]

Communication About Pain

To help doctors and nurses understand your pain, you need to learn how to talk about your pain and communicate that information to them.

It is a start to say "I'm in pain." However, you then need to describe your pain as specifically as you can.

Remember, there is much more happening with your pain than the physical pain. Your own pain is as individual as you are. Recall that Dr. Myron Yaster mentioned that one reason pain is so different in each person is because each person experiences life in a unique manner. For example, two people can listen to the same music and feel differently about it. In Chapter 1, Dr. Ronald Melzack wrote that trying to measure pain just by intensity was like "specifying the visual world in terms of light flux only, without regard to pattern, color, texture and the many dimensions of visual experience." In addition, you bring your own emotional, metabolic, physical, and possibly genetic differences to your pain.

C. Richard Chapman, Ph.D., Director of the Pain and Toxicity Research Program at the Fred Hutchinson Cancer Research Center, writes, "Pain falls into a class of specific sensory experiences such as smell or sounds since we experience pain as a bodily sensation."[38]

You need to learn how to describe your pain with all the richness of detail that you can. For example:

- Where is the pain located?
- Is the pain in one site or many?
- What does the pain feel like?

Sensory Feeling:
- Temporal:
  Beating, pounding, etc.
- Spatial:
  Shooting, radiating, etc.
- Punctate pressure:
  Piercing, stabbing, etc.
- Incisive pressure:
  Cutting, sharp, etc.

- Constrictive pressure:
  Crushing, cramping, etc.
- Traction pressure:
  Pulling, tugging, etc.
- Thermal:
  Burning, searing, etc.
- Brightness:
  Tingling, stinging, etc.

- Dullness: Aching, dull, etc.

Affective Feeling:

- Tension:
  Exhausting, fatiguing, etc.
- Autonomic:
  Sickening, nauseating, etc.

- Fear:
  Terrifying, dreadful, etc.
- Punishment:
  Killing, vicious, etc.

Evaluate Feeling:

- Agonizing, annoying, unbearable, savage, etc.

Brief Pain Inventory

One way to measure pain severity and other questions related to pain is the *Brief Pain Inventory* (BPI) beginning on the next page. *The BPI asks patients to rate the severity of their pain at its worst, least, on the average, and at the time they fill out the questionnaire.*

The BPI also "asks for ratings of how much pain interferes with mood, walking, other physical activity, work, social activity, relations with others, and sleep. The BPI asks patients to represent the location of their pain on a pain drawing, and asks other questions about duration of pain relief and cause of pain, and provides a list of descriptors to help the patient describe pain quality.

"Once you have filled in your answers, it may be helpful to show the BPI to your doctor or nurse. A short form of this scale has recently been developed for daily pain monitoring and for clinical use," write Charles Cleeland, Ph.D., and Karen Syrjala, Ph.D.

The more your doctors and nurses know about your pain, the greater the chance that you will receive individualized pain care.

Mark on the drawings, and answer the questions about how your pain feels now.

Dr. Chapman notes that there are many complex components involved in assessing pain:

> Pain measurement, from the sensory perspective, requires eliciting information from patients about pain intensity via self-report and recording that information. . . . The expression of pain is a socially meaningful communication, and it may involve facial expression, postural change, altered voice, behavioral components as well as the report of the subjective judgment. Ideally, the patient's report should match the nonverbal communication, but *experienced clinicians* know that this is not always the case. Many

Brief Pain Inventory

Date: __ / __ / __
Name: _____ _____ _____
             Last   First   Middle Initial
Phone: ( )_____   Sex: ☐ Female   ☐ Male
Date of Birth: __ / __ / __

1) Marital Status (at present)
    1. ☐ Single   3. ☐ Widowed
    2. ☐ Married   4. ☐ Separated/Divorced

2) Education (Circle only the highest grade or degree completed)
    Grade   0   1   2   3   4   5   6   7   8   9
              10 11 12 13 14 15 16 M.A./M.S.
    Professional degree (please specify) _____

3) Current occupation _____
    (specify titles: if you are not working, tell us your previous occupation)

4) Spouse's Occupation_____

5) Which of the following best describes your current job status?
    ☐ 1. Employed outside the home, full-time
    ☐ 2. Employed outside the home, part-time
    ☐ 3. Homemaker
    ☐ 4. Retired
    ☐ 5. Unemployed
    ☐ 6. Other

6) How long has it been since you first learned your diagnosis?
    _____ months

7) Have you ever had pain due to your present disease?
    1. ☐ Yes   2. ☐ No   3. ☐ Uncertain

8) When you first received your diagnosis, was pain one of your symptoms?
    1. ☐ Yes   2. ☐ No   3. ☐ Uncertain

9) Have you had surgery in the past
month?   1. ☐ Yes   2. ☐ No

10) Throughout our lives, most of us have had pain from time to time (such as minor headaches, sprains, and toothaches). Have

you had pain *other* than these everyday kinds of pain during the *last week?*

1. ☐ Yes   2. ☐ No

IF YOU ANSWERED YES TO THE LAST QUESTION, PLEASE GO ON TO QUESTION 11 AND FINISH THIS QUESTIONNAIRE. IF NO, YOU ARE FINISHED WITH THE QUESTIONNAIRE.

11) On the diagram, shade in the areas where you feel pain. Put an X on the area that hurts the most.

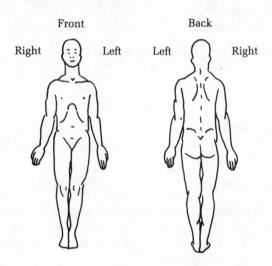

12) Please rate your pain by circling the one number that best describes your pain at its *worst* in the last week.

    0   1   2   3   4   5   6   7   8   9   10
No   Pain as bad as
Pain   you can imagine

13) Please rate your pain by circling the one number that best describes your pain at its *least* in the last week.

    0   1   2   3   4   5   6   7   8   9   10
No   Pain as bad as
Pain   you can imagine

14) Please rate your pain by circling the one number that best describes your pain on the *average.*

    0   1   2   3   4   5   6   7   8   9   10
No   Pain as bad as
Pain   you can imagine

15) Please rate your pain by circling the one number that tells how much pain you have *right now*.

    0   1   2   3   4   5   6   7   8   9   10
    No   Pain as bad as
    Pain   you can imagine

16) What kinds of things make your pain feel better (for example, heat, medicine, rest)?

    _____

    _____

17) What kinds of things make your pain worse (for example, walking, standing, lifting)?

    _____

    _____

18) What treatments or medications are you receiving for your pain?

    _____

    _____

19) In the last week, how much relief have pain treatments or medications provided? Please circle the one percentage that most shows how much relief you have received.

    0% 10% 20% 30% 40% 50% 60% 70% 80% 90% 100%
    No   Complete
    Relief   Relief

20) If you take pain medication, how many hours does it take before the pain returns?

    ☐ 1. Pain medication doesn't help   ☐ 5. Four hours.
         at all.   ☐ 6. Five to twelve hours.
    ☐ 2. One hour.   ☐ 7. More than twelve hours.
    ☐ 3. Two hours.   ☐ 8. I do not take pain
    ☐ 4. Three hours.   medication.

21) Circle the appropriate answer for each item.
    I believe my pain is due to:

Yes ☐   No ☐   1. The effects of treatment (for example, medication, surgery, radiation, prosthetic device).

Yes ☐   No ☐   2. My primary disease (meaning the disease currently being treated and evaluated).

Yes ☐   No ☐   3. A medical condition unrelated to primary disease (for example, arthritis).

22) For each of the following words, check yes or no if that adjective applies to your pain.

Aching	☐ Yes	☐ No
Throbbing	☐ Yes	☐ No
Shooting	☐ Yes	☐ No
Stabbing	☐ Yes	☐ No
Gnawing	☐ Yes	☐ No
Sharp	☐ Yes	☐ No
Tender	☐ Yes	☐ No
Burning	☐ Yes	☐ No
Exhausting	☐ Yes	☐ No
Tiring	☐ Yes	☐ No
Penetrating	☐ Yes	☐ No
Nagging	☐ Yes	☐ No
Numb	☐ Yes	☐ No
Miserable	☐ Yes	☐ No
Unbearable	☐ Yes	☐ No

23) Circle the one number that describes how, during the past week, *pain* has interfered with your:

A. General activity

0   1   2   3   4   5   6   7   8   9   10
Does not   Completely
interfere   interferes

B. Mood

0   1   2   3   4   5   6   7   8   9   10
Does not   Completely
interfere   interferes

C. Walking ability

0   1   2   3   4   5   6   7   8   9   10
Does not   Completely
interfere   interferes

D. Normal work (includes both work outside the home and housework)

0   1   2   3   4   5   6   7   8   9   10
Does not   Completely
interfere   interferes

E. Relations with other people

0   1   2   3   4   5   6   7   8   9   10
Does not   Completely
interfere   interferes

F. Sleep
    0   1   2   3   4   5   6   7   8   9   10
    Does not   Completely
    interfere   interferes
G. Enjoyment of life
    0   1   2   3   4   5   6   7   8   9   10
    Does not   Completely
    interfere   interferes

cancer patients, perhaps because they are aware of the emotional impact of communicating pain, tend to conceal or understate pain during transactions with physicians. Some patients deal with the threat that pain represents (e.g. a signal of disease progression) by denial and inaccurate attribution. In such cases physicians need to recognize other signs of pain and distress and to address them directly with patients and family so that patients can receive appropriate analgesic support.[39]

When a patient is first seen by a doctor, a critical part of the initial medical evaluation must be "Is the patient in pain?" "Assume nothing," says Susan Beck, Ph.D., R.N., professor at the University of Utah Health Sciences Center.[40]

Assessment of cancer pain is the first step toward truly knowing, or individualizing the pain just as the patient is individualized. Patients are not rubber stamps of each other, nor is their pain.

Mark Jensen, Ph.D., who specializes in rehabilitation medicine at the University of Washington, states that there are some important issues to be aware of:

1. Pain assessment is necessary for adequate pain treatment.
2. Cancer pain is complex.
3. Cancer pain is multi-dimensional.
4. Cancer pain comes from many sources.
5. Cancer pain changes over time.
6. Cancer pain must be assessed frequently. Too few assessments result in inadequate pain treatment.
7. Pain affect levels—the emotional and life quality disruptions.
8. Pain intensity levels—how much pain is being felt.[41]

Deborah McGuire, Ph.D., R.N., Director of Nursing Research at the Johns Hopkins University School of Nursing, says, "Pain is a multidimensional phenomenon that has psychosocial dimensions. There is a cognitive, affective and sociocultural result of pain. A holistic viewpoint is needed to treat cancer pain. The patient's perspective is critical."[42]

Biobehavioral Pain Profile

Jo Anne Dalton, Ph.D., R.N., is concerned about the complex behaviors that are a direct result of pain, as mentioned in Chapter 1. The following *Biobehavioral Pain Profile* was designed to measure "patient-reported personal and environmental factors that may be associated with reports of pain intensity, interference of activities due to pain and selection of and outcomes of various treatment methods."[43]

0–10 Numeric Pain Intensity Scale

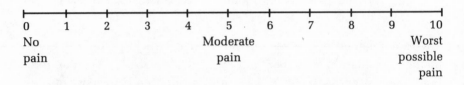

0	1	2	3	4	5	6	7	8	9	10
No pain					Moderate pain					Worst possible pain

In addition, you can use the simple *0–10 Numeric Pain Intensity Scale. Mark your pain level on the horizontal line.*

If you don't have this scale with you in the doctor's office or in the hospital, you can draw one for yourself. You can rate the pain verbally if you are too ill or too immobilized to mark the scale.

In 1991 a study was done to determine whether patients' communication about the intensity of their pain and the health care providers' evaluation of the intensity matched each other. Patients were given the assessment scale. When a patient indicated a 4, for moderate pain, the nurses and doctors made the same assessment. However, when the patient indicated 7 to 10, for severe pain, the doctors and nurses underassessed the pain by up to 75%. The patient's self-report on the scale was quite different from what the doctors and nurses thought the pain was.[44]

This inconsistency must end. Doctors and nurses need to learn and

Biobehavioral Pain Profile

Circle the number that best represents your response. Instructions for each section are listed below.

Indicate how often you engage in the following actions when you have pain:

	never							often
1. Voice frequent complaints	0	1	2	3	4	5	6	7
2. Voice frequent requests for medication	0	1	2	3	4	5	6	7
3. Cancel a diagnostic appointment	0	1	2	3	4	5	6	7
4. Not appear for a diagnostic appointment	0	1	2	3	4	5	6	7
5. Put off making a diagnostic appointment	0	1	2	3	4	5	6	7
6. Cancel a treatment appointment	0	1	2	3	4	5	6	7
7. Not appear for a treatment appointment	0	1	2	3	4	5	6	7
8. Put off making a treatment appointment	0	1	2	3	4	5	6	7
9. Avoid talking/being with family	0	1	2	3	4	5	6	7
10. Avoid talking/being with friends	0	1	2	3	4	5	6	7

Indicate how often you experience the following physical changes when you have pain:

	never							often
11. Muscle tenseness	0	1	2	3	4	5	6	7
12. Increased breathing rate	0	1	2	3	4	5	6	7
13. Perspiration	0	1	2	3	4	5	6	7
14. Nausea	0	1	2	3	4	5	6	7
15. Increased heart rate	0	1	2	3	4	5	6	7

Indicate how often the following thoughts accompany your feelings of pain:

	never						often
16. "Something terrible is happening"	0	1	2	3	4	5	6	7
17. "A tumor is growing"	0	1	2	3	4	5	6	7
18. "My disease is spreading"	0	1	2	3	4	5	6	7
19. "I'm terrified"	0	1	2	3	4	5	6	7
20. "Nobody understands"	0	1	2	3	4	5	6	7

	no fear						great fear
21. In general, how much do you fear pain?	0	1	2	3	4	5	6	7

How much do the following influence how you feel about pain?

	no influence						strong influence
22. Stories about cancer and pain told by family	0	1	2	3	4	5	6	7
23. Stories about cancer and pain told by friends	0	1	2	3	4	5	6	7
24. Family experience with cancer pain	0	1	2	3	4	5	6	7
25. Family experience with other pain	0	1	2	3	4	5	6	7
26. Nurses' descriptions of what your pain will be like	0	1	2	3	4	5	6	7
27. Physicians' descriptions of what your pain will be like	0	1	2	3	4	5	6	7
28. Nurses' facial expression when they ask you about your pain	0	1	2	3	4	5	6	7
29. Physicians' facial expression when they ask you about your pain	0	1	2	3	4	5	6	7
30. Literature (magazines, books, newspapers)	0	1	2	3	4	5	6	7
31. Television/radio	0	1	2	3	4	5	6	7

How much do the following personal factors influence how you feel about pain?

	no influence						strong influence
32. Past and current medical treatment	0	1	2	3	4	5	6	7
33. Not getting enough pain medication	0	1	2	3	4	5	6	7

34. Past and current surgical treatment	0	1	2	3	4	5	6	7
35. Past and current diagnostic treatment	0	1	2	3	4	5	6	7
36. Past personal experience with cancer pain	0	1	2	3	4	5	6	7
37. Past personal experience with other pain (i.e., childbirth, dental pain)	0	1	2	3	4	5	6	7
38. Past personal experience with unrelieved pain	0	1	2	3	4	5	6	7
39. Observing fear of pain in others	0	1	2	3	4	5	6	7
40. Observing pain in others	0	1	2	3	4	5	6	7
41. Knowledge of the causes of pain	0	1	2	3	4	5	6	7
42. Not understanding the cause of my pain	0	1	2	3	4	5	6	7
43. Knowledge that my disease is progressing	0	1	2	3	4	5	6	7
44. Not understanding the course of my disease	0	1	2	3	4	5	6	7
45. Uncertainty about the future	0	1	2	3	4	5	6	7
46. Belief that pain cannot be controlled	0	1	2	3	4	5	6	7
47. Decreased activity due to pain	0	1	2	3	4	5	6	7
48. Feelings about disfigurement	0	1	2	3	4	5	6	7
49. Feelings about incapacity	0	1	2	3	4	5	6	7
50. Feelings about loss of control	0	1	2	3	4	5	6	7
51. Feelings about loss of self-esteem	0	1	2	3	4	5	6	7
52. Feelings about loss of identity	0	1	2	3	4	5	6	7
53. Feelings about loss of role as mother, father, wife, or husband	0	1	2	3	4	5	6	7
54. Feelings about helplessness	0	1	2	3	4	5	6	7
55. Feelings about hopelessness	0	1	2	3	4	5	6	7
56. Feelings about isolation	0	1	2	3	4	5	6	7
57. Feelings about loss of life	0	1	2	3	4	5	6	7

master the tools of pain assessment and use them to help control the patient's pain. There is no way for anyone to know how much pain the patient is in. The only way to know is from the patient's self-report. The patient must be believed.

Memorial Pain Assessment Card

The *Memorial Pain Assessment Card* is a quick, easy-to-use pain assessment tool.[45]

Be Specific About Your Pain

You should write down what *helps* your pain:

• Sitting, lying, heat, cold, music, etc.

Write down what makes your pain *worse:*

• Walking, lifting, sitting, eating, etc.

Keep a *Daily Pain Diary* to help you chart your own pain. Items you will want to keep track of in your *Daily Pain Diary*:

What you could or could not eat.
How many hours you could sleep.
What activities you could or could not engage in.
What time of the day or night you had pain or did not have pain, and for how long.
What pain-relief medication you were taking.
Did it provide relief?
For how long?
What nondrug techniques you used, when, and with what result.

The more accurately you can describe your pain, the better chance you have of obtaining pain relief from your doctor.
You should enlist your family to help you assess your pain. Your well-being is important to them. Let them participate in your care so they can understand your pain.

It is important for you to remember that 85% to 90% of all cancer pain can be controlled well and the remainder can usually be relieved at some level.

Memorial Pain Assessment Card

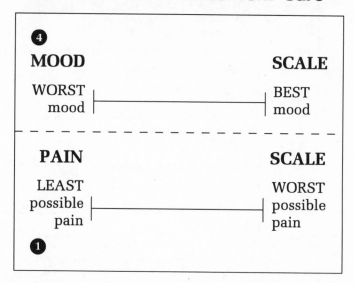

Front side of MPAC. VAS measures of pain intensity and mood. Card is folded along broken line such that each measure is presented to the patient separately, in numbered order.

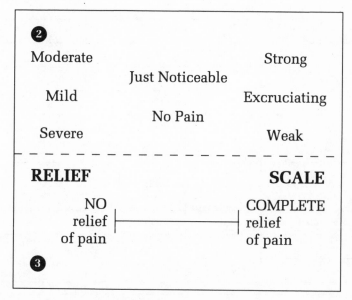

Back side of MPAC. Modified Tursky Pain Descriptors Scale and VAS measure of pain relief.

Permission granted by Kathleen Foley of Memorial Sloan-Kettering Hospital, 1993.

Daily Pain Diary

Name_____Date_____

Time	Pain rating scale	Medication type & amount taken	Other pain relief measures tried or anything that influences your pain	Major activity being done: lying sitting standing/walking
12 MIDNIGHT				
1 A.M.				
2				
3				
4				
5				
6				
7				
8				
9				
10				
11				
12 NOON				
1				
2				
3				
4				
5				
6				
7				
8				
9				
10				
11				

Comments:_____

_____

_____

From McCaffery, M., Beebe, R. N., *Pain: Clinical Manual for Nursing Practice* (St. Louis: C. V. Mosby Co., 1989). Reprinted by permission, 1993.

CANCER PAIN AND SUFFERING
AND THE MEASUREMENT
OF QUALITY OF LIFE

Part of the measurement of pain is directly related to a patient's *Quality of Life*. As Moinpour and Chapman point out, "Medicine has done little to specifically prevent or alleviate suffering." They add:

> Suffering is an enduring state that occurs in response to a chronic or prolonged intensely stressful situation, often with many stressors. Pain from metastatic disease may be a prominent cause of a cancer patient's suffering, but one must look at the whole person over time—personal losses, surgical mutilation, inability to cope with repeated procedural distress or pain, social separation during inpatient stay, etc.—to understand his or her suffering, even when the disease causes severe pain. . . . Suffering often has multiple sustaining determinants that exist in a complex network of cause-and-effect relationships. For example, severe pain impairs human relationships, blocks treasured recreational pursuits, and damages the self-image of normally active, productive persons. These losses foster depression, and this in turn impairs sleep and exacerbates fatigue. Trapped in the vicious cycle of pain and insomnia, patients become increasingly negative, withdrawn, and dispirited.[46]

Dr. Eduardo Bruera notes, *"Cancer pain doesn't come alone, it comes accompanied by devastating symptoms that affect the assessment and treatment of pain and the treatment of pain affects those other symptoms. The inter-relation is extremely profound."*[47]

The World Health Organization

The World Health Organization has defined health on a multidimensional level:

"Health is not only the absence of infirmity and disease but also a state of physical, mental and social well-being." Morris in 1986 defined quality of life as "the prevention and alleviation of physical and mental suffering and the presence of a supportive network of informal relationships."[48]

It is critical to address the hand-in-glove result of pain and the suffering it produces by measuring the patient's quality of life.

Dr. Betty Ferrell comments that the "majority of pain treatments do not accommodate the individual. Health care professionals need to find out what is important to each patient, what can be done to help the patient perform what is important to them, what has meaning for them."[49]

Ferrell has explored the relationship between pain and the quality of life. She notes that "pain is associated with physical symptoms such as fatigue, nausea, and appetite disturbance. It is also associated with psychological symptoms including anxiety, fear and depression. Pain impacts all aspects of the Quality of Life including physical well being, psychological well being, social concerns and spiritual well being."[50]

Dr. Russell Portenoy et al. conducted a study of 218 cancer patients to assess the prevalence and characteristics of symptoms that bothered the patients the most. The following is a list of thirty-three items, from the most to least bothersome.[51]

Prevalence and Characteristics of Symptoms Determined by the Memorial Symptom Assessment Scale in 218 Cancer Patients

Symptom	Overall Prevalence
Lack of energy	73.4
Worrying	72.4
Feeling sad	67.4
Pain	63.1
Feeling nervous	62.4
Feeling drowsy	59.7
Dry mouth	55.3
Difficulty sleeping	52.8
Feeling irritable	47.2
Nausea	44.7
Lack of appetite	44.5
Difficulty concentrating	40.1
Feeling bloated	38.7
Change in the way food tastes	37.2
Numbness/tingling in hands or feet	36.4
Constipation	33.6
Cough	29.4
"I don't look like myself"	28.2
Itching	27.2
Swelling of arms or legs	27.5

Symptom	Overall Prevalence
Weight loss	27.0
Weight gain	25.7
Diarrhea	23.9
Dizziness	23.4
Problems with sexual interest or activity	23.3
Shortness of breath	22.9
Vomiting	21.1
Hair loss	17.1
Problems with urination	15.6
Mouth sores	12.9
Urinary accidents	12.4
Nightmares	11.9
Difficulty swallowing	10.6

© Russell K. Portenoy, Memorial Sloan-Kettering Cancer Center. Reprinted by permission, 1993.

Quality of Life Measuring Tool

Dr. Ferrell et al. constructed a Quality of Life measuring tool. The *quantity* of pain—its intensity—was measured by asking the patient, "How much pain are you having?"

Pain distress was measured by asking, "If you have pain, how distressing is it?"

How pain impacts on the Quality of Life was measured in four dimensions.

The recommendations based on this research can be summarized in this way:

- Quality of Life, like pain, can be best determined by the patient.
- Quality of Life measures enable health care providers to evaluate the patient's overall status.
- Because pain impacts on all dimensions of Quality of Life, pain assessment should be multidimensional.
- Pain treatments should be evaluated based on their impact on all dimensions of Quality of Life, rather than on simple measures of pain intensity.
- Pain is a symptom, but pain greatly impacts on other symptoms, such as sleep disturbance, nausea, anxiety, and depression.
- Use of the Quality of Life model provides a conceptual basis for the

Pain Impacts the
Dimensions of Quality of Life

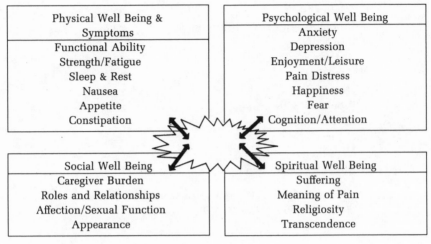

Physical Well Being & Symptoms	Psychological Well Being
Functional Ability	Anxiety
Strength/Fatigue	Depression
Sleep & Rest	Enjoyment/Leisure
Nausea	Pain Distress
Appetite	Happiness
Constipation	Fear
	Cognition/Attention

Social Well Being	Spiritual Well Being
Caregiver Burden	Suffering
Roles and Relationships	Meaning of Pain
Affection/Sexual Function	Religiosity
Appearance	Transcendence

© B. Ferrell. Reprinted by permission, 1993.

relationship between interrelated concepts such as pain and suffering.[52]

The following *Quality of Life Tool* can be filled out by you to assess what is happening to you right now. *"Normal" for you means what was normal for you before you were ill.*

The routine use of pain assessment tools with every patient can change the guesswork of pain assessment into a real system of assessment so that patients can receive better pain management.[53]

Charles Cleeland, Ph.D., professor of Neurology at the University of Wisconsin Medical School, notes, *"Inappropriate or inadequate assessment of patients is the single biggest cause of poor pain management. Physicians aren't asking their patients about the severity of their pain."*[54]

Once assessment has been completed, pain treatment must begin. The goal should be to relieve enough pain so that the patient can return to as normally functioning a life as possible. Although it may not be possible to relieve all pain, "it is possible to attain relief in 80% or more of cancer patients," notes Dr. Russell Portenoy.[55]

Quality of Life Tool
Patient Version

Below are a number of questions pertaining to your well being. Please make an X on the line to indicate what is happening to you at the present. The term "normal for me" means what was normal *prior to illness.*

BELOW IS AN EXAMPLE WHICH MAY HELP YOU IN RESPONDING TO THE QUESTIONNAIRE.

How do you feel about your ability to concentrate?

_____X_____

cannot concentrate   can concentrate
at all   extremely well
(The "X" on the line indicates you are able to concentrate but not 100%.)

1. How easy or difficult is it to adjust to your disease and treatment?
   not at all _____ very easy

2. How much enjoyment are you getting out of life?
   none _____ a great deal

3. Do you worry about the cost of your medical care?
   a great deal _____ not at all

4. If you have pain, how distressing is it?
   extremely _____ not at all
   distressing   distressing

5. How useful do you feel?
   not at all _____ extremely useful
   useful

6. How much happiness do you feel?
   none at all _____ a great deal

7. How satisfying is your life?
   not at all _____ extremely
   satisfying   satisfying

8. Is the amount of affection you give and receive sufficient to meet your needs?
   not at all _____ completely

9. Is your disease or treatment interfering with your personal relationships?
   a great deal _____ not at all

10. Are you worried (fearful or anxious) about the outcome of your disease?

    constantly _____ not at all

11. How much are you able to do the things you like to do such as watch TV, read, garden, listen to music, etc.?

    not at all _____ a great deal

12. How is your present ability to pay attention to what's happening?

    extremely poor _____ excellent

13. How much strength do you have?

    none at all _____ a great deal

14. Do you tire easily?

    a great deal _____ not at all

15. Is the amount of time you sleep sufficient to meet your needs?

    not at all _____ completely

16. How good is your quality of life?

    extremely poor _____ excellent

17. Are you able to take care of your personal needs (dress, hair, toilet, baths, etc.)?

    I can't do _____ I can do
    anything   everything
    by myself   myself

18. How much pain do you have?

    a great deal _____ no pain

19. How much of an appetite do you have?

    none _____ more than usual

20. How is your bowel pattern?

    the worst _____ normal for me
    I've ever had

21. Is the amount you eat sufficient to meet your needs?

    not at all _____ completely

22. Are you worried about your weight?

    a great deal _____ not at all

23. Do you have nausea?

    all the time _____ never

24. Do you vomit?

    all the time _____ never

25. Have you had any changes in taste?

    a great deal _____ none at all

26. Are you able to get around inside your hospital room or home?
completely _____ can get around
bedbound   on my own

27. How satisfied are you with your appearance?
completely _____ completely
dissatisfied   satisfied

28. Are you worried about unfinished business?
extremely _____ not at all

29. Is the support you receive from others sufficient to meet your needs?
not at all _____ completely
sufficient   sufficient

30. Do you feel like you are in control of things, of your life?
I feel totally _____ I feel totally
out of control   in control

MANAGEMENT

The first method of relieving cancer pain is to use anticancer therapy: surgery, chemotherapy, hormone therapy, radiation, palliative surgery, or a combination of therapies.

If pain continues afterward, complete assessment of the patient must take place to locate the pain precisely and develop the best possible pain relief plan. Pain can be acute, chronic, or a combination of both.

Peter Koo, Pharm.D., a pain specialist and professor of Pharmacology at the University of California, San Francisco, notes, "Treatment of chronic cancer pain is often difficult and frustrating for the clinician because there is no definitive formula for success. Much of the difficulty is the result of inadequate training of clinicians in dealing with the complex pharmacologic and psychosocial problems associated with chronic cancer pain."[56]

To assist doctors in the treatment of cancer pain, the World Health Organization has developed a comprehensive "analgesic ladder."

Every doctor should learn and adhere to this ladder. The ladder operates on the concept that it is best for doctors to learn how to use a few drugs well.

The WHO Three-Step Analgesic Ladder

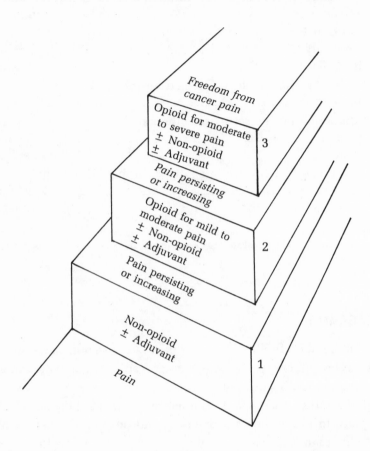

The following points summarize the *WHO Analgesic Ladder for Drug Administration.* It refers to three graduated classes of pain-relieving medications.

1. Systemic analgesics will usually provide good relief from cancer pain, provided the right drugs, the right doses, and the right schedule are applied.
2. Oral administration is the preferred route. Only when an obstacle to this type of administration exists (for example, intestinal occlusion, vomiting) should an alternate delivery method be used (such as subcutaneous, rectal, intravenous).
3. Treatment is begun with a nonopioid drug (such as aspirin, Ty-

lenol, or Advil). The dose is adjusted to optimum level. If necessary, adjuvant (other) drugs are used in addition.

4. If and when this treatment no longer relieves pain, a weak opioid
   (such as codeine) is administered in addition to the nonopioid.
   One or more adjuvants can be combined, if necessary.

5. When a weak opioid no longer relieves pain, strong opioid (such
   as morphine) therapy is begun immediately, along with adjuvant
   drugs and nonopioid analgesics, if necessary (for example, Advil
   is given at the same time as morphine).

6. Dosages are titrated (adjusted) against the patient's pain report
   and administered regularly, at time intervals dictated by the
   drugs' pharmacokinetics (how they work and how long they last
   in the body).

7. Initial ladder treatment is determined according to the previous
   therapy.

Ventafridda et al. found that the "WHO ladder appeared effective,
both chronically, as far as pain relief is concerned, and also in the last
weeks of life. Hours of sleep are greatly improved and the activity of
the patients is not unduly modified."[57]

A Basic Drug List

Start with the nonopioids, such as:

- Aspirin
- Acetaminophen (Tylenol)
- Nonsteroidal anti-inflammatory drugs (NSAIDs), such as an ibu-
  profen (Nuprin, Motrin, Advil)

However, these drugs have a *ceiling effect*—at some point an increase in the dose does not provide any more pain relief.

The rule of thumb is that if pain relief is not achieved by these drugs,
then opioids should be selected. As mentioned, the combination of an
anti-inflammatory drug and a morphine-like drug often achieves excellent pain control.

The *adjuvant* or *enhancing* drugs, such as antidepressants and amphetamines, can be used to enhance pain relief and combat depression,
sedation, or other side effects of pain control treatment (see Chapter 1).

If pain is persistent or severe, opioids are used with nonopioids.
There are opiate receptors, or binding sites, in the brain, spinal cord,

and other areas of the body. An opioid such as morphine provides pain relief by binding to the receptors (see Chapter 1).

Weak opioid: Codeine
Strong opioid: Morphine

WHO, as well as the American College of Physicians and the American Medical Association, *suggests oral medication as the choice for the majority of patients, unless the patient cannot take oral medication or the pain is complex and/or extremely severe. Oral medication is easy to use, can be time-released, and is cost-effective.*

Opioids are the cornerstone of severe cancer pain control. The doctor, nurse, patient, and family often have an uneducated and unreasonable fear of addiction. All need to strive for a new understanding of addiction. As mentioned, when the "Just say no to drugs" campaign was initiated, "Just say yes to drugs for pain relief" was mistakenly left out.

Dr. Kathleen Foley says, "*A cancer patient taking morphine takes morphine for pain relief.* They typically do not become high. The street addict takes heroin, takes morphine, for a high, to feel good. They take it to be knocked out. The cancer patient takes it to function. The differences are so enormous that the only thing in common is the drug."[58]

In 1989 the *Harvard Medical Letter* stated, "*When pain is severe, giving an opioid is as appropriate as giving insulin for diabetes.*"[59]

Opioids are commonly used for pain relief because they are flexible in dosage, formulas, and routes of administration.

Dosage

When administering an opioid, the dose should be flexible. A doctor should not be wedded to a fixed dose for a cancer patient in pain. Dr. Raymond Houde writes, "There is no optimal dose for any type of pain; there are merely recommended starting doses from which the optimal dose is determined by titration and the maximal dose limited only by adverse effects."[60]

It is important to mention again the difference between *psychological dependence,* which is a component of addiction and causes drug-seeking behavior, and *physical dependence,* which does not mean addiction. Physical dependence can take place over weeks after taking opioids and is characterized by physical symptoms if the drug is suddenly withdrawn. Just as a doctor would not suddenly stop giving a patient medications for high blood pressure, he would not suddenly stop giving an opioid. In addition, more than 99% of patients who take opioids for pain do not become addicted.

Dr. Foley states, "The *misconception* by both clinicians and patients that physical dependence and addiction (psychological dependence) are interchangeable terms limits effective use of them."[61]

Some patients will stay on one dose for many months or more. Sometimes the pain-relieving effect diminishes over time. If this occurs, the doctor should increase the dose, give the drug more frequently, or add another, enhancing drug. Some patients need larger doses if the pain keeps getting worse. The goal is to keep the patients comfortable and allow them to live life to the fullest.

It is impossible to predict or guess how much drug a patient will need to achieve pain relief. As Dr. Peter Koo said in an earlier chapter, "The right dose is the right dose." He adds that some patients suffering from cancer pain can tolerate huge doses of opioids with few adverse effects.

As mentioned in Chapter 1, patients should be provided with a *rescue dose* of drug in case they experience a sudden pain breakthrough.

A controlled-release oral morphine for use in moderate to severe pain can provide continuous pain control on a twelve- or eight-hour regimen. MS Contin is the trade name of a timed-release morphine. It is normally given on a fixed schedule.

In addition to nonopioid and opioid drugs, adjuvant drugs can be used to provide pain relief, reduce sedation and nausea, and provide other benefits. Adjuvant drugs include:[62]*

Corticosteroids

Prednisone:
- To potentiate analgesia
- Elevate mood
- Improve appetite

*Adapted from Bonica, J., *The Management of Pain*, second edition (Philadelphia: Lea & Febiger, 1990), vol. 1.

Antidepressants

Elavil:
- Potentiates opioid analgesia   • Elevates mood

Sinequan:
- Induces sleep

Tofranil:
- Antidepressant

Anxiolytics (antianxiety or antinausea)

Vistaril:
- Potentiates opioid analgesia   • Antinausea
- Reduces anxiety   • Sedative

Valium, Tranxene, Xanax:
- Relieves acute anxiety and   • Antinausea
  panic   • Sedative

Ativan:
- Antianxiety   • Sedative

Phenothiazines (often used for antinausea and anxiety)

Levoprome:
- Produces moderate analgesia   • Antinausea

Thorazine:
- Reduces anxiety   • Antinausea

Compazine:
- Antinausea   • No analgesic effect

Prolixin:
- Antinausea   • Reduces anxiety

Haldol:
- Decreases confusion   • Antinausea

Anticonvulsants

Tegretol:
- Anticonvulsant   • Decreases abnormal central
  nervous system neuronal
  activity

Amphetamines

Dexedrine:
- Potentiates opioid analgesia   • Elevates mood

Desoxyn:
- Decreases lethargy   • Increases physical activity

In addition, the moderate use of alcohol might make pain more bearable. It is important to discuss its use with your doctor if you are taking pain-relieving medications. Alcohol also has sedating qualities.

Drug Delivery Systems

Most patients and many doctors and nurses are unaware of how many drug delivery systems are available to the patient.

Oral:
- The preferred route of administration because of convenience, cost, and blood levels produced.

Tablets/capsules:
- Delay in absorption time (thirty to sixty minutes), and 20% to 30% of the dose may not be absorbed. Peak effect occurs one to two hours after dose. Some come in long-acting timed-release doses.

Liquid:
- Helpful for those patients who have trouble with tablets. Can be combined with other medications if necessary.

Mucosal:
- Dissolving tablets on gumline. One to two hours' dissolving time.

Nose spray:
- For patients who cannot take medication orally, or prefer this system. Takes about fifteen to twenty minutes to be absorbed.

Patch:
- An adhesive patch worn for forty-eight to seventy-two hours. Contains a measured dose of pain medication that provides forty-eight-hour relief. *(If patients are on other oral or intravenous pain medications, there is a period of time during which both should be used until the medication in the patch is absorbed to a peak level in the blood.)* Can be worn for widespread pain control. It is called "transdermal" when the drug is delivered across the skin.

Rectal:
- This route provides slow but effective absorption.

Intramuscular:
- A single dose injected into muscle. The injection is painful. There are huge differences in how long it takes the drug to be absorbed by the muscle and how long relief lasts.

Intravenous:
- Single dose injected into a vein. An intravenous line (IV) may be left in place for single, multiple, or continuous (PCA) doses of medication. Takes effect in ten to fifteen minutes. Peak effect is similar.

Subcutaneous:
- Injected under the skin. For patients who cannot take oral medication or whose veins cannot be used. Can also use PCA at the bedside or through portable pumps.

Epidural:
- Tiny tube placed outside the spinal column. Can be used for a single, multiple, or continuous infusion of drug. Can use PCA at bedside or a portable pump.

Spinal:
- Injected directly into the spinal space. Can be single, multiple, or continuous infusion of drug. Can use PCA at bedside or a special implantable pump, which requires a minor surgical procedure.

Side Effects

As mentioned earlier, side effects should be anticipated and aggressively treated. Some of the side effects of opioid therapy are:

Constipation:
- The most frequent side effect. Patients receiving opioids should also receive fluids and laxatives. Patients should eat food high in fiber, such as uncooked fruits, vegetables, and whole-grain breads and cereals. A few tablespoons of bran adds bulk to food. A dietitian can help plan meals that are high in fiber.

Nausea and vomiting:
- These can be controlled by adjusting the drug, switching the drug, or using medications to offset the nausea and vomiting.

Sedation, drowsiness and confusion:

- Can usually be controlled after a few days on the drug with dose adjustment, the more frequent use of smaller doses, or the use of amphetamines to counter sedation.

Respiratory depression:

- This generally is not a problem if the dose is adjusted properly. If it occurs, reducing the dose or administering a slow dose of a drug called Naloxone should alleviate the problem.

Tolerance:

- It is not understood why cancer patients occasionally develop tolerance to opioids quickly while others can remain on the same dose for months.

    Drs. Foley and Inturrisi note that a progression of the cancer rather than the development of tolerance can result in the need to increase the dose. Occasionally tolerance occurs, producing a decreased effect in the absence of progressive disease.

    Drs. Foley and Inturrisi add that *"there appears to be no limit to the development of tolerance, and with appropriate adjustment of dose most patients can continue to obtain pain relief. In cancer patients with severe pain, opioid-type analgesics should not be used sparingly or 'saved to the last' out of the fear that an increasing opioid requirement represents 'loss of control.' "*[63]

Physical dependence:

- Withdrawal symptoms can take place if the opioid is stopped abruptly. This can easily be offset by slowly tapering off the drug.

Psychological dependence:

- A component of addiction. Rarely (if ever) takes place if opioids are given in a dose that relieves pain and are administered on a fixed schedule.

Judith Paice, R.N., M.S., of Rush University's College of Nursing in Chicago, notes that "education is perhaps the most important service nurses can provide in alleviating cancer pain. By recognizing the fear associated with tolerance, physicians and nurses may administer opioids earlier and in necessary dosages. Patients and families should be reassured that many options for pain management are available. Colleagues, patients and families must be convinced that analgesic tolerance is an involuntary physiologic process, separate and distinct from addiction."[64]

Other Pain-Relief Approaches

There are some patients who will not obtain pain relief from drug therapy. In these cases, alternate efforts must be attempted. They are:

Neurostimulation:
- The use of external or implanted devices to enhance the function of certain parts of the nervous system to control pain.
- *TENS* (transcutaneous electrical nerve stimulation): An external device using a battery-powered pulse generator and electrodes which are applied to the skin at predetermined trigger points or acupuncture points.
- *Dorsal Column Stimulation:* An electrode is implanted over the spinal cord through a special needle.

Regional analgesia:
- Pain relief achieved by injecting a local anesthetic, opioid, or other substances near or into a nerve or nerve root. It can block almost any peripheral nerve in the body.
- *Nerve Blocks:* Can provide temporary relief using short- or long-acting anesthetics. Using alcohol or other substances and/or freezing can provide relief for varying lengths of time.
- *Epidural:* Can provide relief for hours, days, or months. Local anesthetic, opioids, steroids, or other substances are injected in a single dose or continuously through a portable or implantable pump.
- *Intrathecal:* Goes into the spinal canal. It can achieve relief for hours, days, or months. Single injection and/or portable pump or implantable pump.
- *Trigger point injections:* Use saline or local anesthetic into a painful joint or trigger point. Sometimes steroids are added.

Non-Drug Techniques

In addition, non-drug pain relieving techniques are the following:

Heat:
- Heat packs or dry/moist heating pads may help to relieve your pain.

Cold:
- Cold packs or ice help to ease pain, lessen edema, and limit muscle spasm. A rubber glove or ziplock bags can be filled with water and

alcohol and put in the freezer. The alcohol keeps the ice mushy, so it can be formed around a body part or small area. Even a bag of frozen peas can be used.

For some painful areas, ice placed directly on the skin can provide fast pain relief.

Sometimes alternating heat and cold can provide relief.

Cryoanalgesia **(extreme cold):**
- Used to destroy peripheral nerves for long-term relief of pain.

Mobilization:
- Stretching or strength-building exercises can aid in pain relief. Special compression devices are used to offset swelling of the extremities.

Counterirritant:
- A substance that causes irritation in one area to decrease pain in that area or in another, distant area. Also, rubbing, pressure, vibration, etc.

PSYCHOLOGICAL ASPECTS

Because pain is part of the total human response to illness, psychological and psychosocial reactions must be considered.

"All patients with cancer fear becoming disabled and dependent, having altered appearance and changed body function and losing the company of those close to them. Although such fears are similar in all patients, the level of psychologic distress is highly variable. This variability is accounted for by three factors: *medical* factors (site, stage, treatment and clinical course of the cancer and the presence of pain); *psychologic* factors, prior adjustment, coping ability, emotional maturity, the disruption of identified goals and ability to modify plans; and *social* factors such as the availability of emotional support offered by family, friends and co-workers," write Mary Jane Massie, M.D., and Jimmie Holland, M.D., of the Psychiatry Service at Memorial Sloan-Kettering Hospital in New York.[65]

Balfour Mount, M.D., professor of Surgery and Director of Palliative Care at McGill University, notes that in the 1960s LeShan spoke of the chronic pain sufferer caught in an awake nightmare of helplessness, hopelessness, and meaninglessness. Mount writes, *"It has become increasingly evident that pain may be most helpfully viewed not as 'physical pain' or 'emotional pain' but as a total experience. . . . To fail to assess all dimensions of the experience—physical, psychosocial and spiritual—is to limit our understanding of the process and thus to doom our therapeutic interventions to suboptimal results.*"[66]

Martha Shawyer, R.N., M.A., of the School of Nursing, Wichita State University, writes this about the psychosocial factors in pain: "Cancer is a stressor in itself." However, cancer is complicated by other stressors:

Loss or Threat of Loss of a Significant Object

A person can lose a body part or function. The mental pain associated with this loss is dependent on how the person and society view that particular part or function. The loss of a breast or uterus may indicate to a woman that she is no longer needed. Men who have had penilectomies often describe themselves as no longer being "a man."

Another loss often experienced as a threat is that of loss of roles previously assumed. Physical pain or weakness may mean that the person is no longer capable of holding his or her previous job. Along with this loss may come a change in relationships with friends.

The imbalance in supply and demand of energy leads to fatigue. Pain is often increased because of the loss of energy adequate to deal with the situation. Fatigue itself can create a vulnerable setting for mental pain to occur, as well as lowering the sufferer's resistance to persistent physical pain.

Injury or Threat of Injury

Injury or threat of injury to the body or mind is ever present. Cancer by nature is a perpetual assault on the body, since it saps the body for its own existence and nutrition. In addition, the treatments for cancer—surgery, radiation, chemotherapy, and immunotherapy—are potential assaults, because they create a system of reactions within the body that can affect not only tumor cells but normal, healthy cells as well.

Frustration of Drives

The patient with cancer lives with many ambiguities that can present problems to the individual and his or her family and caretakers. Will the cancer grow? How far will it extend? How will it be treated? Will the treatment stop the growth? How will he or she feel when he or she is taking the treatment? These questions are faced *every day.*[67]*

A diagnosis of cancer accompanied by pain potentially can produce any one or all of these stressors.

Anxiety

Anxiety is one of the principal contributors to the pain experience.

"Much of the fear experience that characterizes the cancer patient is a function of uncertainty, a factor that has been linked to anxiety. . . . Chronic anxiety is known to result in disturbed autonomic [nervous system] and endocrine function, and it may lead to a variety of well-known psychosomatic symptom complexes such as tension headache, peptic ulcer or spastic colon,"[68] writes Dr. Chapman. He adds that pain feeds the cancer patient's anxiety because it may signal progression of the disease. In turn, the patient becomes hypersensitive to any normal ache and pain as a warning that the disease is changing. Anxiety and pain coexist in a vicious circle.

Depression

Dr. Chapman continues:

> If the patient becomes more and more disengaged from his normal social functioning and increasingly dependent on care-providers and the medical establishment, a sense of helplessness develops. If the disease progresses, the patient typically evolves from repeated bouts of feeling helpless to a general theme of hopelessness and despair. Such depression can be increased by financial problems that face the family because of the patient's inability to work and mounting medical costs . . . current theories hold that environmentally precipitated depression may be associated with the depletion of critical neurotransmitter substances such as serotonin. . . .

Anger

> Because patients perceive and interpret their own suffering and the losses associated with the progress of the disease, many tend to respond with anger that takes many forms. It is not uncommon for patients to ask, "Why me?" Resentment and bitterness may develop

*Adapted from Jacox, A., *Pain: A Sourcebook for Nurses and Other Health Professionals* (Boston: Little, Brown and Co., 1977).

over time as patients develop a sense of hopelessness. Such anger is consequent, in part, to frustration with therapeutic failure. Repeatedly, the patient is given hope by the physicians only to learn that yet another failure has occurred and the disease has again eluded treatment. When anger is turned inward, it feeds depression.

It must be emphasized that the anxiety, depression and anger described are not necessarily abnormal.[69]

COPING STRATEGIES

Dr. Mount notes the coping strategies that are commonly used by a patient with cancer. They are:

1. Seek more information about the situation (rational intellectual)
2. Talk with others to relieve distress (shared concern)
3. Laugh it off; make light of situation (reversal affect)
4. Try to forget; put it out of mind (suppression)
5. Do other things to distract oneself (displacement)
6. Take firm action based on present understanding (confrontation)
7. Accept, but find something favorable (redefinition)
8. Submit to and accept the inevitable (fatalism)
9. Do something, anything, however reckless, impractical (acting out)
10. Negotiate feasible alternatives (if x, then y)
11. Reduce tension by drinking, overeating, drugs (tension reduction)
12. Withdraw socially into isolation (stimulus reduction)
13. Blame someone or something (disowning responsibility)
14. Seek direction from an authority and comply (compliance)
15. Blame yourself, sacrifice or atone (self pity)

Therefore a variety of paths may be utilized as the patient integrates the hard reality at hand.[70]

Providing Control

It has been pointed out that losses beset the patient with cancer. When the patient also has severe pain, there are feelings of helplessness. There are some techniques that can help to reduce pain and provide the patient with some feelings of control.

Relaxation, Mental Imagery, Self-hypnosis

This is mentally going into another setting. It can be a setting from memory, such as a visit to the beach, or one that is made up. Chapter 1 has the basic relaxation technique.

Stephanie Matthews-Simonton writes in her book *Getting Well Again:*

> Many of our patients experience a decrease in pain after beginning to use the relaxation/mental imagery process regularly. We believe this occurs for two reasons. First, the relaxation activity reduces muscle tension, which reduces pain. Second, as the mental imagery process helps the patient develop an increased expectancy that he can recover, his fear is lessened, reducing tension and further decreasing pain.

Visualizing the Pain

1. Prepare yourself by relaxation.
2. Focus on the pain. What color is it? See its color and shape and size clearly. It may be a bright red ball. It may be the size of a tennis ball. It may be the size of a grapefruit or a basketball.
3. Mentally project the ball out into space, maybe ten feet away from your body.
4. Make the ball bigger, about the size of a basketball. Then shrink it to the size of a pea. Now let it become whatever size it chooses to be. Usually it returns to the original size you visualized.
5. Begin to change the ball's color. Make it pink, then light green.
6. Now take the green ball and put it back where you originally saw it. At this point, notice whether or not your pain has been reduced.
7. As you open your eyes, you are now ready to resume your activities.[71]

Simonton notes that sometimes replacing pain with pleasure can help the patient forget for a while that there is pain.

Other techniques designed to achieve a mental and physical state of relaxation are suggested by Baruch Fishman, Ph.D., and Matthew Loscalzo, M.S.W., of the Pain Service at Memorial Sloan-Kettering:

Meditation:
- Involves mentally chanting a word or rehearsing a specific sentence such that attention is withdrawn from distressing feelings and thoughts and a relaxed state is thereby induced.

Music Therapy:
- Usually involves a professional therapist who engages the patients in active or passive musical experiences. Music can have a direct mood-altering effect, as well as an indirect relaxing effect through diversion of attention from stress-provoking stimuli.[72]

  If patients play a musical instrument they should be encouraged to bring their instrument with them. A songwriter had an electric piano brought into his room at the hospital. He used earphones plugged into the piano so he could play and not disturb other patients.

Art Therapy:
- Art therapists are trained to help patients express their feelings through art. It can also be an avenue for relaxation and distraction.

Humor:
- Humor and laughter can help provide pain relief and distraction during illness.

MULTIDISCIPLINARY TEAM

Cancer pain is an intertwined physical, emotional, and psychological event. It is necessary to treat the total pain of the individual. A multi-disciplinary team should include:

Social Worker:
- To provide psychological counseling, insurance and financial assistance, and family counseling

Psychologist or Psychiatrist:
- To address anxiety, depression, or other psychological needs

Clergy
- To help with the spiritual support of patient and family

Physical Therapist:
- To restore or improve physical function or to teach patients how to use crutches, walkers, or braces and how to move from bed to chair.
- Also could include whirlpool, massage, hot or cold therapy, and exercises.

Occupational Therapist:
- To restore or improve such tasks such as dressing, eating, bathing, etc., so as to allow patient an independent life-style.

Dietician:
- To assist with meal planning, calorie intake, alternative food choices, or supplements

Pharmacist:
- To assist with medication doses and evaluation of pain management and/or management of side effects.

FAMILY CAREGIVERS

The diagnosis of cancer not only affects the patient, it affects each family member in varying degrees and has different meanings for each.

Dr. Betty Ferrell et al. have addressed the impact of cancer pain on family caregivers. They write:

> The impact of the disease on the family is multifocal. Caring for a loved one with cancer entails inherent physical and psychosocial burdens. Whether or not they feel competent to do so and despite the stress of incorporating caregiving into their daily lives, family members become active caregivers. . . . family caregiving requires adjustments in daily schedules, imposes financial burdens, and causes individual members to reevaluate their relationships with the patient. Advances in cancer treatment have led to increased survivorship, which in turn has led to caregiving demands that exist for years. . . . there are phases of adjustment to cancer, including shock and strain in the initial phase, living with uncertainty and restructuring family roles in the adaptation phase, and grieving in the dying phase.[73]

The researchers used the *Quality of Life Model.* The questions developed for the study were:

- What are family members' descriptions of pain?
- What impact does pain have on the caregivers?
- What are the roles of family caregivers in the pharmacologic and nonpharmacologic management of cancer pain?
- What are the primary questions and concerns expressed by caregivers about the management of cancer pain?

The answers provided an understanding of the family perspective of pain and the meaning of the experience to the individual.

The results identified four major themes in response to the *caregivers' description of pain.*

1. *Anatomic descriptions:* Many caregivers described simply by location (for example, "It is in his back.").
2. *Hidden pain:* Some caregivers perceived that the patient was hiding or minimizing the pain.
3. *Family fear and suffering:* Caregivers described the pain as frightening to them, and their own suffering was apparent.
4. *Overwhelming/unendurable pain:* Caregivers described the pain as very intense and overwhelming.

Word Descriptors Used by Caregivers to Describe Pain

Aching	Pressure
Agonizing	Pulling
Agony	Pushing
Bad	Radiating
Burning	Searing
Constant	Severe
Continuous	Sharp
Cramping	Sore
Debilitating	Spastic
Exasperating	Squeezing
Excruciating	Stabbing
Extreme	Strong
Horrendous	Tense
Horrible	Terrible
Hot	Throbbing
Hurting	Tightness
Inconceivable	Tingling
Intense	Traveling
Intermittent	Unbearable
Itching	Uncomfortable
Miserable	Uncontrollable
Overwhelming	

© B. Ferrell. Reprinted by permission, 1993.

Families' Descriptions of Pain

ANATOMIC

"She has pain throughout her sternum—pressure pain; pain in the shoulder blades. Her back is essentially broken—spinal compression."

"It's in different spots at different times. It travels around and is not so much where the [metastasis] to hip was found but is now in the ribs."

HIDDEN PAIN

"A lot of the time I can sense what she is going through, but she doesn't want to burden others, so she minimizes."

"She pretends she doesn't have any, but when it really gets

bad she says, 'I just can't stand it.' She doesn't want anyone to know it hurts, but since her hospitalization we've made a pact that she'll tell me when she's hurting. She doesn't express her feelings loudly, so when she said she was hurting, you knew it was bad."

FAMILY FEAR AND SUFFERING

"He was in very severe pain before his surgery, and I'm just waiting for it to start again. I'm so afraid."

"It's scary. It came on so fast, and now it seems to be constant. Sometimes it's worse than others, but it always seems to be there."

"She's hurting, and it makes me cry. It's like a knife twisting in her."

"It was awful watching him being in pain, knowing surely there was something to help him."

"Intense, terrible—I can't take it anymore. The last couple of weeks I thought she was gone because of the pain."

"It is very, very difficult. It is so hard to watch someone you love suffer."

"It is the closest thing to hell I can imagine."

"I don't think I can find the words. Only a mother that has gone through it can describe it."

"It was awful. It was the most awful thing that you can imagine."

OVERWHELMING/UNENDURABLE PAIN

"Horrible pain. Burning with fever inside. Aching, like turning a hot knife. Horrible."

"It's an unbearable pain. He said he just couldn't take it."

"Completely overwhelming. Radiates throughout her body, causing tremors. Sharp pain."

"Really painful; never really goes away. So painful—swollen tongue with sores down his neck. He says it's worse than childbirth."

"A burning sensation like a branding iron. Within the last month, she has been in agonizing pain, with wild eyes. She felt like she was being stabbed with a knife. She felt like her insides were blowing up."

"The pain was unbearable, like a bulldozer was going all through her."

"It is exasperating. She shouts. It is terrible, sharp pain."

There were questions and probes about the caregiver experience of pain:

- Can you describe the patient's pain?
- What is it like for you having someone you love with pain?
- What things, other than giving medications, do you do to help relieve the pain?
- Do you have any questions or concerns or other comments to share regarding your experiences as a caregiver in managing pain?

The caregiver experience of pain resulted in three major themes:

1. *Helplessness:* Caregivers described feelings of helplessness when observing pain and a feeling of being unable to do anything to relieve the pain. Many expressed the wish to share the pain with or endure the pain for their loved one.
2. *Coping by denying feelings:* Caregivers described hiding their emotions, "being strong," and building a defense against watching their loved one in pain. The burden this created was twofold. First, caregivers risked being viewed as insensitive by others; second, hiding their feelings required much energy.
3. *Wish for death:* Subjects described the pain as the worst aspect of the illness and said that, to end the pain, death would be a welcome relief.

"The study findings provided an increased understanding of family caregivers' description of pain," Ferrell stated.[74]

Family Experience of Pain

HELPLESSNESS

"I feel helpless. I wish I could take it from her. It hurts deep within to see her suffer. I'd do anything for her."

"Sometimes he's just fine for hours and hours; then I think I see him wince. It makes me feel so helpless."

"It is really discouraging at times. You feel very bad, helpless. I wish I could share the pain with him. It is pitiful."

"It's terrible to watch her when it gets bad. Sometimes I feel bad, kind of helpless, don't know what to do."

"It's hard. I feel myself in tears, not knowing what to do."

"Helpless. You can't absorb their pain. A word picture would be the man watching his wife have a baby."

"I feel so helpless in front of her; she is in so much pain. Too watch my best friend that I love so much in pain really makes me feel helpless."

COPING BY DENYING FEELINGS

"Frustrating. Hurts. I've built a defense and gotten hard so it won't hurt."

"Hurts. She has gone through enough already! I don't know if I'd go through all this if it were me. I've been brave; I haven't gone and cried."

"I try to keep a happy face on."

"It's hard for me. My sister is falling apart over this. I have to be the strong one and keep things together."

"It's hard to describe. You have to adjust suddenly to a lot of changes. She felt like damaged goods, and I have to be strong, keep the emotion inside of me. My cousin called me 'insensitive' because she didn't see me cry."

WISH FOR DEATH

"Awful not being able to do anything. Heartbreaking. You just think death would be better."

"It is the worst part. Someone told me that it is God's way of making you relieved when she finally dies—because it's so horrible seeing her suffer every day. You just wish she would die so she could finally be comfortable."

© B. Ferrell. Reprinted by permission, 1993.

(Note: Home care is covered in Chapter 7 and nearing the end of life in Chapter 10.)

SUMMARY

Cancer carries with it an emotionally loaded package that other diagnoses do not, even though other illnesses may be more debilitating or cause an early death. There is always fear, anxiety, concern about loss of a body part or loss of a normal life. Unrelieved cancer pain is of the utmost concern to all patients with cancer.

Obviously, the first line of medical defense against cancer and pain is either surgery, radiation, chemotherapy, or immunotherapy. However, one or all of these treatments can diminish the body and the spirit. For patients, pain can signal the return of cancer or indicate a hastening of death.

Systemic analgesics and adjuvant drugs or other pain-relieving techniques should be employed in an aggressive effort to control pain in order for the patient to enjoy his or her life as fully as possible.

Cancer pain is a highly complex, emotionally charged event that each patient experiences uniquely. Each patient should be treated as individually as possible, with exacting attention paid to proper physical workups and assessment of pain and each patient's needs.

Lack of education on the part of the health care team is no longer an excuse for poor pain management.

The amount of pain care literature available to everyone in the health care field must be taken advantage of and integrated into the everyday standard of practice.

There is a moral, ethical, and legal imperative to relieve pain, and every patient has a basic human right to control of his or her pain. Doctors, nurses, and other health care professionals must be held accountable for pain management.

Patient suffering should be addressed and treated. Family caregivers' burdens and suffering should not be overlooked.

The following is a comprehensive list of cancer resources.

CANCER RESOURCES

NATIONAL SUPPORT

National Cancer Institute
Public Inquiries Office, Building 31,
  Room 10A19
9000 Rockville Pike
Bethesda, MD 20892
(800) 4-CANCER
  Ask about "Physician Data Query (PDQ)," which contains information on treatment of cancer, plus information on over 1,000 active clinical trials.

American Cancer Society
1599 Clifton Road, N.E.
Atlanta, GA 30329
(800) ACS-2345

Ask about "CanSurmount," for those who have just been diagnosed to speak to those who have recovered from cancer; "Reach to Recovery," for information about recovery from breast cancer.

Cancer Care
1180 Avenue of the Americas
New York, NY 10036
(212) 302-2400

Cancer Caring Center
4117 Liberty Avenue
Pittsburgh, PA 15224
(412) 622-1212

Pennsylvania Department of Health
Cancer Control Program
P.O. Box 90
Harrisburg, PA 17108
(800) 537-4063
 Excellent national resource.

Cancer Federation
P.O. Box 52109
Riverside, CA 92517

Cancer Guidance Institute
1323 Forbes Avenue
Pittsburgh, PA 15219
(412) 261-2211

Families Against Cancer
P.O. Box 588
DeWitt, NY 13214
(315) 446-5326

National Coalition for Cancer Research
426 C Street, N.E.
Washington, DC 20002
(202) 544-1880

National Coalition for Cancer
 Survivorship
1010 Wayne Avenue, Suite 300
Silver Springs, MD 20910
(301) 585-2616

National Hospice Organization
1901 N. Monroe Street, Suite 901
Arlington, VA 22209
(800) 658-8898

Patient Advocates for Advanced
 Treatments
1143 Parmelee, N.W.
Grand Rapids, MI 49504
(616) 453-1477

Vital Options
4419 Coldwater Canyon Avenue,
 Suite A
Studio City, CA 91604
(818) 508-5687

Cancer Fax
Fax (301) 402-5874 for menu of options

Wisconsin Cancer Pain Initiative
3675 Medical Sciences Center
University of Wisconsin
1300 University Avenue
Madison, WI 53706

Oncology Nursing Society
501 Holiday Drive
Pittsburgh, PA 15220-2749

Collaborating Center for Symptom
 Evaluation
610 Walnut Street
Madison, WI 53705

Collaborating Center for Cancer Pain
 Research and Education
Pain Service, Memorial Sloan-Kettering
 Hospital
1275 York Avenue
New York, NY 10021

Cancer Response Service
(800) ACS-2345

National Association of Oncology Social
 Workers
1275 York Avenue, Room MRI 1107
New York, NY 10021
(212) 639-7015

Cancer Research Institute
National Headquarters
681 Fifth Avenue
New York, NY 10022
(800) 99-CANCE

Cancer Consulting Group
990 Grove
Evanston, IL 60201
(708) 866-7711
(800) 383-4636

CanHelp
3111 Paradise Bay Road
Port Ludlow, WA 98365
(206) 437-2291

Cancervive
6500 Wilshire Boulevard, Suite 500
Los Angeles, CA 90048
(213) 203-9232

Canadian Cancer Society
130 Bloor Street West, Suite 1001
Toronto, Ontario M5S 2V7, Canada

PUBLICATIONS

"Advanced Cancer: Living Each Day" (85-856). National Cancer Institute. A booklet providing practical information to make living with advanced cancer easier.

"Breast Cancer: Understanding Treatment Options" (87-2675). National Cancer Institute. This booklet summarizes options for local treatment.

Cancer Nursing. Published monthly.

"Caring for the Patient with Cancer at Home: A Guide for Patients and Families" (4656-PS, 1988 edition). American Cancer Society. A guidebook providing detailed helpful information on how to care for the patient at home.

"Chemotherapy and You: A Guide to Self Help during Treatment" (88-1136). National Cancer Institute. This booklet addresses problems and concerns of patients receiving chemotherapy.

Coping Magazine. Published quarterly.

Coping with Chemotherapy by Nancy Bruning. Ballantine Books, 1986. A good practical and comprehensive guide to the medical and emotional aspects of chemotherapy treatment. If unavailable from bookstores it can be ordered in hardcover from *Coping* magazine, Book Order Department, P.O. Box 5006, Brentwood, TN 37027, (615) 790-7553.

"Eating Hints: Recipes and Tips for Better Nutrition During Cancer Treatment." Office of Cancer Communications, National Cancer Institute, Building 31, Room 10A18, Bethesda, MD 20205. This cookbook-style booklet includes recipes and suggestions for maintaining optimum realistic nutrition during treatment.

"Good Nutrition: Cookbook for the Cancer Patient" (C-152), Central Pennsylvania Oncology Group, P.O. Box 850, Milton S. Hershey Medical Center, Hershey, PA 17033. Free.

I Can Cope by Judi Johnson and Linda Klein. DCI Publishing, 1988. A co-founder of ACS's eight-week "I Can Cope" program has published a guide to staying healthy with cancer using the experiences of several cancer patients.

Invisible Scars: A Guide to Coping with the Emotional Impact of Breast Cancer by Mimi Greenberg. Walker, 1988. A useful guide which helps you to be in charge of your treatment.

Love, Medicine and Miracles by Bernie Siegel. Perennial Library, 1987. Promotes visualization, meditation, discussion, and positive thinking.

Planetree Health Information Service, 2040 Webster Street, San Francisco, CA 94115, (415) 923-3680. A nonprofit, consumer-oriented resource for health information, including materials on relaxation and visualization techniques. Write or call for a catalogue and price list.

"Questions and Answers about Pain Control: A Guide for People with Cancer and Their Families" (4518-PS, 1986 edition). American Cancer Society. This booklet discusses pain control using both medical and nonmedical methods. The emphasis is on explanation and self-help.

"Radiation Therapy and You: A Guide to Self-Help during Treatment" (88-2227). National Cancer Institute. Written for the patient receiving radiation.

The Relaxation Response, by Herbert Benson. Avon Books, 1985.

The Road Back to Health by Neil Fiore. Bantam Books, 1984. Good explanation on how to make your own visualization tapes, by a psychologist and former cancer patient. This book is out of print but may still be found in some libraries.

"Sexuality and Cancer" (1988 edition). American Cancer Society. A booklet giving information about cancer and sexuality in areas that might concern the patient and her partner.

Something's Got to Taste Good by Joan Fishman and Joey Graham. Andrews & McMeel, 1981.

Surviving Cancer by Danette G. Kauffman. Acropolis Books, 1989. A practical guide to experiencing cancer and its treatment, with an emphasis on lists of resources for managing the medical, emotional, and financial aspects of the disease.

"Taking Time: Support for the People with Cancer and the People Who Care about Them" (87-2059). National Cancer Institute. Addresses the feelings of other people in similar situations and how they coped.

Up Front: Sex and the Post-Mastectomy Woman by Linda Dackman. Viking, 1990. A personal account, with frank details about the intimate challenges faced by a single woman in her thirties.

We Can Weekends. C/o Judi Johnson, North Cancer Center, 3300 Oakdale North, Robbinsdale, MN 55422, (612) 520-5155. Weekend retreats for families dealing with cancer. Provides an opportunity to focus on the problems and concerns that are encountered in living with cancer. Designed for families with children. Scholarships and baby-sitters available. Contact North Cancer Center to learn if there is a local group.

MAIL ORDER

Compcare Publishers
(800) 328-3330

Coping Catalogue
2019 North Carothers
Franklin, TN 37064
(615) 790-2400

National Self-Help Clearinghouse
Graduate School and University Center
    of City University of New York
33 West 42d Street, Room 620N
New York, NY 10036
    Will refer written inquiries to regional self-help services.

EMPLOYMENT

American Cancer Society
1599 Clifton Road, N.E.
Atlanta, GA 30329
(800) ACS-2345
    Ask about "Cancer—Your Job, Insurance and the Law" (4585-ps), a summary of cancer patients' legal rights regarding insurance and employment.

Health Insurance Association of
    America
1025 Connecticut Avenue, N.W.
Washington, DC 20004-3998
(202) 223-7780
    Ask for "What You Should Know about Health Insurance" (731) and "What You Should Know about Disability Insurance" (733).

Barbara Lazarus
Associate Provost for Academic
    Programs
Carnegie-Mellon University,
    Pittsburgh, PA 15213

National Coalition for Cancer
    Survivorship
(505) 764-9956

Phyllis Stein
Radcliffe Career Services
Radcliffe College
10 Garden Street
Cambridge, MA 02138

For more information in your area, contact your local office of vocational rehabilitation, office of employment security, or private employment agencies.

TRANSPORTATION

Corporate Angel Network
Westchester County Airport, Building 1
White Plains, NY 10604
(914) 328-1313

A nationwide program designed to give patients with cancer the use of available seats on corporate aircraft to get to and from recognized treatment centers. There is no cost or any financial need requirement.

Mission Air Transportation Network
77 Bloor Street West, Suite 1711
Toronto, Ontario M5S 3A1, Canada
(416) 924-9333.
Same as above.

National Cancer Institute
Public Inquiries Office, Building 31,
Room 10A19
9000 Rockville Pike
Bethesda, MD 20892
(800) 4-CANCER

National Cancer Institute
Bethesda, MD 20892-4200
(800) 638-6694

Patients who are treated here as part of a clinical study receive their treatment free and may be housed free of charge at the hospital facilities of NCI.

Volunteer transportation services are often available from local churches, organizations, ambulance service, agency on aging, department of public welfare, or American Cancer Society unit.

FINANCIAL ASSISTANCE

American Association of Retired People
Pharmacy Service
Catalogue Department
P.O. Box 19229
Alexandria, VA 22320

Members can use their nonprofit service to save on prescriptions delivered by mail. Good for tamoxifen (Novaldex). Write for a free catalogue.

For financial services in your area, contact your local area agency on aging, county board of assistance, office of vocational rehabilitation, office of the Social Security Administration, American Red Cross, or Veterans' Administration, or the Income Maintenance Help Line at (800) 692-7462.

OTHER RESOURCES

American Society of Clinical Oncology
435 North Michigan Avenue, Suite 1717
Chicago, IL 60611
(312) 644-0828

Will mail to medical professionals a list of member oncologists by geographical area.

Institute for the Advancement of Health
16 East 53d Street
New York, NY 10022
(212) 832-8282

A national organization devoted to promoting awareness of mind-body health interactions. Supplies information on behavioral techniques to promote comfort and health.

National Lymphedema Network
2211 Post Street, Suite 404
San Francisco, CA 94115
(800) 541-3259

Nonprofit organization providing patients and professionals with information about prevention and treatment of this complication of lymph node surgery. Ask for "Lymphedema after Treatment for Breast Cancer," NABCO fact sheet.

Wellness Community
1235 5th Street
Santa Monica, CA 90401
(213) 393-1415

Extensive support and education programs which encourage emotional recovery and a feeling of wellness.

NCI CANCER CENTERS

Comprehensive Care Centers for Cancer

ALABAMA
University of Alabama Comprehensive
  Cancer Center
1918 University Boulevard
Basic Health Sciences Building, Room
  108
Birmingham, AL 35294

ARIZONA
Arizona Cancer Center
University of Arizona Cancer Center
1501 North Campbell Avenue
Tucson, AZ 85724

CALIFORNIA
Jonsson Comprehensive Cancer Center
  (University of California at Los
  Angeles)
10-247 Factor Building
10833 Le Conte Avenue
Los Angeles, CA 90024-1781

Kenneth Norris Jr. Cancer Center
University of Southern California
1441 Eastlake Avenue
Los Angeles, CA 90033-0804

CONNECTICUT
Yale University Comprehensive Cancer
  Center
333 Cedar Street
New Haven, CT 06510-8028

DISTRICT OF COLUMBIA
Vincent T. Lombardi Cancer Research
  Center
Georgetown University Medical Center
3800 Reservoir Road, N.W.
Washington, DC 20007

FLORIDA
Sylvester Comprehensive Cancer Center
University of Miami Medical School
1475 N.W. 12th Avenue
Miami, FL 33136

MARYLAND
Johns Hopkins Hospital
600 North Wolfe Street
Baltimore, MD 21205

MASSACHUSETTS
Dana Farber Cancer Institute
44 Binney Street
Boston, MA 02115

MICHIGAN
Meyer L. Prentis Comprehensive Cancer
  Center
110 East Warren Avenue
Detroit, MI 48201

University of Michigan Cancer Center
101 Simpson Drive
Ann Arbor, MI 48109-0752

MINNESOTA
Mayo Comprehensive Cancer Center
200 First Street, S.W.
Rochester, MN 55905

NEW HAMPSHIRE
Norris Cotton Cancer Center
Dartmouth-Hitchcock Medical Center
2 Maynard Street
Hanover, NH 03756

NEW YORK
Columbia University Cancer Center
College of Physicians and Surgeons
630 West 168th Street
New York, NY 10032

Kaplan Cancer Center
New York University Medical Center
550 First Avenue
New York, NY 10016

Memorial Sloan-Kettering Cancer Center
1275 York Avenue
New York, NY 10021

Roswell Park Memorial Institute
Elm and Carlton Streets
Buffalo, NY 14263

NORTH CAROLINA
Cancer Center of Wake Forest
  University
Bowman Gray School of Medicine
300 South Hawthorne Road
Winston-Salem, NC 27103

Duke University Comprehensive Cancer
  Center
P.O. Box 3843
Durham, NC 27710

Lineberger Cancer Research Center
University of North Carolina School of
  Medicine
Chapel Hill, NC 27599

OHIO
Ohio State University Comprehensive
  Cancer Center
410 West 12th Avenue
Columbus, OH 43210

PENNSYLVANIA
Fox Chase Cancer Center
7701 Burholme Avenue
Philadelphia, PA 19111

Pittsburgh Cancer Institute
200 Meyran Avenue
Pittsburgh, PA 15213

University of Pennsylvania Cancer
  Center
3400 Spruce Street
Philadelphia, PA 19104

TEXAS
University of Texas M. D. Anderson
  Cancer Center
1515 Holcombe Boulevard
Houston, TX 77030

VERMONT
Vermont Cancer Center
University of Vermont
1 South Prospect Street
Burlington, VT 05401

WASHINGTON
Fred Hutchinson Cancer Research
  Center
1124 Columbia Street
Seattle, WA 98104

WISCONSIN
Wisconsin Clinical Cancer Center
University of Wisconsin
600 Highland Avenue
Madison, WI 53792

Clinical Cancer Centers

CALIFORNIA
City of Hope National Medical Center
Beckman Research Institute
1500 East Duarte Road
Duarte, CA 91010

University of California at San Diego
225 Dickinson Street
San Diego, CA 92103

COLORADO
University of Colorado Cancer Center
4200 East 9th Avenue, Box B190
Denver, CO 80262

ILLINOIS
University of Chicago Cancer Research
  Center
5841 South Maryland Avenue, Box 444
Chicago, IL 60637

INDIANA
Purdue Cancer Center
Purdue University
South University Street
West Lafayette, IN 47907

MAINE
Jackson Laboratory
600 Main Street
Bar Harbor, ME 04609-1500

MASSACHUSETTS
Worcester Foundation for Experimental
  Biology
222 Maple Avenue
Shrewsbury, MA 01545

Center for Cancer Research
Massachusetts Institute of Technology
40 Ames Street
Cambridge, MA 02139

NEBRASKA
Eppley Institute
University of Nebraska Medical Center
600 South 42d Street
Omaha, NE 68198-6805

NEW YORK
Albert Einstein College of Medicine
1300 Morris Park Avenue
Bronx, NY 10461

American Health Foundation
320 East 43d Street
New York, NY 10017

Cold Spring Harbor Laboratory
P.O. Box 100
Cold Spring Harbor, NY 11724

Institute of Environmental Medicine
New York University Medical Center
550 First Avenue
New York, NY 10016

University of Rochester Cancer Center
601 Elmwood Avenue, Box 704
Rochester, NY 14642

OHIO
Case Western Reserve University
University Hospitals of Cleveland
Ireland Cancer Center
2074 Abington Road
Cleveland, OH 44106

PENNSYLVANIA
Fels Research Institute
Temple University School of Medicine
3420 North Broad Street
Philadelphia, PA 19140

Wistar Institute
3601 Spruce Street
Philadelphia, PA 19104

RHODE ISLAND
Roger Williams General Hospital
825 Chalkstone Avenue
Providence, RI 02908

TENNESSEE
St. Jude Children's Research Hospital
332 North Lauderdale Street
Memphis, TN 38101

TEXAS
Institute for Cancer Research and Care
8122 Datapoint Drive
San Antonio, TX 78229

UTAH
Utah Regional Cancer Center
University of Utah Medical Center
50 North Medical Drive, Room 2C10
Salt Lake City, UT 84132

VIRGINIA
Cancer Center
University of Virginia Medical Center
Box 234, Health Science Center
Charlottesville, VA 22908

Massey Cancer Center
Medical College of Virginia
Virginia Commonwealth University
1200 East Broad Street
Richmond, VA 23298

WISCONSIN
McArdle Laboratory for Cancer
  Research
University of Wisconsin
1400 University Avenue
Madison, WI 53706

CHILDREN'S CANCER RESOURCES*

FEDERAL GOVERNMENT RESOURCES

National Institutes of Health
9000 Rockville Pike
Bethesda, MD 20892
(301) 496-4000

The National Institutes of Health (NIH) is one of five health agencies of the Public Health Service that fall under the auspices of the United States Department of Health and Human Services (HHS). The NIH is composed of 13 institutes, the National Library of Medicine, and the Fogarty International Center. Its primary focus is to improve the health of the American people through biomedical research.

National Cancer Institute (NCI)
9000 Rockville Pike
Bethesda, MD 20892
(301) 496-4000

One of the federally-funded National Institutes of Health.

Cancer Information Service
National Cancer Institute
Blair Building, Room 414
9000 Rockville Pike
Bethesda, MD 20892
(800) 4-CANCER
(301) 402-5874

Provides immediate access to the latest cancer information, local resources, publications, support, and understanding. Spanish-speaking staff members are available in some areas.

Office of Cancer Communications
9000 Rockville Pike
Building 31, Room 10A24
Bethesda, MD 20892
(301) 496-5583

Provides written answers to specific questions. Produces and distributes medical, psychosocial, and educational publications. Physician Data Query (PDQ) is NCI's computerized database, providing the most up-to-date information available. PDQ contains three files: Cancer Information on major cancers, Protocols of ongoing clinical trials that are accepting new patients, and Directories of physicians and organizations active in cancer treatment.

Warren Grant Magnuson Clinical Center
National Institutes of Health,
Building 10
Bethesda, MD 20892
Pediatric branch (301) 496-4256
Patient referral (301) 402-0696

The NIH research hospital that conducts medical research and patient treatment programs. The NCI Pediatric Branch provides free treatment for children who fit their research protocols and second opinions for families and physicians.

National Library of Medicine
National Institutes of Health
8600 Rockville Pike
Bethesda, MD 20894
(301) 496-6308

Index Medicus. Monthly, with cumulative annual edition. Subject, author index to over 3,000 substantive biomedical journals.

MEDLARS: Medical Literature Analysis and Retrieval System. Computer searches of biomedical literature can be done at most large university and medical libraries. Abstracts are available on-line on request.

CANCERLINE is a database system that provides quick, easy access to cancer literature.

---

*For further children's cancer resources on community/special needs, medical organizations, bone marrow registries, patient air transport, insurance information, financial assistance, home care, camps, and wish-fulfillment organizations, see Pizzo, Philip A., Popluck, David G., *Principles and Practice of Pediatric Oncology,* second edition (Philadelphia: J. B. Lippincott Company, 1993). This listing courtesy of Philip A. Pizzo and David G. Popluck.

International Cancer Research Data
  Bank Program
Superintendent of Documents
U.S. Government Printing Office
Washington, DC 20402
  Collects, stores, and disseminates results of cancer research.
  Cancergrams, a monthly bulletin of abstracts from selected journal articles on
topics such as carcinogenesis, cancer
therapy, diet, and nutrition.
  Oncology Overviews, a specialized bibliography with abstracts on cancer research topics. Includes all significant
current papers.

National Information Center for
  Children and Youth with Disabilities
P.O. Box 1492
Washington, DC 20013
(800) 999-5599
(703) 893-6061
TDD (703) 893-8614
  Clearinghouse on the education of children and youth with handicaps. Also provides information on rare disorders and
chronic health problems and technical assistance to parents, professionals, and
other interested parties. Publishes *News
Digest, Transition Summary,* and other
publications.

U.S. Department of Education
  Educational Resources Information
  Center
1900 Kenny Road
Columbus, OH 43210-1090
(800) 848-4815
Fax (614) 292-1260
  Clearinghouse on adult, career, and vocational education. Provides information
from its educational database and publications, technical assistance, and training
programs.

U.S. Department of Education
  Rehabilitation Services
  Administration
Office of Special Education and
  Rehabilitation Services
330 C Street, S.W.
Washington, DC 20202
(202) 205-5482
  Responsible for ensuring that state re-

habilitation service agencies comply with
federal law.

U.S. Department of Health and Human
  Services
Public Health Service

Health Care Financing Administration
6325 Security Boulevard
Baltimore, MD 21207
(800) 888-1998

Centers for Disease Control
1600 Clifton Road, N.E.
Atlanta, GA 30333
(404) 639-3311
  Responsible for the study and prevention of disease and for promoting health
and healthy life-styles.

Food and Drug Administration
Office of Public Affairs
5600 Fishers Lane
Rockville, MD 20857
(301) 443-1130
  Provides information and responds to
consumer inquiries on the FDA, what it
regulates and approves in food, drugs,
and cosmetics products.

Parklawn Computer Center
5699 Fishers Lane, Room 2B59
Rockville, MD 20857
(301) 443-7318
  Provides information to access the FDA
electronic bulletin board.

Office of Disease Prevention and Health
  Promotion, National Health
  Information Center
P.O. Box 1133
Washington, DC 20013-1133
(800) 336-4797
  Health information resources in the
federal government. Clearinghouse and
directory of offices and projects that provide health information to health care
professionals and the general public.

Clearinghouse on Disability Information
Office of Special Education and
  Rehabilitation Services
Switzer Building, 330 C Street, S.W.,
  Room 3132
Washington, DC 20202
(202) 205-8241

Clearinghouse for Occupational Safety
and Health Information
Technical Information Branch
4676 Columbia Parkway
Cincinnati, OH 45226
(800) 356-4674

National AIDS Information
Clearinghouse
P.O. Box 6003
Rockville, MD 20849-6003
(800) 458-5231

National Center for Education in
Maternal and Child Health
2000 15th Street North, Suite 701
Arlington, VA 22201
(703) 524-7802
Provides information, educational materials, and technical assistance to organizations, agencies, and individuals. Publishes *Reaching Out,* a directory of organizations that provide child health information.

National Information Center for Orphan
Drugs and Rare Diseases
P.O. Box 1133
Washington, DC 20013
(800) 456-3505
Provides referrals to organizations dealing with rare diseases and orphan drugs. Provides list of drug companies that manufacture orphan drugs.

National Library Service, Division of the
Blind and Physically Handicapped
Library of Congress
1291 Taylor Street, N.W.
Washington, DC 20542
(800) 424-8567

National Rehabilitation Information
Center
8455 Colesville Road, Suite 935
Silver Springs, MD 20910
(800) 346-2742
In MD (301) 588-9284
Fax (301) 587-1967
Information service and research library funded by the Department of Education, National Institute on Disability and Rehabilitation Research, to facilitate access to federally funded research reports. Provides information on assistance devices and rehabilitation. ABELDATA, (202) 319-6090, and REHABDATA, (202) 319-5822, databases. Publishes *NARIC Guide to Disability and Rehabilitation Periodicals* and *NARIC Quarterly* Newsletter.

President's Council on Physical Fitness
and Sports
701 Pennsylvania Avenue, N.W., Suite
250
Washington, DC 20004
(202) 272-3430

U.S. CANCER CENTERS AND PEDIATRIC ONCOLOGY UNITS

Children's Cancer Study Group
W. Archie Bleyer, M.D., Group
Chairman
M. D. Anderson Cancer Center, Division
of Pediatrics
1515 Holcombe Boulevard
Houston, TX 77030
(713) 792-6603

Pediatric Oncology Group
Teresa J. Vietta, M.D., Chairman
Operations Office, Del Coronado
4949 West Pine Boulevard, Suite A, 2d
Floor
St. Louis, MO 63108-1498
(314) 367-3446
Fax (314) 367-4916

Sharon Murphy, M.D., Chair Elect
Children's Memorial Hospital
2300 Children's Plaza
Chicago, IL 60614
(312) 880-4584

ALABAMA
Children's Hospital of Alabama
1600 Seventh Avenue South
Birmingham, AL 35233
Robert Castleberry, M.D.
(205) 939-9100

ARIZONA
Barrow Neurological Institute
Pediatric Hematology/Oncology
  Association, P.C.
350 West Thomas Road
Phoenix, AZ 85013
(602) 266-3355
Jesse Cohen, M.D.
(602) 253-5953

Phoenix Children's Hospital
Children's Cancer Center
909 East Brill Street
Phoenix, AZ 85006
Paul Baranko, M.D.
(602) 239-5785

University of Arizona Cancer Center
Department of Pediatrics
1501 North Campbell Avenue
Tucson, AZ 85724
(602) 694-0111
John Hutter, M.D.
(602) 626-7788

ARKANSAS
Arkansas Children's Hospital
Department of Hematology/Oncology
800 Marshall Street
Little Rock, AR 72202
(501) 320-1100
David Becton, M.D.
(501) 320-1494

CALIFORNIA
Southern California Kaiser-Permanente
  Medical Group
Department of Pediatric
  Hematology/Oncology
9449 East Imperial Highway
Downey, CA 90242
Willye B. Powell, M.D.
(310) 803-2360

City of Hope National Medical Center
Division of Pediatrics
1500 East Duarte Road
Duarte, CA 91010
Robert R. Chilcote, M.D.
(818) 301-8434

Valley Children's Hospital
3151 North Millbrook Avenue
Fresno, CA 93703
Vonda L. Crouse, M.D.
(209) 225-3000

Loma Linda University Medical Center
Department of Pediatrics
11234 Anderson Street
Loma Linda, CA 92354
Antranik A. Bedros, M.D.
(714) 796-7311

Jonathan Jacques Children's Cancer
  Center
Memorial Miller Children's Hospital
2801 Atlantic Avenue, P.O. Box 1428
Long Beach, CA 90801-1428
Jerry Z. Finklestein, M.D.
(301) 426-2146

Cedars-Sinai Medical Center
Department of Pediatrics
  Hematology/Oncology
8700 West Beverly Boulevard
Los Angeles, CA 90048
(310) 855-5000
Carole G. Hurvitz, M.D.
(310) 855-4423

Children's Hospital Los Angeles
Division of Hematology/Oncology
4650 Sunset Boulevard
Los Angeles, CA 90054-0700
(213) 660-2450
Stuart E. Siegel, M.D.
(213) 669-2163

UCLA School of Medicine
Division of Pediatric
  Hematology/Oncology
10833 Le Conte Avenue, Room A2410
Los Angeles, CA 90024
Stephen A. Feig, M.D.
(310) 825-5050

Children's Hospital of Oakland
Department of Hematology/Oncology
747 52d Street
Oakland, CA 94609
James Feusner, M.D.
(415) 428-3372

Kaiser Permanente Hospitals
Department of Pediatric
  Hematology/Oncology
280 West MacArthur Boulevard
Oakland, CA 94611
(510) 596-1000
Stacy Month, M.D.
(510) 596-6592

Children's Hospital of Orange County
Department of Pediatric
  Hematology/Oncology
455 South Main Street, P.O. Box 5700
Orange, CA 92668
(714) 997-3000
Geni A. Bennetts, M.D.
(714) 532-8636

Packard Children's Hospital
Children's Hospital Stanford
Division Hematology/Oncology
725 Welch Road
Palo Alto, CA 94305
Michael Link, M.D.
(415) 853-3378

University of California at Davis
USC Medical Center Ticon II
Pediatric Hematology/Oncology
2515 Stockton Boulevard
Sacramento, CA 95817
(916) 734-2450
Jonathan Ducore, M.D.
(916) 734-2782

Balboa Naval Hospital
Department of Pediatric
  Hematology/Oncology
San Diego, CA 92134-5000
Capt. William J. Thomas, M.D.
(619) 532-6875

University of California at San Diego
225 Dickinson Street
San Diego, CA 92103-8447
Faith Kung, M.D.
(619) 543-6844

Children's Cancer Research Institute
2351 Clay Street, Suite 512
San Francisco, CA 94115
Jordan R. Wilbur, M.D.
(415) 923-3535

University of California, San Francisco
  Medical Center
Division of Pediatric Oncology, Room
  M647
505 Parnassus Street
San Francisco, CA 94143-0106
Katherine K. Matthey, M.D.
(415) 476-3831

Kaiser Permanente Santa Clara
900 Kiely Boulevard
Santa Clara, CA 95051
Lily Young, M.D.
(408) 236-5067

Harbor/UCLA Medical Center
Department of Pediatrics
  Hematology/Oncology
1124 West Carson Street, J4
Torrance, CA 90502
Lance Sieger, M.D.
(310) 212-4154

David Grant USAF Medical Center
Department of Pediatrics
Travis AFB, CA 94535
Maj. Peter J. Chenaille
(707) 423-5323

COLORADO
Fitzsimmons Army Medical Center
Department of Pediatrics
Colfax and Peoria
Aurora, CO 80045-5001
Maj. George Maher, M.D.
(303) 361-3837

Children's Hospital of Denver
University of Colorado School of
  Medicine
Department of Hematology/Oncology
1056 East 19th Avenue, Box B145
Denver, CO 80218
(303) 861-8888
Laurie Odom, M.D.
(303) 861-6470

University of Colorado Cancer Center
4200 Cedar Street
Denver, CO 80262
(303) 270-7235

CONNECTICUT
University of Connecticut Health Center
Department of Pediatric
  Hematology/Oncology
263 Farmington Avenue
Farmington, CT 06032
Arnold J. Altman, M.D.
(203) 679-2221

Yale University School of Medicine,
Pediatrics
333 Cedar Street, Box 3333
New Haven, CT 06510
G. Peter Beardsley, M.D.
(203) 785-4640

DELAWARE
Medical Center of Delaware
Pediatric Hematology/Oncology
4755 Ogletown Road
Newark, DE 19718
(302) 733-1000
Rita S. Meek, M.D.
(302) 633-1020

DISTRICT OF COLUMBIA
Children's National Medical Center
Department of Pediatric
  Hematology/Oncology
111 Michigan Avenue, N.W.
Washington, DC 20010
Gregory H. Reaman, M.D.
(202) 745-2140

Georgetown University Medical Center
Vincent Lombardi Cancer Research
  Center
3800 Reservoir Road, N.W.
Washington, DC 20007
Joseph E. Gootenberg, M.D.
(202) 687-2224

Howard University Hospital
Department of Pediatrics and Child
  Health
2041 Georgia Avenue, N.W.
Washington, DC 20060
Sohail R. Rana, M.D.
(202) 865-1595

Pediatric Branch, NCI
Building 10, 13N240
Bethesda, MD 20892
Philip Pizzo, M.D.
(301) 402-0696

Walter Reed Army Medical Center
Building 2, K Section, Pediatric Clinic
Georgia Avenue
Washington, DC 20307
David Maybee, M.D.
(202) 576-0421

FLORIDA
University of Florida
Shands Teaching Hospital
Box 100-296, JHMHC, Archer Road
Gainesville, FL 32610
Samuel Gross, M.D.
(904) 392-4470

Memorial Hospital Pediatric Specialty
4340 Sheridan Street, Suite 102
Hollywood, FL 33021
Philippa Sprinz, M.D.
(305) 964-9553

University of Florida
Nemours Children's Clinic
807 Nira Street
Jacksonville, FL 32207
Paul Pitel, M.D.
(904) 390-3789

Miami Children's Hospital
Division of Hematology/Oncology
6125 S.W. 31st Street
Miami, FL 33155
Charles August, M.D.
(305) 662-8360

University of Miami School of Medicine
Jackson Memorial Hospital
Pediatric Hematology/Oncology
1611 N.W. 12th Avenue
Miami, FL 33136
Stuart Toledano, M.D.
(305) 549-7752

Orlando Cancer Center
85 West Miller Street
Orlando, FL 32806
Vincent Giusti, M.D.
(407) 648-3800

Sacred Heart Children's Hospital
Hematology/Oncology
5190 Bayou Boulevard
Pensacola, FL 32503
Thomas Jenkins, M.D.
(904) 477-4861

All Children's Hospital
801 Sixth Street South
St. Peterburg, FL 33701
Jerry Barbosa, M.D.
(813) 892-4176

St. Joseph's Cancer Institute
Children's Center
3001 West Drive, M. L. King Boulevard
Tampa, FL 33607
Cameron Tebbi, M.D.
(813) 870-4252

University of South Florida Medical
 Center
H. Lee Moffitt Cancer Center
12902 Magnolia Drive
Tampa, FL 33612
Eva Hvizdala, M.D.
(813) 972-8430

GEORGIA
Emory University School of Medicine
Trail Annex Pediatrics
2040 Ridgewood Drive, N.E.
Atlanta, GA 30322
Abdel Ragab, M.D.
(404) 727-3970

Scottish Rite Children's Medical Center
1101 Johnson Ferry Road
Atlanta, GA 30342
Elizabeth Kurczynski, M.D.
(404) 256-5252

Medical College of Georgia
Pediatric Hematology/Oncology
1120 15th Street, Room CK 146
Augusta, GA 30912
P. Charlton Davis, M.D.
(404) 721-3626

HAWAII
Tripler Army Medical Center
Department of Pediatrics HSHK-PE-GP
Tripler, HI 96859-5000
Shirley E. Reddock, M.D.
(808) 433-6057

Kapiolani Medical Center for Women
 and Children
1319 Punahou Street
Honolulu, HI 96826
Robert Wilkinson, M.D.
(808) 973-8511

IDAHO
Mountain State's Tumor Institute
151 East Bannock
Boise, ID 83712-6297
Bonita Vestal, M.D.
(208) 386-2711

ILLINOIS
Children's Memorial Hospital
Division of Hematology/Oncology
2300 Children's Plaza
Chicago, IL 60614
Sharon Murphy, M.D.
(312) 880-4584

Cook County Children's Hospital
700 South Wood Street
Chicago, IL 60612
(312) 633-1000
Sudha Rao, M.D.
(312) 633-6526

Rush–Presbyterian–St. Luke's Medical
 Center
1753 West Congress Parkway
Chicago, IL 60612
Alexander Green, M.D.
(312) 942-8114

University of Chicago Medical Center
Pediatric Hematology/Oncology
5841 South Maryland, Box 97
Chicago, IL 60637
F. Leonard Johnson, M.D.
(312) 702-6808

University of Illinois at Chicago
Department of Pediatrics
840 South Wood Street MC856, Room
 1245
Chicago, IL 60612
Helen S. Johnstone, M.D.
(312) 996-6413

Loyola University Medical Center
Department of Pediatric
 Hematology/Oncology
2160 South First Avenue
Maywood, IL 60153
Carlos R. Suarez, M.D.
(708) 216-6319

Lutheran General Children's Medical
 Center
Department of Pediatric
 Hematology/Oncology
1775 Dempster Street
Park Ridge, IL 60068-1174
Jong Kwon
(708) 696-7682

University of Illinois, Rockford
College of Medicine
Pediatric Hematology/Oncology
1400 Charles Street
Rockford, IL 61104
Torrey L. Mitchell, M.D.
(815) 987-1845

INDIANA
Indiana University, Riley Hospital
Pediatric Hematology/Oncology
702 Barnhill Drive
Indianapolis, IN 46202-5225
Phillip Breitfield, M.D.
(317) 274-8784

Methodist Hospital
Department of Hematology/Oncology
1701 North Senate Boulevard
Indianapolis, IN 46206
Arthur Provisor, M.D.
(317) 927-5770

IOWA
Iowa Methodist Medical Center
Raymond Blank Children's Hospital
1200 Pleasant Street
Des Moines, IA 50308
Stephen C. Elliott, M.D.
(515) 241-6230

University of Iowa Hospitals and
    Clinics
Pediatric Hematology/Oncology
200 Hawkins Drive
Iowa City, IA 52242
C. Thomas Kisker, M.D.
(319) 356-3422

KANSAS
University of Kansas Medical Center
39th and Rainbow Boulevard
Kansas City, KS 66160
Tribhawan Vats, M.D.
(913) 588-6340

St. Francis Regional Medical Center
929 North St. Francis Street
Wichita, KS 67214
(316) 268-5000
David Rosen, M.D.
(316) 263-4311

KENTUCKY
University of Kentucky
A. B. Chandler Medical Center
Department of Pediatrics
800 Rose Street
Lexington, KY 40536-0284
Martha Greenwood, M.D.
(606) 233-5694

Kosair Children's Hospital
Pediatric Hematology/Oncology
231 East Chestnut Street
Louisville, KY 40202
(502) 629-6000
Salvatore J. Bertolone, M.D.

LOUISIANA
Children's Hospital of New Orleans
200 Henry Clay Avenue
New Orleans, LA 70118
Rafael Ducos, M.D.
(504) 896-9740

Tulane University Medical School
Department of Pediatrics, Division of
    Hematology/Oncology
1430 Tulane Avenue
New Orleans, LA 70112
James R. Humbert, M.D.
(504) 588-5412

MAINE
Eastern Maine Medical Center
Pediatrics Specialty Clinic
489 State Street
Bangor, ME 04401
Sam W. Lew, M.D.
(207) 945-7554

Maine Children's Cancer Program
685 Congress Street
Portland, ME 04102
Stephen Blattner, M.D.
(207) 775-5481

MARYLAND
Johns Hopkins Oncology Center
Clinical Research Administration
550 North Broadway, Suite 1121
Baltimore, MD 21205
Brigid Leventhal, M.D.
(301) 955-7224

University of Maryland Medical System
Pediatrics, Room N5W77
22 South Green Street
Baltimore, MD 21201
Christopher Frantz, M.D.
(301) 328-2808

National Cancer Institute
Pediatric Branch, Building 10, 13N240
Bethesda, MD 20892
Philip Pizzo, M.D.
(301) 402-0696

National Naval Medical Center
Pediatric Clinic, Building 9
8901 Wisconsin Avenue
Bethesda, MD 20889-5000
Bertrand Duval-Arnould, M.D.
(301) 295-4900

MASSACHUSETTS
Boston Floating Hospital for Infants and
   Children
Pediatric Hematology/Oncology, Box 14
750 Washington Street
Boston, MA 02111
Lawrence C. Wolfe, M.D.
(617) 956-5535

Dana Farber Cancer Institute
44 Binney Street
Boston, MA 02115
Holcombe Grier, M.D.
(617) 732-3971

Children's Hospital and Medical Center
300 Longwood Avenue
Boston, MA 02115
Stephen Sallan, M.D.
(617) 732-3971

Massachusetts General Hospital
32 Fruit Street, ACC 707, 7th Floor
Boston, MA 02114
William Ferguson, M.D.
(617) 726-2737

Baystate Medical Center, Children's
   Hospital
Pediatrics Hematology/Oncology
759 Chestnut Street
Springfield, MA 01199
John F. Kelleher, M.D.
(413) 784-5378

University of Massachusetts Medical
   Center
Pediatrics
55 Lake Avenue North
Worcester, MA 01655
(508) 865-0011
Peter Newburger, M.D.
(508) 856-4225

MICHIGAN
University of Michigan
Mott Children's Hospital
Pediatric Hematology/Oncology F6515,
   Box 0238
1500 East Medical Center Drive
Ann Arbor, MI 48109-0238
Lawrence Boxer, M.D.
(313) 763-9293

Children's Hospital of Michigan
Wayne State University
3901 Beaubien Boulevard
Detroit, MI 48201
Jeanne Lusher, M.D.
(313) 745-5649

St. John Hospital and Medical Center
22201 Moross
Detroit, MI 48236
(313) 343-4000
Hadi Sawaf, M.D.
(313) 343-7979

Michigan State University
Pediatric and Human Development
   Department
Life Sciences B240
East Lansing, MI 48824-1317
Roshi Kulkarni, M.D.
(517) 355-5039

Hurley Medical Center
One Hurley Plaza
Flint, MI 48502
Susumu Inoue, M.D.
(313) 257-9585

Grand Rapids Clinic and Oncology
   Program
100 Michigan, N.E.
Grand Rapids, MI 49503
James B. Fahner, M.D.
(616) 774-1230

William Beaumont Hospital
Division of Pediatric
  Hematology/Oncology
3601 West Thirteen Mile Road
Royal Oak, MI 48072
(313) 551-5000
Charles A. Main, M.D.
(313) 551-0360

MINNESOTA
Duluth Clinic
Department of Hematology/Oncology
400 East 3d Street
Duluth, MN 55805
Robert D. Niedringhaus, M.D.
(218) 722-8364

Minneapolis Children's Medical Center
Medical Office Building
2525 Chicago Avenue South, Room 402
Minneapolis, MN 55404
Maura C. O'Leary, M.D.
(612) 863-5940

University of Minnesota Medical Center
Pediatric Hematology/Oncology
Harvard and East River Road
Minneapolis, MN 55455
(612) 626-3000
Mark Nesbit, M.D.
(612) 626-2778

Mayo Clinic
Department of Pediatric
  Hematology/Oncology
200 First Street, S.W.
Rochester, MN 55905
Gerald S. Gilchrist, M.D.
(507) 284-2922

St. Paul Children's Hospital
345 North Smith
St. Paul, MN 55102
John R. Priest, M.D.
(612) 220-6732

MISSISSIPPI
University of Mississippi Medical
  Center
2500 North State Street
Jackson, MS 39216
Jeanette Pullen, M.D.
(601) 984-5220

Kessler AFB Medical Center
Pediatric Hematology/Oncology
KTTC Medical Center
Kessler AFB, MS 39534
Thomas Abshire, M.D.
(601) 377-6626

MISSOURI
University of Missouri Health Sciences
  Center
Child Health
1 Hospital Drive
Columbia, MO 65212
Nasrollah Hakami, M.D.
(314) 882-4929

Children's Mercy Hospital
Department of Pediatric
  Hematology/Oncology
24th and Gillham Road
Kansas City, MO 64108
Arnold I. Freeman, M.D.
(816) 234-3265

Cardinal Glennon Children's Hospital
1465 South Grand Avenue
St. Louis, MO 63104
Dennis M. O'Connor, M.D.
(314) 577-5638

Washington University Medical Center
St. Louis Children's
Pediatric Hematology/Oncology
400 South Kingshighway Boulevard
St. Louis, MO 63110
Alan Schwartz, M.D.
(314) 454-6209

NEBRASKA
Children's Memorial Hospital, Omaha
Pediatric Hematology/Oncology
8301 Dodge Street
Omaha, NE 68114
David J. Gnarra, M.D.
(402) 390-5400
(402) 390-5549

University of Nebraska Medical Center
Department of Pediatric
  Hematology/Oncology
600 South 42d Street
Omaha, NE 68198-2165
Peter F. Coccia, M.D.
(402) 559-4000
(402) 559-7257

NEVADA
Humana Children's Hospital
Department of Pediatric
  Hematology/Oncology
3186 Maryland Parkway
Las Vegas, NV 89109
(702) 731-8000
Ronald S. Oseas, M.D.
(702) 737-0017

NEW HAMPSHIRE
Dartmouth-Hitchock Medical Center
Norris Cotton Cancer Center
Pediatric Hematology/Oncology
2 Maynard Street
Hanover, NH 03756
(603) 650-5000
Eric Larsen, M.D.
(603) 646-5541

NEW JERSEY
University of Medicine and Dentistry of
  New Jersey
Cooper Hospital, Department of
  Pediatrics
3 Cooper Plaza
Camden, NJ 08103
(609) 342-2000
Milton H. Donaldson, M.D.
(609) 342-2264

Hackensack Medical Center
Tomorrow's Children's Institute
30 Prospect Avenue
Hackensack, NJ 07601
(201) 996-2000
Michael Harris, M.D.
(201) 996-3231

Newark Beth Israel Medical Center
Valerie Fund Children's Center
Department of Pediatrics
201 Lyons Avenue
Newark, NJ 07112
Peri Kamalakar, M.D.
(201) 926-7161

Overlook Hospital
Valerie Fund Children's Center
99 Beauvoir Avenue
Summit, NJ 07901-0220
Steven L. Halpern, M.D.
(201) 522-2353

NEW MEXICO
University of New Mexico School of
  Medicine
Surge Building, Department of
  Pediatrics
2701 Frontier, N.E.
Albuquerque, NM 87131
Marilyn Duncan, M.D.
(505) 272-4461

NEW YORK
Albany Medical Center
Department of Pediatrics
48 New Scotland Avenue
Albany, NY 12208
(518) 445-3125
Andre Lascari, M.D.
(518) 445-5513

Montefiore Hospital and Medical Center
111 East 210th Street
Bronx, NY 10467
Eva Radel, M.D.
(212) 519-3816

Brookdale Hospital Medical Center
Pediatric Hematology
Linden Boulevard at Brookdale Plaza
Brooklyn, NY 11212
Joel A. Wolk, M.D.
(718) 240-5904

Downstate Medical Center
Department of Pediatrics
450 Clarkson Avenue
Brooklyn, NY 11203
(718) 270-1625
Sreedhar P. Rao, M.D.
(718) 245-3131

Roswell Park Memorial Institute
Department of Pediatrics
Elm and Carlton Streets
Buffalo, NY 14263
Martin Brecher, M.D.
(716) 845-2333

North Shore University Hospital
Pediatric Hematology/Oncology
300 Community Drive
Manhasset, NY 11030
Joseph A. Kochen, M.D.
(516) 562-0100

Columbia Presbyterian Medical Center
of Physicians and Surgeons
Babies Hospital, Division of Pediatric
Hematology/Oncology
3959 Broadway, Room 517N
New York, NY 10032
(212) 305-2500
Sergio Piomelli, M.D.
(212) 305-5808

Memorial Sloan-Kettering Cancer Center
Department of Pediatric
Hematology/Oncology
1275 York Avenue
New York, NY 10021
(212) 639-7900
Peter G. Steinherz, M.D.
(212) 639-7978

Mount Sinai School of Medicine
Pediatric Hematology/Oncology
One Gustave L. Levy Place
New York, NY 10029
Jeffrey Lipton, M.D.
(212) 241-6031

New York Hospital, Cornell Medical
Center
Department of Pediatrics N-740
525 East 68th Street
New York, NY 10021
Margaret W. Hilgartner, M.D.
(212) 472-5454

New York University Medical Center
Department of Pediatric
Hematology/Oncology
550 First Avenue
New York, NY 10016
Aaron R. Rausen, M.D.
(212) 263-7144

University of Rochester Medical Center
Pediatric Box 777
601 Elmwood Avenue
Rochester, NY 14642
(716) 275-2222
Harvey Cohen, M.D.
(716) 275-2981

State University of New York
Health Science Center, Syracuse
Pediatric Hematology/Oncology,
Room 5C
750 East Adams Street
Syracuse, NY 13210
Ronald Dubowy, M.D.
(315) 464-5294

New York Medical College
Pediatric Hematology/Oncology
Munger Pavillion, Room 110
Valhalla, NY 10595
(914) 285-7000
Somasundaram Jayabose, M.D.
(914) 285-7997

NORTH CAROLINA
University of North Carolina Memorial
Hospital
Department of Pediatric
Hematology/Oncology
509 Burnett-Womack Building, 229 H
Chapel Hill, NC 27514
(919) 966-4131
Herbert A. Cooper, M.D.
(919) 966-1178

Presbyterian Hospital
200 Hawthorne Lane
Charlotte, NC 28233
(704) 384-4000
Barry Golembe, M.D.
(704) 372-8750

Duke University Medical Center
Duke Hospital North, Room 5413
Box 2916, Erwin Road
Durham, NC 27710
John Falletta, M.D.
(919) 684-3401

East Carolina University School of
Medicine
P.C.M.H., 288W, Pediatric
Hematology/Oncology
200 Stantonsburg Road
Greenville, NC 27858
C. Tate Holbrook, M.D.
(919) 551-4676

Bowman Gray School of Medicine
Department of Pediatrics
Medical Center Boulevard
Winston-Salem, NC 27157-1081
Allen Chauvenet, M.D.
(919) 716-4085

NORTH DAKOTA
Dakota Hospital
720 South University Drive
Fargo, ND 58103
(701) 280-4100
Janet P. Tillisch, M.D.
(701) 280-3429

Fargo Clinic
Roger Maris Cancer Center
820 4th Street North
Fargo, ND 58122
Nathan Kobrinsky, M.D.
(701) 234-7544

St. Luke's Hospital
Children's Hospital Meritcare
5th Street and Mills Avenue
Fargo, ND 58102
(701) 234-6000

OHIO
Children's Hospital Medical Center of
  Akron
Department of Pediatric
  Hematology/Oncology
281 Locust Street
Akron, OH 44308
Carl E. Krill, Jr., M.D.
(216) 379-8730

Children's Hospital Medical Center
Pediatric Hematology/Oncology
Elland Avenue and Bethesda
Cincinnati, OH 45229-2899
(513) 599-4200
Ralph A. Gruppo, M.D.
(513) 559-4266

Cleveland Clinic Foundation
Department of Pediatric
  Hematology/Oncology
9500 Euclid Avenue, Desk S-35
Cleveland, OH 44195
Karen Bringlesen, M.D.
(216) 444-5517

Metro Health Medical Center
Department of Pediatric
  Hematology/Oncology
2500 Metro Health Drive
Cleveland, OH 44109
Elizabeth H. Danish, M.D.
(216) 459-5801

Rainbow Babies' and Children's
  Hospital
Pediatric Hematology/Oncology
2074 Abington Road
Cleveland, OH 44106
Susan B. Shurin, M.D.
(216) 844-3345

Children's Hospital of Columbus
Department of Pediatric
  Hematology/Oncology
700 Children's Drive
Columbus, OH 43205
Frederick B. Ruymann, M.D.
(614) 461-2678

Children's Medical Center Dayton
One Children's Plaza
Dayton, OH 45404
Robert D. Stout, M.D.
(513) 226-8432

Medical College of Ohio
Department of Pediatrics
P.O. Box 10008
Toledo, OH 43699-0008
Emel Bayar, M.D.
(419) 381-4483

Western Reserve Care System
Tod Children's Hospital
500 Gypsy Lane
Youngstown, OH 44501
(216) 740-4948
Mustafa Barudi, M.D.
(216) 740-3955

OKLAHOMA
Oklahoma University Health Sciences
  Center
Children's Hospital of Oklahoma
940 N.E. 13th Street
Oklahoma City, OK 73104
Ruprecht Nitschke, M.D.
(405) 271-5311

OREGON
Oregon Health Sciences University
Doernbecher Children's Hospital
Pediatric Oncology
3181 S.W. Sam Jackson Park Road
Portland, OR 97201
Robert C. Neerhout, M.D.
(503) 494-8194

PENNSYLVANIA
Geisinger Medical Center
Hematology/Oncology
100 North Academy Avenue
Danville, PA 17822
Narayan R. Shah, M.D.
(717) 271-6848

Hershey Medical Center
Department of Pediatric
  Hematology/Oncology
Box 850, University Drive, Room C616A
Hershey, PA 17033
John E. Neely, M.D.
(717) 531-6012

Children's Hospital of Philadelphia
Division of Oncology
34th and Civic Center Boulevard
Philadelphia, PA 19104
(215) 590-1000
Anna T. Meadows, M.D.
(215) 590-2804

St. Christopher's Hospital for Children
Erie Avenue at Front Street
Philadelphia, PA 19134-1095
(215) 427-5336
Edwin C. Douglas, M.D.
(215) 427-5174

Children's Hospital of Pittsburgh
Department of Pediatric
  Hematology/Oncology
3705 Fifth Avenue
Pittsburgh, PA 15213
Joseph Mirro, M.D.
(412) 692-5055

PUERTO RICO
University of Puerto Rico
Medical Sciences Campus, Room B340,
  Third Floor
San Juan, PR 00936
Luis Clavell, M.D.
(809) 754-8783

RHODE ISLAND
Rhode Island Hospital
Pediatric Hematology/Oncology MPS-1
593 Eddy Street
Providence, RI 02903
(401) 277-5435
Edwin Forman, M.D.
(401) 444-5171

SOUTH CAROLINA
Medical University of South Carolina
Children's Hospital
Pediatric Hematology/Oncology,
  Room 514
171 Ashley Avenue
Charleston, SC 29425
(803) 792-2300
Joseph Laver, M.D.
(803) 792-2957

Richland Memorial Hospital
Children's Center for Cancer and Blood
  Disorders
7 Richland Medical Park
Columbia, SC 29203
Robert S. Ettinger, M.D.
(803) 765-6484

Greenville Hospital System
CTC Pediatric Hematology/Oncology
701 Grove Road
Greenville, SC 29605
Cary Stroud, M.D.
(803) 455-8898

SOUTH DAKOTA
Sioux Valley Hospital
1100 South Euclid Avenue
Sioux Falls, SD 57105
(605) 333-1000
Marwan D. Hanna, M.D.
(605) 339-1000

TENNESSEE
East Tennessee Children's Hospital
2018 Clinch Avenue, S.W.
P.O. Box 15010
Knoxville, TN 37901-5010
(615) 541-8000
Ray C. Pals, M.D.
(615) 541-8266

St. Jude Children's Research Hospital
Hematology/Oncology
332 North Lauderdale Street
Memphis, TN 38105
William Crist, M.D.
(901) 522-0335

Vanderbilt University Medical Center
T-3311 Medical Center North
Pediatric Hematology/Oncology
1161 21st Avenue South
Nashville, TN 37232-2588
John N. Lukens, M.D.
(615) 322-7475

TEXAS
Texas Tech University Health Sciences
  Center
1400 Wallace Boulevard
Amarillo, TX 79106
Ihpan Al-Khalil, M.D.
(806) 354-5522

University of Texas Southwestern
  Medical Center
Children's Medical Center
1935 Motor Street
Dallas, TX 75235
George Buchanan, M.D.
(214) 920-2382

William Beaumont Army Medical
  Center
Department of Pediatrics
El Paso, TX 79920
Jerry Swaney, M.D.
(915) 569-2263

Brooke Army Medical Center
Beach Pavilion HSHE-DP
Hematology/Oncology Service
Stanley Road, Building 2376
Fort Sam Houston, TX 78234-6200
Allen Potter, M.D.
(512) 221-0531

Cook–Fort Worth Children's Medical
  Center
Department of Hematology/Oncology
Carter Building
801 Seventh Avenue
Fort Worth, TX 76104-9958
W. Paul Bowman, M.D.
(817) 885-4006

University of Texas Medical Branch at
  Galveston
Pediatric Hematology/Oncology
Market and 9th Streets
Galveston, TX 77555
Blanche P. Alter, M.D.
(409) 772-2341

Baylor College of Medicine
Texas Children's Hospital,
  Hematology/Oncology
6621 Faunin Avenue
Houston, TX 77030
C. Philip Steuber, M.D.
(713) 770-4200

M. D. Anderson Cancer Center
Division of Pediatrics
1515 Holcombe Boulevard, Box 87
Houston, TX 77030
(713) 792-6620
W. Archie Bleyer, M.D.
(713) 792-6604

Wilford Hall USAF Medical Center
Pediatric Oncology
USAF Medical Center
Lackland AFB, TX 78236
Daniel McMahon, M.D.
(512) 670-6642

Southwest Texas Methodist Hospital
Division of Pediatric
  Hematology/Oncology
7700 Floyd Curl Drive
San Antonio, TX 78229
Kenneth H. Lazarus, M.D.
(512) 616-0800

University of Texas Health Sciences
  Center, San Antonio
Pediatric Hematology/Oncology,
  Room 540F
7703 Floyd Curl Drive
San Antonio, TX 78284-7810
(512) 567-7000
Richard Parmley, M.D.
(512) 567-5265

Scott and White Memorial Hospital
2401 South 31st Street
Temple, TX 76508
(817) 774-2006
Lawrence Frankel, M.D.
(817) 774-2111

UTAH
Primary Children's Medical Center
Pediatric Hematology/Oncology
100 North Medical Drive
Salt Lake City, UT 84113
Richard T. O'Brien, M.D.
(801) 588-2680

VERMONT
University of Vermont College of
  Medicine
Given Medical Building, Pediatrics
Colchester Avenue
Burlington, VT 05405
Joseph Dickerman, M.D.
(802) 656-2296

VIRGINIA
University of Virginia Children's
  Medical Center
Department of Pediatrics, Room 3002,
  MR-4 Building
300 Park Place
Charlottesville, VA 22908
Peter E. Waldron, M.D.
(804) 924-5105

Fairfax Hospital
3300 Gallows Road
Falls Church, VA 22046
Jay Greenberg, M.D.
(703) 876-9111

Children's Hospital King's Daughters
601 Children's Lane
Norfolk, VA 23507
Rebecca L. Byrd, M.D.
(804) 628-7242

Virginia Commonwealth University
Pediatric Hematology/Oncology
12th and Marshall Street
Richmond, VA 23298
Harold Mauer, M.D.
(804) 786-9602

WASHINGTON
Children's Hospital and Medical Center
Pediatric Hematology/Oncology, Room
  D600M, MS ZC-10
4800 Sand Point Way, N.E.,
  P.O. Box 5371
Seattle, WA 98105
James Miser, M.D.
(206) 526-2107

Fred Hutchinson Cancer Research
  Center
1124 Columbia Street
Seattle, WA 98104
(206) 467-5000

Group Health Cooperative
Department of Pediatrics
200 15th Avenue East
Seattle, WA 98112
Philip Herzog, M.D.
(206) 326-3163

Deaconess Medical Center
Pediatric Oncology Office 5C
West 800 Fifth Avenue
Spokane, WA 99210-0248
Frank A. Reynolds, M.D.
(509) 458-7230

Madigan Army Medical Center
Department of Pediatrics
Fort Lewis
Tacoma, WA 98431
Bruce Cook, M.D.
(206) 967-6946

Mary Bridge Hospital
311 South L Street
Tacoma, WA 98405
(206) 594-1415
Daniel Niebrugge, M.D.
(206) 383-5777

WEST VIRGINIA
Charleston Area Medical Center
Pediatric Hematology/Oncology
3200 MacCorkle Avenue, S.E.
Charleston, WV 25304
Kenneth A. Starling, M.D.
(304) 347-1341

West Virginia University Health
  Sciences Center
Health Sciences North Pediatrics
Morgantown, WV 26506
A. Kim Ritchey, M.D.
(304) 293-4451

WISCONSIN
Webster Clinic
900 South Webster Avenue
Green Bay, WI 54301
Dorothy Ganick, M.D.
(414) 437-0431

Gundersen Clinic
Department of Pediatrics
1836 South Avenue
La Crosse, WI 54601
L. Gilbert Thatcher, M.D.
(608) 782-7300

University of Wisconsin Medical Center
Department of Pediatric
Hematology/Oncology
600 Highland Avenue
Madison, WI 53792
Paul S. Gaynon, M.D.
(608) 263-8554

Marshfield Clinic
Department of Pediatric
Hematology/Oncology
1000 North Oak
Marshfield, WI 54449
H. James Nickerson, M.D.
(715) 387-5018

Children's Hospital of Wisconsin
9000 West Wisconsin Avenue
P.O. Box 1997
Milwaukee, WI 53201
(414) 266-2000
Bruce Camitta, M.D.
(414) 266-4170

COMMUNITY RESOURCES AND SUPPORT GROUPS

Community Resources—General

AMC Cancer Research Center
Cancer Information and Counseling
Line
Cancer Intervention Division
1600 Pierce Street
Denver, CO 80214
(800) 525-3777
In CO (303) 233-6501

American Association of Blood Banks
8101 Glenbrook Road
Bethesda, MD 20814
(301) 907-6977

American Association of Cancer
Education
Educational Research and Development
University of Alabama–Birmingham
401 CHSD University Street
Birmingham, AL 35294
A multidisciplinary organization that
provides education and training for pro-
fessionals involved in cancer care.

American Cancer Society
1599 Clifton Road, NE
Atlanta, GA 30329
(800) ACS-2345
In GA (404) 320-3333
National office, state divisions, and
local units. Provides funds for research,
professional education and training, and
conferences. Produces and distributes
publications and audiovisuals. Service
and Rehabilitation Divisions provide ed-

ucation, information, in-hospital information centers, direct family aid such as
home-care item loans, transportation services, housing near treatment centers, vis-
itor programs, and support and self-help
groups.

American Red Cross
18th and D Street, N.W.
Washington, DC 20006
(202) 737-8300
Provides community services, blood
bank, and bone marrow donor programs.
Publications. Local chapters.

American Self-Help Clearinghouse
St. Clare's–Riverside Medical Center
25 Pocono Road
Denville, NJ 07834
(800) 367-6274
In NJ (201) 625-7101
Provides referrals to regional clearing-
houses and support groups. Publishes
The Self-Help Sourcebook and a news-
letter.

Association for the Care of Children's
Health
7910 Woodmont Avenue, Suite 300
Bethesda, MD 20814
(301) 654-6549
Fax (301) 986-4553
A multidisciplinary organization of
health care professionals and parents promoting the psychosocial health and well-

being of children and their families in health care settings. Sponsors conferences. Publishes *Children's Health Care, ACCH News,* and *ACCH Network* newsletters and booklets. Local affiliates.

Association of Community Cancer
  Centers
11600 Nebel Street, Suite 201
Rockville, MD 20852
(301) 984-9496
  Provides a mechanism for the exchange of information among health care professionals to help make high-quality cancer care available in the community. Publishes *Community Cancer Programs in the United States* and newsletter *Oncology Issues.*

Cancer Federation
21250 Box Springs Road, Suite 209
Morena Valley, CA 92387
(714) 682-7989
Fax (714) 682-0169
  Provides funds for research, hospice program, scholarships for professionals in oncology, and some financial aid to cancer patients. Referrals. Newsletter *The Challenger.*

Cancer Fund of America
2901 Breezewood Lane
Knoxville, TN 37921
(615) 938-5281
  Provides financial assistance to cancer patients and grants for hospice programs. Nationwide.

Candlelighters Childhood Cancer
  Foundation
7910 Woodmont Avenue, Suite 460
Bethesda, MD 20814
(800) 266-2223
(301) 657-8401
Fax (301) 657-8319
  Clearinghouse, advocacy, and educational arm of international network of over 400 self-help groups of parents of children with cancer and health care professionals. Promotes development of educational materials, conducts surveys, and seeks solutions to problems and needs of patients and families. Publishes *CCCF Quarterly Newsletter* and *CCCF Youth*

Newsletter. Provides guidelines to help form new groups. Foundation office and local groups provide peer-support, practical assistance, and information.

Center for Attitudinal Healing
19 Main Street
Tiburon, CA 94920
(415) 435-5022
  A national organization for children or adults facing a catastrophic illness. Publications.

Center for Medical Consumers
237 Thompson Street
New York, NY 10012
(212) 674-7105
  Provides referrals to health organizations. Newsletter *Health Facts.*

Centers for Disease Control
1600 Clifton Road, N.E.
Atlanta, GA 30329
(404) 639-3311

Chemotherapy Foundation
183 Madison Avenue, Room 403
New York, NY 10016
(212) 213-9292
  Supports research and develops educational materials for professionals and general public. Conferences.

Children in Hospitals
31 Wilshire Park
Needham, MA 02192
(617) 482-2915
  Promotes hospital policies that are sensitive to the needs of all family members. Educates consumers about ways to prepare for and cope with hospitalization and other medical situations.

Community Health Accreditation
  Program
350 Hudson Street
New York, NY 10014
(800) 669-1656
  Listing of home care agencies that are accredited or nonaccredited.

Consumer Health Information Research
  Institute
3521 Broadway
Kansas City, MO 64111-2501
(800) 821-6671

Provides information about question-able medical practices, including unorthodox cancer treatment.

Healing the Children
North 1603 Belt
Spokane, WA 99205
(509) 327-4281

Helps underprivileged children around the world gain access to medical treatment in the United States.

Innercare
100 West Franklin Avenue, Suite 200
Minneapolis, MN 55404
(612) 872-6622
(800) 257-7914

Developed "Imagine Me" program for children with chronic illnesses to help them manage stressful situations.

Joint Commission on Accreditation of
  Healthcare Organizations
Public Information Coordinator
Department of Corporate Relations
One Renaissance Boulevard
Oakbrook Terrace, IL 60181
(708) 916-5632

The commission accredits hospitals that meet its standards. Listing available.

The Kids on the Block
9385-C Gerwig Lane
Columbia, MD 21046
(800) 368-5437
In MD (410) 290-9095

Creates and provides specially designed educational puppet programs to teach children and adults how to deal with specific illnesses or handicapping conditions.

Laughter Therapy
P.O. Box 827
Monterey, CA 93940
(408) 625-3788

Provides old *Candid Camera* video-tapes to patients.

Leukemia Society of America
600 Third Avenue
New York, NY 10017
(212) 573-8484

Provides funding for research in leuke-mia, lymphomas, and Hodgkin's disease, and sponsors symposia and conferences. Produces and distributes publications. Local chapters provide free use of audio-visuals and publications and some financial assistance for drugs, laboratory costs associated with blood transfusions, radiation therapy, and transportation.

Leukemia Research Foundation
899 Skokie Boulevard, Suite LL14
Northbrook, IL 60062
(708) 480-1177

Provides funds for leukemia research.

Love Letters
P.O. Box 416875
Chicago, IL 60641
(708) 515-9501

Mails free newsletters with jokes and puzzles to chronically ill children.

National Association of Hospital
  Hospitality Houses
P.O. Box 8022
Muncie, IN 47304
(800) 542-9730
In IN (317) 288-3226

Provides housing and support services for families from out of town while patient receives medical treatment. National directory for referrals.

National Cancer Care Foundation and
  Cancer Care
1180 Avenue of the Americas,
  2d Floor
New York, NY 10036
(212) 221-3300

Provides referrals to nonmedical resources. Provides financial assistance and support groups primarily in Connecticut, New Jersey, and New York.

National Coalition for Cancer
  Survivorship
1010 Wayne Avenue
Silver Spring, MD 20910
(301) 585-2616

Coalition of independent groups, referrals, information and resources, advocacy, and speakers' bureau. Publishes *NCCS Network*.

National Council Against Health Fraud
  Resource Center
3521 Broadway
Kansas City, MO 64111
(800) 821-6671

Collects and disseminates publications on questionable health practices and organizations.

National Health Information Center
P.O. Box 1133
Washington, DC 20013-1133
(800) 336-4797
In MD (301) 565-4167

Provides referrals to organizations dealing with various health issues. Publications.

National Organization for Rare
  Disorders
P.O. Box 8923
New Fairfield, CT 06812-1783
(800) 999-6673

Pediatric Projects
P.O. Box 571555
Tarzana, CA 91357
(800) 947-0947
(818) 705-3660

Distributes mental health publications and medically oriented toys to help families cope with health care. Newsletter *Pediatric Mental Health.*

Research America
99 Canal Center Plaza, Suite 250
Alexandria, VA 22314
(703) 739-2577

Advocacy organization for medical research.

Ronald McDonald Children's Charities
One McDonald's Plaza
Oak Brook, IL 60521
(708) 575-7048

Provides grants for development and support programs in health care, research and educational projects and start-up funds for Ronald McDonald Houses and rehabilitation centers.

Ronald McDonald Houses
Henry N. W. Lienau, Coordinator
c/o Golin Harris Communications
500 North Michigan Avenue
Chicago, IL 60611
(312) 836-7104

"Homes away from home" for families of pediatric patients from out of town while child receives medical treatment. Moderate cost.

Sick Kids Need Involved People
990 Second Avenue, 2d Floor
New York, NY 10022
(212) 421-9160

A national organization of parents and professionals that provides education, referrals to resources, and advocacy to families dealing with complex and specialized issues of pediatric home health care for technology-dependent children. Local chapters.

United Way of America
701 North Fairfax Street
Alexandria, VA 22314-2045
(703) 836-7100

NOTES

[1]Stehlin, J., "A Cancer Surgeon Talks with Patients and Families," Stehlin Foundation for Cancer Research, Houston, 1976.

[2]American Cancer Society, "Cancer Facts and Figures," 1992.

[3]Joranson, D., Cleeland, C., Weissman, A., Gilson, A., "Opioids for Chronic Cancer and Non-cancer Pain: A Survey of State Medical Board Members," *Federation Bulletin: The Journal of Medical Licensure and Discipline,* vol. 79, no. 4 (June 1992), 15–45.

Twycross, R., Ventafridda, V., *The Continuing Care of the Terminal Cancer Patient* (New York: Oxford Pergamon Press, 1980), 15–45.

[4]Ventafridda, V., Tamborini, A., Caraceni, F., et al., "A Validation Study of the WHO Method for Cancer Pain Relief," *Cancer,* vol. 59, no. 4 (1987), 850–56.

[5]Foley, K. M., "The Treatment of Cancer Pain," *New England Journal of Medicine,* 1985, 11: 313(2):84–95.

[6]Moinpour, C. M., Chapman, C. R., *Pain Management and Quality of Life in Cancer Patients* (Berlin: Springer-Verlag), Transdermal Fentanyl, September 27–28, 1991, 45.

[7]Bonica, J., *The Management of Pain*, second edition (Philadelphia: Lea & Febiger, 1990), vol. 1, 410.

[8]Public Health Service, Agency for Health Care Policy and Research, "Cancer Pain Guidelines." In press.

[9]Bonica, J., "Effective Pain Management for Cancer Patients," monograph for Pharmacia Deltec, March 1992.

[10]McCaffery, M., Ferrell, B., "Opioid Analgesics: Nurses' Knowledge of Doses and Psychological Dependence," *Journal of Nursing Staff Development*, March–April 1992, 7783.

Ferrell, B., McCaffery, M., "Pain and Addiction: An Urgent Need for Change in Nursing Education," *Journal of Pain and Symptom Management*, vol. 7, no. 2 (February 1992), 117–24.

[11]Weissman, D., Dahl, J., "Attitudes About Cancer Pain: A Survey of Wisconsin's First-Year Medical Students," *Journal of Pain and Symptom Management*, vol. 5, no. 6 (December 1990), 345.

[12]Donovan, M., Dillon, P., "Incidence and Characteristics of Pain in a Sample of Hospitalized Cancer Patients," *Cancer Nursing*, vol. 10, no. 2 (1987), 85–92.

[13]Dahl, J., Joranson, D. E., Engber, D., Dosch, J., "The Cancer Pain Problem: Wisconsin's Response. A Report on the Wisconsin Cancer Pain Initiative," *Journal of Pain and Symptom Management*, 3 (1988), S1–5.

[14]Von Roen, J., personal communication, 1992.

[15]Price, D., Harkins, S., "The Affective-Motivational Dimension of Pain," *Journal of the American Pain Society*, vol. 1, no. 4 (Winter 1992) 231.

[16]Ferrell, B., Wisdom, C., Wenzl, C., "Quality of Life as an Outcome Variable in the Management of Cancer Pain," *Cancer*, 63 (1989), 2327.

[17]Grossman, S. A., personal communication, 1992.

[18]Grossman, S. A., "When Pain Strikes," *20/20* interview, ABC News, August 18, 1989.

[19]Max, M., "Improving Outcomes of Analgesic Treatment: Is Education Enough?" *Perspective, Annals of Internal Medicine*, 113 (1990), 885–89.

[20]Portenoy, R., personal communication, 1989.

[21]Foley, K., "Medical Progress: The Treatment of Cancer Pain," *New England Journal of Medicine*, vol. 313, no. 2 (July 1985), 84–93.

[22]Daut, R., Cleeland, C., "The Prevalence and Severity of Pain in Cancer," *Cancer*, 50 (1982), 1913–18.

[23]Foley, K., "Medical Progress: The Treatment of Cancer Pain," *New England Journal of Medicine*, vol. 313, no. 2 (July 1985), 84–93.

[24]Bonica, J., *The Management of Pain*, second edition (Philadelphia: Lea & Febiger, 1990), vol. 1, 410.

[25]Bonica, J., *The Management of Pain*, second edition (Philadelphia: Lea & Febiger, 1990).

[26]Foley, K., "Medical Progress: The Treatment of Cancer Pain," *New England Journal of Medicine*, vol. 313, no. 2 (July 1985), 84–93.

[27]Foley, K., Sundaresan, N., "Supportive Care of the Cancer Patient," *The Management of Cancer Pain*, second edition, ed. Bonica, J. (Philadelphia: Lea & Febiger, 1990), section 3, 1940–61.

28Foley, K., Sundaresan, N., "Supportive Care of the Cancer Patient," *The Management of Cancer Pain,* second edition, ed. Bonica, J. (Philadelphia: Lea & Febiger, 1990), section 3, 1940–61.

29Donaldson, G., "Issues in Quantifying and Analyzing Individual Differences," 3rd Annual Bristol-Myers Squibb Symposium on Pain Research, Seattle, Washington, July 23–26, 1992.

30Mehta, M., *Intractable Pain* (London: W. B. Saunders, 1973), 152.

31Liebeskind, J., "Studies of Pain, Stress and Immunity," 3rd Annual Bristol Myers–Squibb Symposium on Pain Research, Seattle, Washington, July 1992.

32McCaffery, M., Beebe, R. N., *Pain: Clinical Manual for Nursing Practice* (St. Louis: C. V. Mosby Co., 1989), 235.

33Smith, R., personal communication, 1992.

34Smith, R., "Ethical Issues Surrounding Cancer Pain," in "Current and Emerging Issues in Cancer Pain." In press.

35Bonica, J., *The Management of Pain,* second edition (Philadelphia: Lea & Febiger, 1990), vol. 1, 410.

36Bonica, J., *The Management of Pain,* second edition (Philadelphia: Lea & Febiger, 1990), vol. 1, 416.

37Gonzales, G., Elliott, K., Portenoy, R., Foley, K., "The Impact of a Comprehensive Evaluation in the Management of Cancer Pain," *Pain,* 47 (1991), 141–44.

38Chapman, R., "The Emotional Aspect of Pain," in "Current and Emerging Issues in Cancer Pain." In press.

39Chapman, R., "The Emotional Aspect of Pain," in "Current and Emerging Issues in Cancer Pain." In press.

40Beck, S., "Innovation in Cancer Pain: Assessment and Treatment," Nursing's Contribution to Cancer Pain Management, University of Washington, July 22, 1992.

41Jensen, M., "Current and Emerging Issues in Cancer Pain: Research and Practice," 3rd Annual Bristol-Myers Squibb Symposium on Pain Research, Seattle, Washington, July 23–26, 1992.

42McGuire, D., "Innovation in Cancer Pain: Assessment and Treatment," Psychosocial Components of Cancer Pain, University of Washington, Seattle, July 22, 1992.

43Dalton, J., "Biobehavioral Pain Profile: Development and Psychometric Properties." In press.
  Dalton, J., personal communication, 1992.

44Grossman, S. A., Scheidler, V. R., Swedeen, K., Mucenski, J., Piantadosi, S., "The Correlation of Patient and Caregiver Ratings of Cancer Pain," *Journal of Pain and Symptom Management,* vol. 6 (February 1992), 53.

45Memorial Pain Assessment Card, Memorial Sloan-Kettering Cancer Center, New York, New York.

46Moinpour, C. M., Chapman, C. R., *Pain Management and Quality of Life in Cancer Patients* (Berlin: Springer-Verlag), Transdermal Fentanyl, September 27–28, 1991, 46.

47Bruera, E., American Pain Society, 11th annual scientific meeting, San Diego, California, October 22–25, 1992.

48Morris, J., Suissa, S., Sherwood, S., et al., "Last Days: A Study of the Quality of Life of Terminally Ill Cancer Patients," *Journal of Chronic Disease,* vol. 34, no. 1 (1986), 47–62.

[49]Ferrell, B., "Pain and the Quality of Life: Nursing Implications," Innovations in Cancer Pain: Assessment and Treatment, University of Washington, July 22, 1992.

[50]Ferrell, B., personal communication, 1993.

[51]Portenoy, R., "Prevalence and Characteristics of Symptoms Determined by the Memorial Symptom Assessment Scale in 218 Cancer Patients." In press.

[52]Ferrell, B., "Pain and the Quality of Life: Nursing Implications," Innovations in Cancer Pain: Assessment and Treatment, University of Washington, July 22, 1992.

[53]Grossman, S. A., personal communication, 1992.

[54]Cleeland, C., "Documenting Barriers to Cancer Pain Management," 3rd Annual Bristol–Myers Squibb Symposium on Pain Research, Seattle, Washington, July 23–26, 1992.

[55]Portenoy, R., personal communication, 1989, 1992.

[56]Koo, P., "Management of Cancer Pain," *Highlights on Antineoplastic Drugs,* vol. 6, no. 2 (May–June 1988), Adria Laboratories.

[57]Vettafridda, V., Tamburini, M., Caraceni, A., et al., "A Validation Study of the WHO Method for Cancer Pain Relief," *Cancer,* 59 (1987), 850–56.

[58]Foley, K., "When Pain Strikes," *20/20* interview, ABC News, August 18, 1989.

[59]*Harvard Medical School Letter,* vol. 14, no. 8 (June 1989).

[60]Houde, R., Kosterlitz, H. W., Terenius, C. Y., *Advances in Pain Research and Therapy.* Dahlem Konferenzen (Weinheim: Verlag Chemie, 1980), 396.

[61]Foley, K., "The Treatment of Pain in the Patient with Cancer," *CA—A Cancer Journal for Clinicians,* vol. 36, no. 4 (July–August 1986), 194–215.

[62]Adapted from Bonica, J., *The Management of Pain,* second edition (Philadelphia: Lea & Febiger, 1990), vol. 1.

[63]Foley, K., Inturrisi, C., "Analgesic Drug Therapy in Cancer Pain: Principles and Practice," *Medical Clinics of North America,* vol. 71, no. 2 (March 1987), 208.

[64]Paice, J., "The Phenomenon of Analgesic Tolerance in Cancer Pain Management," *Oncology Nursing Forum,* vol. 15, no. 4 (1988), 455–60.

[65]Massie, M. J., Holland, J., "The Cancer Patient with Pain: Psychiatric Complications and Their Management," *Medical Clinics of North America,* vol. 71, no. 2 (March 1987), 243.

[66]Mount, B., "Psychological and Social Aspects of Cancer Pain," *The Textbook of Pain,* ed. P. Wall and R. Melzack (London: Churchill Livingstone, 1984), 460.

[67]Adapted from Jacox, A., *Pain: A Source Book for Nurses and Other Health Professionals* (Boston: Little, Brown and Co., 1977), 378–79.

[68]Chapman, R., in Bonica, J., Ventafridda, V., *International Symposium on Pain of Advanced Cancer* (New York: Raven Press, 1979), vol. 2, 45–58.

[69]Chapman, R., in Bonica, J., Ventafridda, V., *International Symposium on Pain of Advanced Cancer* (New York: Raven Press, 1979), vol. 2, 45–58.

[70]Mount, B., "Psychological and Social Aspects of Cancer Pain," *The Textbook of Pain,* ed. Wall, P., Melzack, R. (London: Churchill Livingstone, 1984), 460.

[71]Simonton, S., *Getting Well Again* (New York: Bantam Books, 1992), 139.

[72]Fishman, B., Loscalzo, M., "Cognitive-Behavioral Interventions in Management of Cancer Pain: Principle and Applications," *Medical Clinics of North America,* vol. 71, no. 2 (March 1987).

[73]Ferrell, B., Rhiner, M., Zichi Cohen, M., Grant, M., "Pain as a Metaphor for Illness. Part I: Impact of Cancer Pain on Family Caregivers," *Oncology Nursing Forum,* vol. 18, no. 8 (1991), 1303–1309.

Ferrell, B., personal communication, 1992.

[74]Ferrell, B., Rhiner, M., Zichi Cohen, M., Grant, M., "Pain as a Metaphor for Illness. Part I: Impact of Cancer Pain on Family Caregivers," *Oncology Nursing Forum,* vol. 18, no. 8 (1991), 1303–1309.

6

HIV AND AIDS-RELATED PAIN

The diagnosis of HIV infection and AIDS carries with it the overwhelming fears of a life compromised by unrelenting medical and psychological challenges, dependency, loss, potential pain, and the possibility of an untimely death. Unrelieved pain can cause further anxiety, anger, depression, and feelings of helplessness and hopelessness.

William S. Breitbart, M.D., of the Psychiatry Service, Neurology Department at Memorial Sloan-Kettering Cancer Center, says, "Clinicians have neglected pain management in HIV-infected/AIDS patients, focusing instead on treating life-threatening opportunistic infection, cancer and neuropsychiatric syndromes such as AIDS dementia complex. There are few systematic studies that examine the prevalence of pain, describe specific pain syndromes or examine the relationship of the pain experience and psychological factors in the AIDS population."[1]

Christine Miaskowski, R.N., Ph.D., F.A.A.N., of the University of California School of Nursing, San Francisco, writes, "Persons with cancer and HIV-related pain pose numerous challenges for health care personnel."[2]

Richard Payne, M.D., Chief of the Pain and Symptom Management Service at M. D. Anderson Cancer Center in Houston, notes, "Estimates of the prevalence of pain in patients with HIV infection and AIDS range from 15% to 50% in the hospitalized, ambulatory or terminally ill patient. Like the patient with cancer, pain syndromes in the HIV-infected individual can be classified as those which are directly related to the disease; directly related to therapy; and those unrelated to disease or therapy. A major clinical issue which arises in the patient with AIDS associated with intravenous drug abuse is the responsible and humane treatment of pain with opioids [morphine-like drugs] in such individuals."[3]

In the preceding chapter, cancer pain syndromes were explained in detail. In addition, HIV and AIDS patients may have pain specifically related to their diagnosis. Drs. Payne and Breitbart note the following AIDS-associated pain syndromes:

A. Pain related to AIDS
   HIV neuropathy
   HIV myelopathy
   Kaposi's sarcoma
   Secondary infection
   Organomegaly
   Myositis
B. Pain related to AIDS therapy
   Antivirals (AZT, DDi, DDC)
   Biological modifiers (GM-CSF)
   Chemotherapy (Vincristine)
   Radiation
   Surgery
   Procedures (e.g., bronchoscopy)
C. Pain unrelated to AIDS or therapy
   Disk disease
   Diabetic neuropathy
   Others[4]

PREVALENCE OF PAIN

Researchers at Memorial Sloan-Kettering examined the prevalence and characteristics of pain in a population of HIV-infected persons receiving medical care in an *ambulatory* setting.

Pain in HIV-Infected Patients in an Ambulatory Setting:
- 38% reported significant pain. Patients had an average of two or more pains at any given time.
- 50% comprised painful sensory neuropathy.
- 45% of those with Kaposi's sarcoma had lower extremity pain.

Pain in AIDS Patients in a Hospital:
- 50% of hospitalized AIDS patients required treatment for pain.
- 22% had chest pain (pneumocystis carinii pneumonia, procedures, tumor, etc.).

- 13% had headache pain (herpes, fever, meningitis, tension, infection, radiation, etc.).
- 11% had oral cavity pain (thrush, herpes simplex and zoster, ulcers, Kaposi's sarcoma, chemotherapy, etc.).
- 9% had abdominal pain (tumor involvement, bowel obstruction, ulcer, infections, diarrhea, chemotherapy, Kaposi's sarcoma, etc.).
- 6% had peripheral neuropathy (nervous system disease or abnormality: chronic inflammation, herpes zoster, toxic, or metabolic abnormalities, surgery, etc.) [5, 6, 7]

ASSESSMENT

As discussed throughout the book, *assessment of pain is paramount to relieving pain.* Inadequate pain management is often due to such factors as health professionals not believing the patient; a focus on treating the disease only; lack of knowledge of pain syndromes; lack of knowledge of state-of-the-art pain-relieving techniques; poor understanding of the pharmacology of drugs; fears of respiratory depression and patient addiction.

Peter Koo, Pharm.D., notes that "Most M.D.s are trained to be captain of the ship when it comes to pain management and often underutilize the skills of other health care professionals. M.D.s need to learn how to access pharmacists, physical therapists, psychologists, occupational therapists, and nurses when it comes to pain."[8]

The methods of assessment are the same for HIV-infected and AIDS patients as they are for cancer patients or patients suffering acute pain. However, HIV and AIDS patients may encounter more severe emotional distress at diagnosis because of their fear of a potentially rapid physical decline, disability, lack of support, financial burdens, the impact of treatments, fears of abandonment, and the possibility of an early death.

In the Memorial Sloan-Kettering study of ambulatory patients, depression was "significantly correlated with the presence of pain. In addition to being significantly more distressed and depressed, those with pain were twice as likely to have suicidal ideation (40%) as those without pain (20%). HIV-infected patients with pain were more functionally impaired, and this was highly correlated to levels of pain intensity and depression. Those who felt that pain represented a threat to their health reported more intense pain than those who did not see pain as a threat. Patients with pain were more likely to be unemployed or disabled, and reported less social support."[9]

Health care professionals and loved ones should be aware of the possible early onset of psychological distress, and encourage psychiatric intervention and possibly psychopharmacologic therapies. As discussed earlier, tricyclic antidepressants have pain-relieving properties, enhance the analgesic effect of morphine-like drugs, and decrease depression. Other drugs can enhance analgesia and reduce side effects and sedation. Psychological support can be helpful in time of crisis, ongoing illness, and loss, and can assist patients in seeking substance abuse programs.

Reducing depression, anxiety, anger, helplessness, and hopelessness can lower the perception of pain. As with other patients experiencing chronic pain and/or pain as a result of progressive disease, health care professionals should encourage *active coping styles,* using the tools of relaxation techniques, hypnosis, biofeedback, and imagery for the patient with mild to moderate pain.

Some patients may not be able to take advantage of these methods because of psychiatric disorders. These patients require exceptional diligence and constant assessment to ensure that they are not in pain. They suffer from poor pain management, just like any patient who cannot act for himself or herself, such as infants, children, the elderly, and those who cannot speak English. *If a patient cannot respond due to diminished capacity to communicate, health care professionals are not absolved of their responsibility for relieving pain.*

HIV AND AIDS PATIENTS SHOULD BE TREATED FOR PAIN

HIV-infected and AIDS patients who experience severe pain should be treated with opioids in the same manner in which acute or cancer patients should be treated. For the *majority* of these patients, fears of addiction are unfounded.

In addition, patients should have the advantage of the same dosing and drug delivery systems available to other patients, including round-the-clock dosing if pain is moderate to severe. Intravenous, subcutaneous, epidural, and spinal continuous infusion methods can be used. PCA (patient-controlled analgesia) allows the patient control and unburdens the nursing or at-home caregivers.

Dr. Peter Koo notes that "the dose must be guided by the patient's clinical response. The dose that works is the dose that works."[10]

HIV-infected and AIDS patients often are plagued with opportunistic infections. Dr. Ronnie Hurtz, Director of Pain Management at St. Luke's/Roosevelt Hospital in New York, urges *"caution* in using continuous infusions with patients not near the end of life because of the potential for infection at the site."[11] For patients who are at risk for infection and/or cannot take oral opioids, Dr. Hurtz often makes use of the fentanyl transdermal patch called Duragesic. The patch provides forty-eight to seventy-two hours of pain control.

ACTIVE DRUG ABUSERS OR THOSE WITH A HISTORY OF DRUG ABUSE

Some patients are active drug abusers and/or have had a history of drug abuse. Dr. Breitbart writes:

> More problematic, however, is managing pain in the growing segment of HIV-infected people who are actively using intravenous drugs. Such use, specifically of intravenous narcotics, raises several pain treatment questions, including how to treat pain in people who have a high tolerance to narcotic analgesics; how to mitigate this population's drug-seeking and potentially manipulative behavior; how to deal with patients who may offer unreliable medical histories or who may not comply with treatment recommendations; and how to counter the risk of patients spreading HIV while high and disinhibited.
>
> In addition, clinicians must rely on a patient's subjective report, which is often the best or only indication of the presence and intensity of pain, as well as the degree of pain relief achieved by an intervention. Physicians who believe they are being manipulated by drug-seeking patients often hesitate to use appropriately high doses of opioid analgesics to control pain.
>
> Most clinicians experienced in working with these patients recommended that practitioners set clear and direct limits. While this is an important aspect of the care of intravenous drug-using people with HIV disease, it is by no means the whole answer. As much as possible, clinicians should attempt to eliminate the issue of drug abuse as an obstacle to pain management by dealing directly with the problems of narcotic withdrawal and drug treatment.
>
> Clinicians should err on the side of believing patients when they

complain of pain, and should utilize knowledge of specific HIV-related pain syndromes to corroborate the report of a patient perceived as being unreliable.

Psychiatrists may be the physicians who have the final opportunity to advocate for adequate pain control on the patient's behalf. The more we know about pain in AIDS, the better we can fulfill such a role.[12]

Dr. Hurtz states, *"No AIDS patient in pain should be denied adequate pain management because of drug abuse, and if the patient is near the end of life, everything possible should be done to help control his or her pain."*[13] Dr. Hurtz comments that AIDS patients are living longer and presenting with extremely complicated pain management issues.

NONDRUG PAIN MANAGEMENT

Nondrug techniques include physical therapy, occupational therapy, nutritional counseling, heat, cold, TENS, and other methods that should be considered for pain relief if the patient can benefit from them (see Chapter 1).

Therapeutic Touch

Gayle Newshan, M.A., the former Clinical Administrator of Pain Management at St. Luke's/Roosevelt Hospital Center in New York, notes that the use of therapeutic touch to manage physical symptoms in persons with AIDS may be helpful:

> Therapeutic Touch is derived from the ancient art of the laying on of hands. It is the intentional transfer of energy through the nurse to the client. The nurse acts as an instrument to mentally and physically focus and direct energy from the environment to the client. This is done in such a way as to positively influence change —in this case, to alleviate physical symptoms. Through Therapeutic Touch, energy is directed with an intent to help the ill person. The energy follows the intent.
>
> The steps of the Therapeutic Touch include: assessment, clearing or unruffling, treatment of balancing, and finishing.[14]

The technique has been used for respiratory gastrointestinal ailments, hiccups, fever, anxiety, and pain.

SUMMARY

HIV-related and AIDS-related pain should be managed within the same guidelines followed for other acute and cancer pain management. There are many special medical problems that cause pain for these patients and require diligent assessment and compassionate care. Many of these patients have an overlay of anxiety, depression, or hopelessness grounded in their fears of impaired life and the possibility of an untimely death. Psychological symptoms need to be treated aggressively.

The patient who has no history of drug use should have no fears of addiction when opioids are prescribed. The patient who has a history of past or active drug abuse should not be denied pain-relieving drugs, but must be treated for substance abuse, assessed within the framework of his or her disease and followed by one doctor to ensure adequate pain management.

The following are resources for HIV and AIDS patients. It is recommended that the resources located at the end of Chapter 5 be used also.

HIV/AIDS RESOURCES

CDC National AIDS Hotline
(800) 342-2437 (7 days, 24 hours)
Spanish (800) 344-7432 (7 days, 8
A.M.–2 P.M.)
TDD (800) 243-7889 (Mon.–Fri., 10
A.M.–10 P.M.)
  Offers general information about HIV/AIDS and gives national referrals for support in your area.

CDC National AIDS Clearinghouse
(800) 458-5231 (Mon.–Fri., 9 A.M.–
7 P.M.)
  Provides information on literature about HIV/AIDS.

Gay Men's Health Crisis
New York
(212) 807-6655
  Offers grief and healing workshops and bereavement support for people with AIDS and their families, friends, and caregivers.

National Association of People with AIDS
(800) 898-0414
  Support and referral service.

Project Inform
(800) 822-7422
In San Francisco (415) 558-9051

NOTES

[1]Breitbart, W. S., "Pain in AIDS Multidisciplinary Issue, Why Do We Care?, Pain and Symptom Control, Psychiatric Issues and Ethical Dilemmas in the Care of Patients with Cancer," postgraduate course, Memorial Sloan-Kettering Cancer Center, April 2–4, 1992.

[2]Miaskowski, C., "Managing Cancer and HIV-Related Pain: Current Concepts and Future Directions," University of California at San Francisco School of Medicine and Nursing, December 3, 1992.

[3]Payne, R., "Differential Diagnosis of Cancer and HIV-Related Pain Syndromes," 1992, lecture notes.

Payne, R., personal communication, 1993.

[4]Breitbart, W. S., "Pain in AIDS Multidisciplinary Issue, Why Do We Care?, Pain and Symptom Control, Psychiatric Issues and Ethical Dilemmas in the Care of Patients with Cancer," postgraduate course, Memorial Sloan-Kettering Cancer Center, April 2–4, 1992.

Payne, R., "Differential Diagnosis of Cancer and HIV-Related Pain Syndromes," 1992, lecture notes.

Payne, R., personal communication, 1993.

[5]Breitbart, W. S., "Pain in AIDS Multidisciplinary Issue, Why Do We Care?, Pain and Symptom Control, Psychiatric Issues and Ethical Dilemmas in the Care of Patients with Cancer," postgraduate course, Memorial Sloan-Kettering Cancer Center, April 2–4, 1992.

[6]Lewis, M., Warfield, C., "Management of AIDS," *Hospital Practice*, October 30, 1990, 51–54.

[7]Lebovits, A., Lefkowitz, M., McCarthy, D., et al., "The Prevalence and Management of Pain in Patients with AIDS: A Review of 134 Cases," *Clinical Journal of Pain*, vol. 5, no. 3, 245–48, 1098.

Kelly, J. B., Payne, R., "Pain Syndromes in the Cancer Patient," *Neurologic Clinics*, September, 1991, 937–53.

Barone, J., Gingold, B., Arvanitis, M., Nealon, T., "Abdominal Pain in Patients with Acquired Immune Deficiency Syndrome," *Annals of Surgery*, vol. 204, no. 6 (December 1986), 619–23.

[8]Koo, P., personal communication, 1993.

[9]Breitbart, W. S., "Pain in AIDS Multidisciplinary Issue, Why Do We Care?, Pain and Symptom Control, Psychiatric Issues and Ethical Dilemmas in the Care of Patients with Cancer," postgraduate course, Memorial Sloan-Kettering Cancer Center, April 2–4, 1992.

[10]Koo, P., Managing Cancer and HIV-Related Pain: Current Concepts and Future Directions, 1993.

[11]Hurtz, R., personal communication, 1993.

[12]Breitbart, W. S., "Pain in AIDS Multidisciplinary Issue, Why Do We Care?, Pain and Symptom Control, Psychiatric Issues and Ethical Dilemmas in the Care of Patients with Cancer," postgraduate course, Memorial Sloan-Kettering Cancer Center, April 2–4, 1992.

[13]Hurtz, R., personal communication, 1993.

[14]Newshan, G., "Therapeutic Touch for Symptom Control in Persons with AIDS," *Holistic Nurs. Pract.*, vol. 3, no. 4 (1989), 45–51.

HOME CARE

Up to six million Americans received home care in 1987, from a variety of providers. The Agency for Health Care Policy and Research of the U.S. Department of Health and Human Services found that about half of the home care recipients were older than sixty-five. More than $13 billion was spent on home care in 1991.[1]

Until the late nineteenth century, the home was the primary location for treatment of the sick. Patients were placed in the hospital only when they were impoverished and didn't have access to medical care, which was defined as not having a personal physician. Hospitals were run then (and continue to be run) at a pace that benefitted the hospital schedule. As Norman Cousins said, "A hospital is no place for a person who is ill."[2]

Today, home care is again an option for the patient who is ill. It is appropriate for patients who suffer chronic conditions requiring long-term care, such as diabetes, high blood pressure, emotional problems, Alzheimer's, and HIV-related illness, or patients recovering from heart attacks, strokes, or accidents. In addition, cancer patients, as well as infants and children in need of medical and nursing care, can be cared for in the home. (Hospice care is discussed in Chapter 10).

There are currently twelve thousand home care agencies in the United States.

HOME-BASED CARE SERVICES

Some of the care services that are available in the home setting are:

Doctors' visits
Nursing

Physical, speech, and occupational therapy
Nutritionist
Social worker
Clergy visits
Home health aides
Mental health services
Intravenous therapy
Injections
Enteral nutrition
Parenteral nutrition
Chemotherapy
Antibiotic therapy
Laboratory tests
EKG
X-rays
Pain management
Oxygen, medical equipment, supplies
Dental care
Catheter care
Diabetic care
Ostomy care
Wound care
High-tech care
Pregnancy care
Newborn care
Chronic care for children
Traction
Stroke rehabilitation
Housekeeping
Transportation
Companion care
Cooking, laundry, marketing, etc.
Child-care
Meal delivery
Personal emergency response systems
Respite care to provide time off for family members

HOME CARE IS COST-EFFECTIVE

"Home care is not only the most humane manner of delivering care, and the one most preferred by the patient, but often it is the most cost effective. For example, Blue Cross/Blue Shield of Harrisburg, Pennsylvania, this year agreed to exchange a ventilator-dependent pediatric patient's hospital care benefit for home care services at a cost savings of $2000 a day. Instead of paying for hospitalization in an intensive care unit at nearly $3000 per day, Blue Cross will provide 16 hours per day of home services at a cost of less than $800 per day."[3]

Lewin/ICF in Washington, D.C., reported a cost difference between hospital and home care for three medical problems. Hip-fracture patients reduced their costs by $2,300 per day, amyotrophic lateral sclerosis patients with pneumonia by $300, and those with chronic obstructive pulmonary disease by $520. Maternity discharges to home care, reducing a three-day stay in the hospital to two and a half days, could save $40 million to $50 million annually.[4]

The following examples demonstrate the monthly savings of home care compared to hospital care:

Condition	Hospital	Home	Savings
Infant born with breathing/feeding problems	$60,000	$20,000	$40,000
Nutrition infusion	23,670	9,000	14,670
Patient requiring respiratory support	24,715	9,267	15,448
Ventilator-dependent patient	22,569	1,766	20,803[5]

The National Association for Home Care reports, "The Nursing Home Without Walls program in New York State, which has been operating since 1978, has shown that the cost of services for patients treated in the home has consistently been about half the cost of corresponding institutional care. In cases where the patients would otherwise be in acute care hospitals, rehabilitation hospitals or other facilities with higher costs than skilled nursing or other health-related facilities, the program has resulted in greater savings."[6]

LOCATING HOME CARE AGENCIES

Local hospital discharge planner
United Way
Visiting Nurse Association

Churches
Doctors
Social service agencies
County public health departments
Friends
Social Security Administration

WHO PAYS FOR HOME CARE?

Private insurance
Medicare
Medicaid
Veterans' Administration
CHAMPUS (military dependents)

EVALUATING THE QUALITY OF HOME CARE

It is far more difficult to monitor the quality of home care services than that of services in a hospital or other health care institution. There are no uniform or standard laws or review procedures. And, as in nursing home services, most care is provided by aides, who often have little training or supervision, reports the American Association of Retired Persons (AARP) in Washington, D.C.

There is evidence that some home care agencies have poorly trained staff with little supervision, resulting in poor patient care, and in some cases abuse.

Currently, there are three ways that outside organizations monitor home care quality. The AARP notes the following monitoring measures:

1. State licensure: Thirty-nine states, including Washington, D.C., license home health care agencies. Standards vary from state to state. In general, agencies that provide nursing and one other therapeutic service must be licensed. If nonskilled or only one high-technology service is provided (e.g., intravenous therapy), a license may not be required.
2. Certification for Medicare: In order to receive Medicare-covered services, the provider must be certified.
3. Accreditation: Accreditation programs are offered by private, nongovernmental organizations to agencies providing either skilled or nonskilled care. Programs are not monitored by the government, but

may be an indicator of an agency that has attempted to meet some standards.[7]

PAIN MANAGEMENT IN THE HOME

As mentioned, acute and chronic pain are undertreated by 50% in the hospital setting, and chronic pain often is not treated in a multidisciplinary model.

"Home care is where so much of patient care takes place, not the hospital," reports Anna Williams, M.N., R.N., C.S., of the Pain Management Service, Swedish Hospital Tumor Institute, in Seattle, Washington. "It is important to make certain that pain is not keeping a patient from being able to achieve the highest level of functional ability possible in their home. They should be able to carry out activities of daily living. Pain interferes with those activities."[8]

The greatest problem for patients who suffer pain in the home care setting is the difficulty of assessing pain levels and pain relief. Other problems are side effects, lack of monitoring of patients, misunderstandings about doses and schedules, patient and nursing fears of addiction and respiratory depression, and patients not reporting their pain levels.

Bruce Ferrell, M.D., and Betty Ferrell, Ph.D., F.A.A.N., note, "Pain management at home remains an understudied problem. Heavy reliance on family members, logistic access to diagnostic facilities, and often limited pharmacy services, can all influence the effectiveness of pain management at home. Patients, families, and health care professionals often promote long-term care at home, assuming that patients are more comfortable there. Pain, however, may not be substantially better managed at home, and barriers have been described that actually hindered pain management at home." They note that "clinical experience suggests that pain management is a common problem in home care."[9]

"Most of the home care is delivered by community doctors and nurses who do not know how to manage patients with pain. There is a gap from the pain care in the hospital to home care," notes Nessa Coyle, M.S., R.N., A.N.P, the Director of Supportive Care of the Pain Service at Memorial Sloan-Kettering in New York.[10]

Ferrell and Ferrell note:

> Hospitals typically provide highly technical equipment and services for acutely ill patients. For patients with severe pain, this often

amounts to a variety of aggressive or invasive strategies for definitive treatment of the underlying conditions. Home care, by contrast, relies heavily on low-tech strategies, concentrating mostly on symptom management. For pain management nonpharmacologic strategies are often used. Patients are often reluctant to use narcotic medications in the home, and this reluctance is compounded by limited patient education, the fear of addiction, and misunderstanding about proper dosages. Over-the-counter analgesics, alcohol, liniments, and homeopathic potions are frequently used.[11]

SUMMARY

As discussed earlier, a burden falls on the family caregivers, which can greatly impair the normal function of the spousal and family interaction. Seeing a loved one in pain takes its toll on emotions, intimacy, physical strength, sleep, and work.

It is important to make use of the pain assessment tools found throughout other chapters. The simplest to use for adults is the *0–10 Numeric Pain Intensity Scale.* As pointed out, tools to assess functional status, impairment, goals, family caregiving impact, Quality of Life measurements, Biobehavioral Pain Profile, and other areas have an important role in the home and should not be left inside a hospital or a doctor's office. However, each instrument must be individualized. Some patients may not have the cognitive ability to respond to some of the assessment tools.

If patients cannot tolerate oral and/or long-acting oral medication, other modalities of continuous intravenous, intraspinal, or subcutaneous infusion with an option for patient-controlled analgesia (PCA) are available in the home.

In addition, use of over-the-counter drugs and nondrug therapies such as relaxation techniques, heat/cold therapy, massage, and other pain relievers mentioned earlier can be employed.

The goal is to assess and relieve pain so that patients can return to the highest level of functioning ability. Home care requires a team effort, with close supervision by doctors, nurses, and other home care specialists.

The following is a list of home care resources that will enable the patient to find the most qualified care.

HOME CARE RESOURCES

NATIONAL ASSOCIATION

National Association for Home Care
Hospice Association of America
Center for Health Care Law
Home Care Aide Association of
America
All located at:
519 C Street
N.E. Stanton Park
Washington, DC 20002-5809
(202) 547-7424
Fax (202) 547-3540

American Federation of Home Health
Agencies
1320 Fenwick Lane, Suite 100
Silver Spring, MD 20910
(800) 368-5927

American Hospital Association
Division of Ambulatory and Home Care
Services
840 North Lake Shore Drive
Chicago, IL 60611
(312) 280-6000

Community Health Accreditation
Program
National League of Nursing
10 Columbus Circle
New York, NY 10019
(212) 582-1022

Home Health Services and Staffing
Association
815 Connecticut Avenue, N.W., Suite
206
Washington, DC 20006
(202) 331-4437

Joint Commission on the Accreditation
of Healthcare Organizations
One Renaissance Boulevard
Oakbrook Terrace, IL 60181

Visiting Nurse Associations of America
3801 East Florida Avenue, Suite 806
Denver, CO 80210
(303) 753-0218

American Association of Retired
Persons
601 East Street, N.W.
Washington, DC 20049
(202) 434-2277

Royal Victoria Hospital Palliative Care
Service
687 Pine Avenue West
Montreal, Quebec H3A 1A1, Canada
(514) 843-1542
An independent national organization
of groups providing palliative care and
hospice in Canada.

PUBLICATIONS

These publications are free from the American Association of Retired Persons, 601 East Street, N.W., Washington, DC 20049, (202) 434-2277.

"Before You Buy: A Guide to Long-Term Care Insurance" (D12893).
"Care Management: Arranging for Long Term Care" (D13803).
"Checklist of Concerns and Resources for Caregivers" (12895).
"Coping and Caring: Living with Alzheimer's Disease" (D12441).
"Handbook About Care in the Home" (D955).
"Insurance Checklist" (D1032). Guide for the individual to help determine personal insurance needs.
"Knowing Your Rights" (D12330). Information on Medicare's prospective payment system, with emphasis on patient's rights.
"A Matter of Choice: Planning Ahead for Health Care Decisions" (D12776).
"Medicare: What It Covers, What It Doesn't" (D13133).
"Miles Away and Still Caring: A Guide for Long Distance Caregivers" (12748).
"Nursing Home Life: A Guide for Residents and Families" (13063).
"A Path for Caregivers" (D12957).

"Personal Emergency Response System (PERS): Meeting the Need for Security and Independence" (D12905).

"Tomorrow's Choices: Preparing Now for Future Legal, Financial and Health Care Decisions" (D13479).

"Your Home, Your Choice: A Workbook for Older People and Their Families" (D12143).

The following publications are available from the National Association for Home Care, 519 C Street, N.E. Stanton Park, Washington, DC 20002-5809, Attn.: Publications, (202) 547-7424, fax (202) 547-3540.

"Home Care Brochure" (C-001).
"How to Choose a Home Care Agency" (C-005).
"What Are They Saying About Home Care?" (C-003).
"Why Home Care?" (C-004).
All About Home Care: A Consumer's Guide (#4203).
Caring magazine. $45 per year.
The Crisis of Chronically Ill Children in America: Triumph of Technology—Failure of Public Policy (#4229).
HomeCare News. $18 per year.
No One Prepared Me for This (#4239).

PRIVATE SERVICES

Option Care
34012 Ninth Avenue, South Building C
Federal Way, WA 98003
(206) 838-3232
In WA (800) 624-0226
　　JCAHO-accredited provider of home IV and nutritional therapies. Clinical staff available 7 days, 24 hours.

Caremark
455 Knightsbridge Parkway
Lincolnshire, IL 60069
(800) 323-8083
(708) 215-3300
　　Provides home care patient services, including chemotherapy, diet, pain management, and advocacy. Nationwide network. Newsletter *Caring for People.*

Critical Care America
50 Washington Street
Westborough, MA 01581-5030
(800) 344-5500
In MA (508) 836-3610
　　Provides professional home infusion therapy, including chemotherapy, TPN, antibiotics, and growth hormone. Offers a pediatric patient education program for children on IV therapy. Nationwide network.

Home Intensive Care
150 Northwest 168th Street, 2d Floor
North Miami Beach, FL 33169
(800) 344-3181
In FL (305) 653-0000
Fax (305) 651-2147
　　Provides professional home care patient services, including chemotherapy, total parenteral nutrition, and pain management. Nationwide network.

Pediatric Services of America
5834 C Peach Corners East
Narcross, GA 30092
(800) 950-1580
　　Provides pediatric home nursing services and equipment.

To find medical equipment, look in the yellow pages under "Hospital Equipment and Supplies" and "Pharmacies."

HOME-HEALTH HOTLINE NUMBERS

The government has established these state-run toll-free numbers to collect information on home health agencies certified by Medicare. Each state is to conduct surveys on complaints about patient care and whether any problems were found during the survey.

REGION I
Connecticut	(800) 828-9769
Maine	(800) 621-8222
Massachusetts	(800) 462-5540
New Hampshire	(800) 621-6232
Rhode Island	(800) 228-2716
Vermont	(800) 698-4683

REGION II
New Jersey	(800) 792-9770
New York	(800) 628-5972
Puerto Rico	(800) 782-8013

REGION III
Delaware	(800) 942-7373
District of Columbia	(800) 727-7873
Maryland	(800) 492-6002
	(800) 492-6005
Pennsylvania	(800) 222-0989
Virginia	(800) 985-1819
West Virginia	(800) 442-2888

REGION IV
Alabama	(800) 356-9596
Florida	(800) 962-6014
Georgia	(800) 869-1150
Kentucky	(800) 635-6290
Mississippi	(800) 227-7308
North Carolina	(800) 624-3004
South Carolina	(800) 922-6735
Tennessee	(800) 541-7367

REGION V
Illinois	(800) 252-4343
Indiana	(800) 227-6334
Michigan	(800) 882-6006
Minnesota	(800) 369-7994
Ohio	(800) 342-0553
Wisconsin	(800) 642-6552

REGION VI
Arkansas	(800) 223-0340
Louisiana	(800) 327-3419
New Mexico	(800) 752-8649
Oklahoma	(800) 234-7258
Texas	(800) 228-1570

REGION VII
Iowa	(800) 383-4920
Kansas	(800) 842-0078
Missouri	(800) 877-6485
Nebraska	(800) 245-5832

REGION VIII
Colorado	(800) 842-8826
Montana	(800) 762-4618
North Dakota	(800) 472-2180
South Dakota	(800) 592-1861
Utah	(800) 999-7739
Wyoming	(800) 548-1367

REGION IX
Arizona	(800) 221-9968
California	
Northern Region:	
Sacramento	(800) 554-0354
Chico	(800) 554-0350
Santa Rosa	(800) 554-0349
Berkeley	(800) 554-0352
San Francisco	(800) 554-0353
Southern Region:	
San Jose	(800) 554-0343
Fresno	(800) 554-0351
Ventura	(800) 547-8267
Santa Ana	(800) 228-5234
San Diego	(800) 824-0613
San Bernadino	(800) 344-2896
Hawaii	(800) 548-6577
Nevada	(800) 225-3414

REGION X
Alaska	(800) 563-0037

NOTES

[1]National Association for Home Care (NAHC), *Basic Statistics about Home Care 1992,* Washington, D.C.

[2]Cousins, N., personal communication, 1982.

[3]Center for Health Care Law, Washington, D.C., in NAHC report #447, January 31, 1992.

[4]Lewin/ICF, "Economic Analysis of Home Medical Equipment Services," Washington, D.C., May 29, 1991.

[5]Aetna Life & Casualty Co., May 28, 1984, *Business Week* magazine; American Association for Respiratory Therapy, February 1984, *Wall Street Journal;* July 1990, OTA May report, "Technology Dependent Children: Hospital v. Home Care, A Technical Memorandum."

[6]National Association for Home Care (NAHC), *Basic Statistics about Home Care 1992,* Washington, D.C.

[7]"Guide to Homecare," American Association of Retired Persons (Washington, D.C.), 1992.

[8]Williams, A., "Functional Status in Cancer Pain Patients: The Use of Observation Methods in Research," Innovations in Cancer Pain: Assessment and Treatment, First International Nursing Research Symposium on Cancer Pain, Seattle, Washington, July 22, 1992.

[9]Ferrell, B., Ferrell, B. R., "Pain Management at Home," *Clinics in Geriatric Medicine,* vol. 7, no. 4 (November 1991), 765–75.

[10]Coyle, N., "The Nature of Terminal Illness in the Cancer Patient: Pain and Other Symptoms in the Last Weeks of Life," Innovations in Cancer Pain: Assessment and Treatment, University of Washington School of Nursing, Seattle, Washington, July 22, 1992.

[11]Ferrell, B., Ferrell, B. R., "Pain Management at Home," *Clinics in Geriatric Medicine,* vol. 7, no. 4 (November 1991), 765–75.

8

ELDER PAIN CARE

More than 31 million Americans are sixty-five years of age or older. It is projected that in the year 2030 65.6 million will be over sixty-five.

Aging is more than a biological process. "Aging is a time of losses: loss of social role (usually through retirement), loss of income, loss of friends and relatives (through death and mobility). It can also be a time of fear: fear for personal safety, fear of financial insecurity, fear of dependency,"[1] according to Kane, Ouslander, and Abrass in *Essentials of Clinical Geriatrics.*

Pain studies in this older population have been neglected. This is surprising, since up to 80% of this age group suffer from at least one chronic disorder. Donald Schienle, Ph.D., and John Eiler, Ph.D., of the University of Southern California, note:

> If the definition of "chronic condition" is restricted to include only those disorders that impose some limitation on the person having them, then 53 percent of older men and 41 percent of older women are limited in activity to some extent by chronic disabling conditions. About 41 percent of the older population are severely limited by chronic disabling conditions. Heart disease, cancer, cerebrovascular disease, and respiratory disease are the most prevalent physical diseases of old age, limiting daily functioning. Arthritis, rheumatism, and sensory impairment (such as loss of vision and hearing) are also responsible for limiting the activities of well over 25 percent of older adults. In addition to these physical disabilities, approximately 5 percent of older adults suffer some type of organic damage to the brain that

can result in chronic impairment of cognitive functioning. This damage may result from a specific disease process such as arteriosclerosis, heart disease, or a cerebrovascular accident [stroke] or senile dementia of the Alzheimer's type.[2]

Arthritis, cancer, postherpetic pain, low back pain, cardiac disorders, fractures, surgery, and other medical problems can result in moderate to severe pain. As mentioned earlier, undertreated pain can result in increased pain levels, fatigue, sleeplessness, inactivity, depression, deconditioning, and feelings of anger, anxiety, helplessness, or hopelessness.

Research about the true prevalence of pain in the elder population is difficult, for a wide variety of reasons. "They are more diverse in personality, psychologic characteristics, medical problems and socioeconomic characteristics than other population segments," report Drs. Harkins, Kwentus, and Price.[3]

There is a misconception that the elderly do not feel pain, just as there is a common misconception that infants and children do not feel pain. They do.

Barbara Shapiro, M.D., and Betty Ferrell, Ph.D., F.A.A.N., note that "similarities between children and the aged lie in the areas of the physical, developmental, and emotional characteristics of patients; characteristics of healthcare professionals; interactional issues with families, medical caretakers, and society; and issues involving research."[4]

As described earlier, pain is a unique experience for each individual. Pain perception is influenced by what the pain means to each person, as well as cultural, social, metabolic, emotional, age, and possibly genetic and other factors.

Research has shown that undertreated pain in the elderly is significant. Drs. Bruce and Betty Ferrell found that *70% of patients in a nursing home population who could speak had major pain complaints, and one-third of those patients were in constant pain.*[5]

Ferrell and Ferrell surveyed sixty-five nursing home residents about how pain affects them.

How Elders Say Pain Affects Them[6]

Problems	Number of Residents*
Enjoyable activities (recreation, social events) impaired	35 (54%)
Ambulation (walking, transfers) impaired	34 (53%)
Posture impaired	32 (49%)
Sleep disturbance	29 (45%)
Depression	21 (32%)
Anxiety	17 (26%)
Constipation	10 (15%)
Appetite impaired	9 (14%)
Memory impaired	8 (12%)
Incontinence	5 (8%)
Grooming or dressing impaired	5 (8%)
None of the above	15 (23%)

*Numbers total more than 100% because some residents indicated more than one problem.

ASSESSMENT

Assessment of the pain levels of older patients is as important as it is in other age groups. The *Short-Form McGill Pain Questionnaire* can be used successfully with the older patient. Researchers at the National Research Institute of Gerontology and Geriatric Medicine in Parville, Victoria, and Ferrell and Ferrell found that up to 80% were able to complete the scale.

Ferrell and Ferrell found that *patients did not talk about their pain unless someone took the time to ask them—and the question of pain had to be asked in the right format.* For example:

"Do you have pain?" Answer: "No."
"Do you hurt?" Answer: "Yes! I'm miserable."

As reported in the Introduction, some patients don't tell anyone they are in pain; they think that pain may come with illness or age, are afraid to bother anyone, or may have cultural attitudes that affect the reporting of pain. In addition, a patient can be sleeping, smiling, playing cards, or watching TV and still be in pain.

Other problems, such as diminished hearing, eyesight, or cognitive skills, may require frequent assessment. The older patient must be

Short-Form McGill Pain Questionnaire

PATIENT'S NAME: _____ DATE: _____

	NONE	MILD	MODERATE	SEVERE
THROBBING	0)_____	1)_____	2)_____	3)_____
SHOOTING	0)_____	1)_____	2)_____	3)_____
STABBING	0)_____	1)_____	2)_____	3)_____
SHARP	0)_____	1)_____	2)_____	3)_____
CRAMPING	0)_____	1)_____	2)_____	3)_____
GNAWING	0)_____	1)_____	2)_____	3)_____
HOT–BURNING	0)_____	1)_____	2)_____	3)_____
ACHING	0)_____	1)_____	2)_____	3)_____
HEAVY	0)_____	1)_____	2)_____	3)_____
TENDER	0)_____	1)_____	2)_____	3)_____
SPLITTING	0)_____	1)_____	2)_____	3)_____
TIRING–EXHAUSTING	0)_____	1)_____	2)_____	3)_____
SICKENING	0)_____	1)_____	2)_____	3)_____
FEARFUL	0)_____	1)_____	2)_____	3)_____
PUNISHING–CRUEL	0)_____	1)_____	2)_____	3)_____

NO |_____| WORST
PAIN   POSSIBLE
                                          PAIN

PPI [Present Pain Intensity]

0 NO PAIN   _____
1 MILD   _____
2 DISCOMFORTING   _____
3 DISTRESSING   _____
4 HORRIBLE   _____
5 EXCRUCIATING   _____

© R. Melzack. Reprinted by permission, 1993.

monitored for side effects of drugs: constipation, urinary retention, fogginess, cognitive impairment, etc.

Activities of Daily Living

The *Katz Activities of Daily Living* (ADL) assessment provides a simple means of summarizing a person's ability to carry out the basic tasks of self-care:

> Data usually come from the patient or from a caregiver (e.g., nurse or family member) who has had a sufficient opportunity to observe the patient. In some cases, it may be more useful to have the patient actually perform key tasks. Grading of performance is usually divided into three levels of dependency:
>
> (1) Ability to perform the task without human assistance (one may wish to distinguish those persons who need mechanical aids like a walker but are still independent).
>
> (2) Ability to perform task with some assistance.
>
> (3) Inability to perform even with assistance.
>
> Sometimes the latter two classes can be collapsed to form a single category—dependent—which would be contrasted with independent functioning (with or without mechanical assistance).[7]

Some examples of measure of *physical function* are basic activities of daily living:

- Feeding
- Dressing
- Ambulation
- Toileting
- Bathing

- Transfer (from bed to toilet)
- Continence
- Grooming
- Communication

Instrumental activities include:

- Writing
- Reading
- Cooking
- Cleaning
- Shopping
- Doing laundry
- Climbing stairs
- Using a telephone

- Managing medication
- Managing money
- The ability to perform paid employment duties or outside work (such as gardening)
- The ability to travel (use public transportation, go out of town)

However, Kane et al. put forth a few caveats about the usefulness of their assessment:

1. A functional assessment of a patient in an acute state is likely to be invalid (e.g., a patient transferred from a natural environment to the alien world of the hospital, particularly at a time of stress).
2. With the ADL scale, the patient's motivation and the environmental structure are important determinants of performance.
3. It is critical to distinguish what a patient can do under proper circumstances and what is actually done during the patient's daily life. For example, it is not realistic to expect a nursing home patient to show self-care in bathing if the nursing home's policy forbids unattended bathing, or independence in dressing if the staff insists on dressing them as a matter of expectancy.[8]

Many older patients have been seen by a variety of specialists for their various ailments. Often they are not being followed by any one doctor, and they may suffer from polypharmacy as a consequence. *It is important to have an older patient treated by one doctor, if possible, or at least have one doctor who coordinates care.*

TREATMENT

Pharmacological Pain Management

Useful drugs include over-the-counter medications, prescription drugs (opioid [morphine-like] and nonopioid), and other analgesic or enhancing drugs. (See Chapter 1 for drugs and forms of administration.)

It should be noted that older patients often have a problem with taking medication. They may be taking many medications, find side effects unpleasant, not understand the directions, etc.

Older patients often suffer from the same unfounded fears of addiction as the general population. Time must be spent with the patient to be certain they can manage taking medication. Time must be spent to ensure that there is adequate assessment after the medication has been administered. Many older patients will not complain of pain unless asked.

Nonpharmacological Pain Management

Physical techniques include ice, heat, massage, TENS, physical therapy, and occupational therapy.

Psychological techniques include individual and group therapy, biofeedback, relaxation, distraction, hypnosis, etc. (See Chapter 1.)

SUMMARY

The older patient faces the likelihood of one or more forms of chronic illness. Pain is present in the majority of these patients. They often do not complain about having pain. Many older patients are seen by multiple doctors for various ailments, so they often suffer from polypharmacy. These patients need to be evaluated carefully and followed by one doctor or at least need one doctor who oversees their care.

Pain assessment, using standard pain measurement tools, can be effective with the older patient. ADL measurements should also be evaluated.

Pain affects the activity of patients and, if not relieved, can lead to feelings of depression, helplessness, and hopelessness. The goal is to allow the older patient to achieve as high a level of functioning as possible.

The following are elder resources.

ELDER RESOURCES

National Council on the Aging
Department 5087
Washington, DC 20061-5087
  Write for publication #2010, costing $7, which includes a directory of nearly 500 support groups.

Gerontological Society
Clinical Medicine Section
1 Dupont Circle
Washington, DC 20036

American Geriatric Society
10 Columbus Circle, Suite 1470
New York, NY 10019
  Also see Home Care and Nursing Home Resources.

NOTES

[1]Kane, R., Ouslander, J., Abrass, I., *Essentials of Clinical Geriatrics,* second edition, (New York: McGraw-Hill, 1989), 11.

[2]Schienle, D., Eiler, J., "Clinical Intervention with Older Adults," *Chronic Illness and Disability through the Life Span,* ed. Eisenberg, M., Sutkin, L., Jansen, M. (New York: Springer Publishing, 1984), 246.

[3]Harkins, S., Kwentus, J., Price, D., "Pain and Suffering in the Elderly," *The Management of Pain,* ed. Bonica, J., second edition (Philadelphia: Lea & Febiger, 1990), vol. 1, 552.

[4]Shapiro, B., Ferrell, B., "Pain in Children and the Frail Elderly: Similarities and Implications," *American Pain Society Bulletin,* October–November 1992, 11–14.

[5]Ferrell, B., Ferrell, B., "Easing the Pain," *Geriatric Nursing,* July–August 1990, 175.

[6]Shapiro, B., Ferrell, B., "Pain in Children and the Frail Elderly: Similarities and Implications," *American Pain Society Bulletin,* October–November 1992, 11–14.

[7]Kane, R., Ouslander, J., Abrass, I., *Essentials of Clinical Geriatrics,* second edition (New York: McGraw-Hill, 1989), 11.

[8]Adapted from Kane, R., Ouslander, J., Abrass, I., *Essentials of Clinical Geriatrics,* second edition (New York: McGraw-Hill, 1989), 11.

9

NURSING HOMES

Shocking stories about nursing homes abound. Often they are guilty of poor staffing and poor patient care. Some residents are restrained, are not fed balanced or timely meals, have no access to activities, are not clothed, and lack the basics of medical and pain care.

Approximately 31 million Americans are over sixty-five years of age. Up to 6 million older Americans need long-term care today. Most receive care in their homes, but 1.5 million are in nursing homes. More than 50% of nursing home residents suffer from mental or behavioral problems.[1]

Every person in a nursing home has the right to good care under the laws that apply to nursing home care. In addition, as discussed in other chapters, everyone, regardless of age, has the right to adequate pain control. Obviously, a nursing home that does not provide a high quality of care for the individual will not provide quality pain assessment and management.

Pain in the nursing home is understudied by medical care researchers. Bruce Ferrell, M.D., Betty Ferrell, Ph.D., F.A.A.N., and Dan Osterweil, M.D., of the City of Hope, conducted a 1990 survey about pain in the nursing home. The researchers studied 97 residents in a 311-bed multilevel teaching nursing home. They reported:

> The residents were interviewed and charts were reviewed for pain problems and management strategies. Functional status, depression, and cognitive impairment were also evaluated. Results indicate that 71% of the residents had at least one pain complaint (range 1–4). Of subjects with pain, 34% described constant (continuous) pain and 66% described intermittent pain. Of 43 subjects with intermittent pain, 51% described pain on a daily basis. Only 15% of

the residents with pain had received medication within the previous 24 hours. The findings suggest that pain is a major problem in long-term care.[2]

They also found that patients, on the average, had eight medical problems and were taking seven medications. In addition, patients did not talk about their pain unless they were prodded. Doctors were 44% accurate in charting patients' pain, and nurses were 49% accurate. *Up to 37% of patients' pain was not documented at all.*

Choosing a nursing home carefully can ensure proper care of the individual resident. *Recently the Senate Special Committee on Aging found that more than one-third of the nineteen thousand nursing homes in America did not comply with federal regulations, and one out of ten nursing homes was guilty of outright neglect, abuse, or practices that led to death.*

In Chapter 1 you read about a patient whose cancer had spread to his bones. When he left the hospital for a nursing home, his doctor prescribed morphine to be given to him every three to four hours for excruciating pain. The nurse in charge took it upon herself to progressively cut his dose of morphine, until he was receiving only over-the-counter pain medication. After suffering intolerable pain for months, he died. *This should never have happened. Thousands of nursing home patients across the nation are victims of poor pain management.* His family took legal action against the nursing home for failure to provide adequate pain management as ordered by his doctor. The court found the nursing home and the nurse in violation of state and federal laws and awarded the family $7.5 million in punitive damages and $7.5 million for pain and suffering.

The most important considerations when you select a nursing home for yourself or for a loved one are "quality and payment issues," notes the National Citizens' Coalition for Nursing Home Reform in Washington, D.C., which has issued "How Residents and Their Families Can Participate in Care Planning," guidelines concerning quality of care. (For their address, see the resources at the end of this chapter.)

There is a vast difference in the quality of care between one nursing home and the next. Start your education process by:

- Asking your doctor for a referral.
- Talking to Social Services at your local hospital.
- Consulting other families.
- Consulting your church.

- Contacting the State Office on Aging.
- Contacting your local long-term-care ombudsman (see the resources at the end of this chapter). He or she is a legal representative of the law and is an advocate for nursing home residents.

VISIT THE HOME

On your first visit, check the following, which are required by law:

Is the home licensed?

Ask to see the resident assessment chart for each resident's needs and the plan of care to assure that he or she can achieve the highest practicable physical, mental, and psychosocial functioning.

The resident assessment should cover functional abilities such as each resident's ability to walk, talk, eat, dress, bathe, see, hear, communicate, understand, and remember.

The staff should ask in detail about a resident's interests, hobbies, activities, and family relationships.

Plan of Care

How does the staff form a plan of care to address the medical and nonmedical needs of each person?

How often are those needs reviewed?

What changes can the staff make if there are problems such as eating difficulties, lack of socialization, lack of harmony with roommate, etc.?

How often do care planning conferences with staff and residents' families take place? All members of the staff who have contact with residents should participate in this conference.

Care planning must occur every three months, or anytime there is a change in the resident's medical, social, or mental status.

Assessment must take place within fourteen days after admission and at least once a year thereafter, with a review every three months if a resident's condition changes (or more frequently if changes occur more frequently).

Issues that could be discussed at these meetings would be about routine activities related to personal care, eating, staff interaction, medications, and medical treatment options.

A resident advocate should be available through the local ombuds-man or other advocacy groups.

ARE RESIDENTS' RIGHTS POSTED?

Is there access to an ombudsman, should any problem arise?

What access is there to doctors (resident on call, etc.)?

How often do they visit? Most nursing home doctors visit only once a month.

Is there access to psychological or psychiatric assistance? How often?

What kind of follow-up care is there?

Do residents have access to a dentist, optometrist, other?

What access is there to a pharmacy? Is is on a timely basis?

Is there round-the-clock R.N.-licensed nursing?

STAFFING

If the home has more than 120 beds, is there a social worker?

Is there a dietitian?

Is there an activities director?

Is there access to the social worker, physical therapist, occupational therapist?

Is there access to clergy?

Who are the members of the home's quality-assurance committee? It should include a physician, nurses, and other health care profes-sionals.

When was the home last inspected by state and federal agents? Ask to see if inspections include assessment of the actual care of residents.

Check the Staffing

How many staff members work only on weekdays?

Who is there on weekends?

How often does the staff turn over?

Talk to various staff members. Do they seem happy with their work?

Find out how long they have been at the home.

What kind of training do they have?

EVALUATING CARE

Look at the residents' level of care and talk with them.

Is the home clean?

Does it smell bad?

Is it cheerful and homelike in the common areas and in the residents' rooms?

Are residents physically restrained?

Are they drugged?

Are the residents dressed? Out of bed?

Are they in the common rooms?

Are there activities taking place?

What are the meals like? Eat one.

Are the residents eating?

What do they think about the food?

Is there staff to help residents eat if they have problems?

Is help offered in a timely fashion, or does the resident just sit and wait?

Do the residents look depressed, angry, sad?

What do they say?

Visit on a weekend or for an evening meal for a second look.

Talk to other families that are visiting. What do they think?

What is the visiting policy?

What personal belongings can the resident bring into the home?

If you or your loved one is bedridden, take a look at those residents who are bedridden. Are they comfortable?

Are they well groomed? Do they smell fresh?

Does the staff turn the patients in bed to avoid bedsores? Are there bedsores?

How are food, activities, and visitors handled for those who are bedridden?

Are there restraints?

Are they drugged?

PAYMENT

Many residents of nursing homes enter as private-paying individuals but run out of money due to high costs. It is important to select a home that accepts Medicaid payments. Federal law requires that the home provide a list of items and services included in the basic Medicaid or private rate, and any extra charges.

What is the cost?

What is the cost of extras—laundry, wheelchairs, drugs, etc.?

PAIN MANAGEMENT

What is the pain management goal of the home?

Does the home make pain management a priority?

How does the staff assess pain?

Who makes the assessment?

Do they use pain assessment instruments?

Do they chart pain as they do vital signs such as blood pressure and temperature?

How do they assess pain in patients who have lowered cognitive abilities? (See Chapter 8.)

Who will be accountable for pain management?

What action is taken if pain is not controlled?

Who can be called to change medication?

Is nondrug pain management available (massage, heat, cold, physical therapy, exercise, etc.)?

Ferrell and Ferrell reported that:

> . . . 85% of the patients had a prescription for acetaminophen, but it was difficult to distinguish on the patient's chart whether the prescription was routine or for treating pain. Codeine was prescribed; however, the triplicate prescription forms that California doctors had to fill out for morphine had a profoundly deleterious effect on the accessibility of morphine. Patients would not use heating pads, even if they were prescribed. The patients complained that the pads never got hot enough. The reason for the low heat was because administrators do not want to be liable for injuries or mishaps with the heating pads.[3]

In 1987 Congress enacted reforms for nursing homes. "Those laws encompass the rights of residents to dignity, choice, self-determination, quality services and activities, and participation in nursing home administration. They refer specifically to privacy, access to records, freedom from abuse and restraints, visitors, involvement in transfer and discharge plans, safeguarding of personal funds, and protection against discrimination based on income or race.''[4]

If the nursing home staff restricts you from asking questions, or restricts you from speaking to other staff or residents, or the quality of care is lacking, it is not a facility that you or a loved one should consider.

Look for another facility, and report your findings to the local ombudsman. The nursing home could well be in violation of state and federal laws. Ask the hard questions before making any commitment or signing a contract.

The following is a checklist for finding an adequate nursing home and a nursing home resource list.

Nursing Home Checklist

When you visit a nursing home, you should carry this checklist with you. It will help you to compare one facility with another, but remember to compare facilities certified in the same category; for example, a skilled nursing facility with another skilled nursing home. Because nursing homes may be licensed in more than one category, always compare similar types of service among facilities.

	Home A		Home B	
Look at Daily Life	Yes	No	Yes	No
1. Do residents seem to enjoy being with staff?	☐	☐	☐	☐
2. Are most residents dressed for the season and time of day?	☐	☐	☐	☐
3. Does staff know the residents by name?	☐	☐	☐	☐
4. Does staff respond quickly to resident calls for assistance?	☐	☐	☐	☐
5. Are activities tailored to residents' individual needs and interests?	☐	☐	☐	☐
6. Are residents involved in a variety of activities?	☐	☐	☐	☐
7. Does the home serve food attractively?	☐	☐	☐	☐
8. Does the home consider personal food likes and dislikes in planning meals?	☐	☐	☐	☐

	Home A Yes No	Home B Yes No

9. Does the home use care in selecting room-mates? ☐ ☐ ☐ ☐

10. Does the nursing home have a resident's council? If it does, does the council influence decisions about resident life? ☐ ☐ ☐ ☐

11. Does the nursing home have a family council? If it does, does the council influence decisions about resident life? ☐ ☐ ☐ ☐

12. Does the facility have contact with community groups, such as pet therapy programs and Scouts? ☐ ☐ ☐ ☐

Look at Care Residents Receive

1. Do various staff and professional experts participate in evaluating each resident's needs and interests? ☐ ☐ ☐ ☐

2. Does the resident or his or her family participate in developing the resident's care plan? ☐ ☐ ☐ ☐

3. Does the home offer programs to restore lost physical functioning (for example, physical therapy, occupational therapy, speech and language therapy)? ☐ ☐ ☐ ☐

4. Does the home have any special services that meet your needs? For example, special care units for residents with dementia or with respiratory problems? ☐ ☐ ☐ ☐

5. Does the nursing home have a program to restrict the use of physical restraints? ☐ ☐ ☐ ☐

6. Is a registered nurse available for nursing staff? ☐ ☐ ☐ ☐

7. Does the nursing home have an arrangement with a nearby hospital? ☐ ☐ ☐ ☐

Look at How the Nursing Home Handles Payment

1. Is the facility certified for Medicare? ☐ ☐ ☐ ☐
2. Is the facility certified for Medicaid? ☐ ☐ ☐ ☐

3. Is the resident or the resident's family informed when charges are increased? ☐ ☐ ☐ ☐

Look at the Environment

1. Is the outside of the nursing home clean and in good repair? ☐ ☐ ☐ ☐

	Home A		Home B	
	Yes	No	Yes	No
2. Are there outdoor areas accessible for residents to use?	☐	☐	☐	☐
3. Is the inside of the nursing home clean and in good repair?	☐	☐	☐	☐
4. Does the nursing home have handrails in hallways and grab bars in bathrooms?	☐	☐	☐	☐
5. When floors are being cleaned, are warning signs displayed, or are areas blocked off to prevent accidents?	☐	☐	☐	☐
6. Is the nursing home free from unpleasant odors?	☐	☐	☐	☐
7. Are toilets convenient to bedrooms?	☐	☐	☐	☐
8. Do noise levels fit the activities that are going on?	☐	☐	☐	☐
9. Is it easy for residents in wheelchairs to move around the home?	☐	☐	☐	☐
10. Is the lighting appropriate for what residents are doing?	☐	☐	☐	☐
11. Are there private areas for residents to visit with family, visitors, or physicians?	☐	☐	☐	☐
12. Are residents' bedrooms furnished in a pleasant manner?	☐	☐	☐	☐
13. Do the residents have some personal items in their bedrooms (for example, family pictures, souvenirs, a chair)?	☐	☐	☐	☐
14. Do the residents' rooms have accessible storage areas for residents' personal items?	☐	☐	☐	☐

Other Things to Look For

	Home A		Home B	
1. Does the nursing home have a good reputation in the community?	☐	☐	☐	☐
2. Does the nursing home have a list of references?	☐	☐	☐	☐
3. Is the nursing home convenient for family or friends to visit?	☐	☐	☐	☐
4. Does the local ombudsman visit the facility regularly?	☐	☐	☐	☐

© U.S. Department of Health and Human Services, Health Care Financing Administration.

NURSING HOME RESOURCES

NATIONAL ASSOCIATIONS

National Citizens' Coalition on Nursing
Home Reform
1224 M Street, N.W.
Suite 301
Washington, DC 20005-5183
(202) 393-2018
This national resource has an abundance of excellent literature and can refer you to state and local resources. Membership: individual $40, age 65 and older $10, nursing home residents $2.

American Association of Retired
Persons
601 East Street, N.W.
Washington, DC 20049
(202) 434-2277

PUBLICATIONS

The American Association of Retired Persons (address above) offers the following publications.

"Encountering Problems in Nursing Homes" (D13714).
"Long-Term Care Ombudsman Program" (D13717).
"Medicaid Discrimination and Consumer Rights" (D13715).
"New Protection of Nursing Home Residents' Rights" (D13713).
"Nursing Home Life: A Guide for Residents and Family" (D13063).
"The Nursing Home Regulatory System" (D13716).
"A Practical Guide to Nursing Home Advocacy" (D13878).

STATE RESOURCES

Your state Medicaid Agency establishes the rates the states pay nursing facilities for their services. They receive annual cost reports from facilities, which are made available to the public.

Your state Medicaid Fraud Control Unit is authorized by the federal Social Security Act to investigate fraud and abuse by providers that receive payments from Medicare and Medicaid. Most units are within the office of the State Attorney General. They have broad investigative powers and can bring criminal cases against providers.

Your state Board of Examiners for Nursing Home Administrators oversees the federally mandated practice of licensing nursing home administrators. States establish boards to set standards for other professional personnel, including registered nurses, physical therapists, social workers, physicians, dentists, and optometrists, all of whom might come in contact with nursing home residents.

Your state Peer Review Organization is a nonprofit board of physicians that contracts with federal and state governments to handle quality and cost complaints involving physicians paid by the Medicare program, and often Medicaid and private payers as well.

Your state Adult Protection and Advocacy System has offices to assist the mentally ill and developmentally disabled. Staff of this program may enter a facility and take action to protect a resident in danger.

NOTES

[1]Anderson-Ellis, E., *Aging Parents and You* (New York: MasterMedia, 1993).

[2]Ferrell, B., Ferrell, B., Osterweil, D., "Pain in the Nursing Home," *Journal of the American Geriatric Society,* 38 (1990), 409–14.

[3]Ferrell, B., Ferrell, B., "Epidemiology of Pain in the Nursing Home Population," American Pain Society 11th Annual Scientific Meeting, San Diego, October 22–25, 1992.

[4]National Citizens' Coalition for Nursing Home Reform, 1993.

10

NEAR THE END OF LIFE

Dying in pain . . . It is a horrifying thought. The reality is deplorable, but many patients in fact do die in pain. Their suffering is needless, and can almost always be avoided.

Every patient can achieve some level of pain relief or, in the majority of cases, total pain relief. State-of-the-art pain management techniques that are available to patients today leave doctors, nurses, and health care professionals with no excuse for inadequate pain control.

As mentioned, unrelieved pain can lead to anxiety, depression, inactivity, helplessness, hopelessness, and sometimes thoughts of suicide.

If health care professionals were to imagine themselves in the place of the patient with months or weeks to live, and ask themselves, "How would I want to be treated if this were my circumstance?" perhaps more attention would be given to the control of pain.

It is ethically, morally, medically, and legally wrong to deny dying patients pain control.

Pain-relieving drugs should be administered for an acceptable level of patient comfort, without regard to irrational fears of addiction or respiratory depression or misconceptions that pain-relieving drugs such as morphine must be doled out or that there is a ceiling dose beyond which no more drug can be given.

Pain control near the end of life, hospices, and family support are subjects that are rarely covered in medical, nursing, or health care professional school curricula or in hospital training programs. Admitting that dying is part of life is an idea that is often opposed by members of the medical community, who are trained in the medical-technical mode. To allow a patient to die is to admit failure. Somewhere along the line, compassion has not kept pace with technology. *The technology is there, so it must be used.* We are a nation of extended life and medical miracles that often exclude preparation for and attention to the dying process.

Elisabeth Kübler-Ross, who has written extensively on death and dying, notes that fear of dying translates into a denial of death by professionals and patients alike. Because of the denial, there is reluctance to be involved with the dying patient and his or her needs. As Dr. Betty Ferrell says, "The reason we do such a pathetic job of pain control is because we do a pathetic job with dying."[1]

Robert G. Twycross, D.M., F.R.C.P., the Macmillan Clinical Reader in Palliative Medicine at Oxford University, notes that for the patient near the end of life

> . . . the primary aim is no longer to prolong life but to make the life that remains as comfortable and as meaningful as possible. Thus, what may be appropriate treatment in the acutely ill patient may be inappropriate in the dying patient. Cardiac resuscitation, artificial respiration, intravenous infusion, nasogastric tubes and antibiotics are all primarily supportive measures for use in acute non-chronic illnesses to assist a patient through the initial period toward recovery of health. To use such measures in patients who are clearly close to death, and who have no expectancy of a return to health, is generally inappropriate, and therefore "bad" medicine. We have no right or duty, legal or ethical, to prescribe a lingering death.[2]

Earlier, the guidelines for acute, cancer, and chronic pain management were discussed. There are also *unique pain guidelines for the patient near the end of life.*

PLANNING AHEAD OF ILLNESS

One of the most effective means to help ensure that unrelieved pain will not be a terrifying reality for the patient approaching death is to plan ahead.

Legally and medically, it is possible to let family, friends, doctor, and attorney know exactly how aggressively you want to be treated in the hospital if you are in a life-threatening medical crisis or are actively dying. Whether you can or cannot act for yourself, you will have provided your doctors, nurses, and family with a blueprint of to what lengths you want medical technology to be employed to maintain your life, such as the use of mechanical breathing machines, hydration, nutrition, and pain control.

The goal is to give you as much autonomy as possible, to ensure that your final days will reflect your right to self-determination and dignity.

The cases of Karen Ann Quinlan and Nancy Cruzan stick in the mind like a hot ember as examples of what happens when patients are unable to act in their own behalf and have not indicated in advance what level of medical intervention they want if they become hopelessly ill.

State, Federal, and Medical Laws and Recommendations

There are state and federal laws that permit patients the right of self-determination through such instruments as a "Living Will," "Durable Power of Attorney," and hospital admission "Patient Directives." However, if you don't plan ahead for the day when an accident leaves you unconscious, you have a major heart attack, or you are in the last stages of cancer, you could be another Karen Ann Quinlan—with your family saying, "She would never want to live like this," and the medical and legal community saying, "Show us proof of what her wishes were." It is not comforting to think that perfect strangers can make life decisions about you. *You need to let your wishes be known to your family and your lawyer, and make sure that your doctor has a copy of your statement of intent.* It is even recommended that you carry a one-page synopsis of your wishes with your driver's license. Currently less than 15% of all adult patients make Living Wills or Proxy Directives.

There are national recommendations in place regarding ethical guidelines for the use of life-sustaining medical technologies. The Office of the President, Congress, the American Medical Association, and the American Nurses' Association, among others, have all put forth recommendations. The recommendations are based on the law.

Court cases have recognized the power of patients' Advance Directives, Treatment Directives, and Proxy Appointments through legislation, court decisions, or both. In 1990 the Supreme Court noted in the *Cruzan* decision that constitutional protection of the right to refuse treatment could be inferred from the Court's earlier decisions. In 1990

Congress passed the Federal Patient Self-Determination Act, which ties Medicaid and Medicare reimbursement to hospitals and other health care facilities to the requirement that patients be informed about their right to accept or refuse medical or surgical treatment and the right to formulate advance directives.

"The consensus manifested in these rulings and laws is also reflected in hospital accreditation standards. The Joint Commission's 1992 Accreditation Manual for Hospitals requires institutions to have mechanisms for supporting patients' rights and participation in health care decision-making, and requires that institutions have a system for educating staff about the appropriate use of advance directives," write the researchers in a 1993 study on "Decisions Near the End of Life: Professional Views on Life-Sustaining Treatments" for the *American Journal of Public Health.*[3]

It is clear that there is widespread literature, health care policy, federal law, and hospital regulations that agree that patients have the right of self-determination. However, there is a serious question about how faithfully those recommendations are being implemented in hospitals by doctors and nurses.

Lack of Pain Care Near the End of Life

A survey was conducted by Mildred Z. Solomon, Ed. D., et al. to assess the knowledge and practice of guideline recommendations of 687 physicians and 759 nurses in five hospitals. The results were disturbing. Almost 50% of all respondents and 70% of the house officers reported that they had acted against their conscience in providing care to the dying.

The majority of doctors and nurses were "disturbed by the degree to which technological solutions influence care during the final days of a terminal illness and by the undertreatment of pain."

Lack of adequate pain control was reported by 81% of all doctors and nurses as "the most common form of 'narcotic abuse' in the care of the dying patient. Up to 44% of nurses believed that "clinicians give inadequate pain medications most often out of fear of hastening a patient's death."[4]

Arthur David Charap, Ph.D., M.D., conducted a survey to assess the knowledge, attitudes, and experience of medical personnel in the care of the dying. The results showed a lack of knowledge not only of the newer methods of pain management but also of the fundamental principles governing analgesic therapy. He noted a hit-or-miss manner in which dying patients were cared for. In his experience, many patients seemed to be continually complaining of varying degrees of pain and claiming that their pain could have been controlled by opioids [morphine-like drugs]. *He found the care of dying patients to be "haphazard and insensible at best but in many instances exceedingly cruel and inhuman."*[5]

Medical Directives

Below is a Medical Directive that states your wishes regarding various types of medical treatment in several representative situations, so that your desires might be respected. It becomes effective only if you are incapable of making decisions or expressing your wishes. You will be able to designate a person (called a proxy decision maker) to make decisions for you if a situation arises that is not covered in the directive.

- You can also make a personal statement about things that you feel are important to you.
- You will need to sign and date it in the presence of two witnesses, who must sign and date it. You don't need to have it notarized.
- To know the specific law in your state, call the office of the state attorney general or consult a lawyer.
- When the directive is completed, give a copy of it to your doctor(s), your proxy or proxies, and anyone else you want to know about it.
- Do not stash it away where it is not accessible.

You can change your proxy at any time or change your wishes on the form if you desire. Some individuals fear that making out a medical directive is an indication that they don't want to live, or that somehow they are giving up control of their lives. However, considering the alternative—having strange doctors or nurses making decisions about your life without your participation—the medical directive is certainly the more desirable option. It is recommended that everyone, even young men and women in their twenties, make out a directive.

The following is an example of a Medical Directive.

The Medical Directive*

Introduction. As part of a person's right to self-determination, every adult may accept or refuse any recommended medical treatment. This is relatively easy when people are well and can speak. Unfortunately, during severe illness people are often unconscious or otherwise unable to communicate their wishes—at the very time when many critical decisions need to be made.

The Medical Directive states your wishes regarding various types of medical treatment in several representative situations so that your desires can be respected. It comes into effect only if you become incompetent (unable to make decisions or to express your wishes), and you can change it at any time until then. As long as you are competent, you should discuss your care directly with your physician.

The Medical Directive also lets you appoint someone to make medical decisions for you if you should become unable to make your own; this is a proxy or durable power of attorney. Additionally, it contains a statement of your wishes concerning organ donation.

The following pages contain a Medical Directive form on which you can record your own desires. Since such wishes usually reflect personal, philosophical, and religious views, you may want to discuss the issues with your family, friends, or religious mentor before completing the form.

Completing the Form. First you will be asked to consider four different situations that involve mental incompetence: an irreversible coma or a persistent vegetative state (situation A); a coma with very slight and uncertain chance of recovery (situation B); irreversible brain damage or brain disease together with a terminal illness (situation C); and irreversible brain damage or disease but with no terminal illness (situation D). For each of these situations, you will be asked to indicate your wishes concerning possible medical interventions ranging from pain medications to resuscitation. You can refuse a certain treatment or request that it definitely be used, should it be medically appropriate. Alternatively, you can state that you are unsure about your preference for the treatment, or that you would like it tried for a while but discontinued if it does not result in definite improvement. This phase of completing the Medical Directive is best done in discussion with your physician.

Next you will be given the opportunity to designate a proxy decision-maker. This person would be asked to make decisions under circumstances in which your wishes are unclear—for example, if your situation is not covered in this

*© 1990 by the American Medical Association. All rights reserved. Adapted with permission from Emanuel, L. L., Emanuel, E. J., "The Medical Directive: A New Comprehensive Advance Care Document," *JAMA* 261:3288–3293, June 9, 1989. Published as a supplement to the *Harvard Medical School Health Letter*, June 1990. Reprint permission granted by L. L. Emanuel and E. J. Emanuel, 1993.

document or if your preference is undecided. (It is expected, in the former case, that the proxy would be significantly guided whenever possible by your choices in situations A–D.) You can indicate whether the proxy's decisions should override (or be overridden by) your wishes. And, should you name more than one proxy, you can state who is to have the final say if there is disagreement.

Then you will be able to express your preference concerning organ donation. Do you wish to donate your body or some or all of your organs after your death? If so, for what purpose(s) and to which physician or institution?

Before recording a personal statement in the Medical Directive, you may find it helpful to consider the following question. What kind of medical condition, if any, would make life hard enough that you would find attempts to prolong it undesirable? None? Intractable pain? Permanent dependence on others? Irreversible mental damage? Another condition you would regard as intolerable? Under circumstances such as these, medical intervention may include only securing comfort; it may involve using ordinary treatments while avoiding more invasive ones; or employing those that offer improved function; or trying anything appropriate to prolonging life—regardless of quality. You should record here anything you feel is necessary to clarify your personal values concerning the limits of life and the goals of medical intervention.

What to Do with the Form. Finally, to make the Medical Directive effective you will need to sign and date it in the presence of two witnesses. They must sign and date the form as well. You don't need to have it notarized. States vary in the details of legislation covering documents of this sort. If you wish to know the laws in your state, you should call the office of its attorney general or consult a lawyer privately. If your state has a statutory document, you may want to complete the Medical Directive and append it to this form.

You should give a copy of the completed document to your personal physician, as well as to a family member or a friend, to ensure that it will be available if it is needed. Your physician should have a copy of it placed in your medical records and should flag it so that anyone who might be involved in your care can be aware of its presence.

WHAT ARE THE ALTERNATIVES?

The first goal is to recognize the inherent dignity of the human being, the right to a quality of life, and the right to adequate pain management.

The basis and importance of the quality of life has been addressed in Chapter 5. William M. Lamer, Jr., M.D., of the Bresler Center in Santa Monica, California writes, "It appears to me that the concept we call quality of life knows no national boundaries, no social or ethnic distinction, no age limits. No matter who they are or where they are, persons

	SITUATION A	SITUATION B:
MY MEDICAL DIRECTIVE This Medical Directive expresses, and shall stand for, my wishes regarding medical treatments in the event that illness should make me unable to communicate them directly. I make this Directive, being 18 years or more of age, of sound mind, and appreciating the consequences of my decisions.	If I am in a coma or a persistent vegetative state and, in the opinion of my physician and several consultants, have no known hope of regaining awareness and higher mental functions no matter what is done, then my wishes regarding use of the following, if considered medically reasonable, would be:	If I am in a coma and, in the opinion of my physician and several consultants, have a small likelihood of recovering fully, a slightly larger likelihood of surviving with permanent brain damage, and a much larger likelihood of dying, then my wishes regarding use of the following, if considered medically reasonable, would be:

	I want	I want treatment tried. If no clear improvement, stop.	I am undecided	I do not want	I want	I want treatment tried. If no clear improvement, stop.	I am undecided	I do not want
Cardiopulmonary Resuscitation: if at the point of death, using drugs and electric shock to keep the heart beating; artificial breathing.		Not applicable				Not applicable		
Mechanical Breathing: breathing by machine.								
Atificial Nutrition and Hydration: giving nutrition and fluid through a tube in the veins, nose, or stomach.								
Major Surgery, such as removing the gall bladder or part of the intestines.		Not applicable				Not applicable		
Kidney Dialysis: cleaning the blood by machine or by fluid passing through the belly.								
Chemotherapy: using drugs to fight cancer.								
Minor Surgery, such as removing some tissue from an infected toe.		Not applicable				Not applicable		
Invasive Diagnostic Tests, such as using a flexible tube to look into the stomach.		Not applicable				Not applicable		
Blood or Blood Products, such as giving transfusions.								
Antibiotics: using drugs to fight infection.								
Simple Diagnostic Tests, such as performing blood tests or x-rays.		Not applicable				Not applicable		
Pain Medications, even if they dull consciousness and indirectly shorten my life.		Not applicable				Not applicable		

SITUATION C

If I have brain damage or some brain disease that in the opinion of my physician and several consultants cannot be reversed and that makes me unable to recognize people or to speak understandably, *and I also have a terminal illness,* such as incurable cancer, that will likely be the cause of my death, then my wishes regarding use of the following, if considered medically reasonable, would be:

I want	I want treatment tried. If no clear improvement, stop.	I am un-decided	I do not want
	Not appli-cable		
	Not appli-cable		
	Not appli-cable		
	Not appli-cable		
	Not appli-cable		

SITUATION D

If I have brain damage or some brain disease that in the opinion of my physician and several consultants cannot be reversed and that makes me unable to recognize people or to speak understandably, *but I have no terminal illness,* and I can live in this condition for a long time, then my wishes regarding use of the following, if considered medically reasonable, would be:

I want	I want treatment tried. If no clear improvement, stop.	I am un-decided	I do not want
	Not appli-cable		
	Not appli-cable		
	Not appli-cable		
	Not appli-cable		
	Not appli-cable		

DURABLE POWER OF ATTORNEY

I understand that my wishes expressed in these four cases may not cover all possible aspects of my care if I become incompetent. I also may be undecided about whether I want a particular treatment or not. Consequently, there may be a need for someone to accept or refuse medical interventions for me in consultation with my physicians. I authorize

_____

_____

as my proxy(s) to make the decision for me whenever my wishes expressed in this document are insufficient or undecided.

Should there be any disagreement between the wishes I have indicated in this document and the decision favored by my above-named proxy(s),
> *(Please delete one of the following two lines.)*
I wish my proxy(s) to have authority over my Medical Directive.
> *(or)*
I wish my Medical Directive to have authority over my proxy(s).

Should there be any disagreement between the wishes of my proxies,
_____ shall have final authority.

Organ Donation

I hereby make this anatomical gift to take effect upon my death.
> *(Please check boxes and fill in blanks where appropriate.)*
I give
- ☐ my body;   ☐ any needed organs or parts;
- ☐ the following organs or parts_____

_____

to
- ☐ the following person or institution:_____

_____

- ☐ the physician in attendance at my death;
- ☐ the hospital in which I die;
- ☐ the following named physician, hospital, storage bank, or other medical institution:_____

_____

for the following purposes:
- ☐ any purpose authorized by law;   ☐ transplantation;
- ☐ therapy of another person;   ☐ research;
- ☐ medical education.

MY PERSONAL STATEMENT (use another page if necessary)

_____

_____

_____

Signed_____Date_____
Witness_____Date_____
Witness_____Date_____

with advanced, incurable illness seek relief, comfort, assurance, and support. They desire the familiar over the new, friend over stranger, calm over turmoil, hope over fear, constancy over change. They want meaning, clarity, and purpose in the midst of confusion and pain. They fear losing their identity, the sense of control, the personal contact."[6]

Near the end of life, the most important aspect of the quality of life is what can be done to help the patient feel more comfortable.

It is a time for doctors, nurses, and health care professionals to lay aside the aggressive "cure" behavior, to stop "treating" the patient according to the results of tests, and to look to the patient for direction. What is most important to the patient? What do they most want to do? What has meaning for them—to be able to play cards with a friend, work in the garden, go to church, sit up and visit with friends or family, spend quality time with children?

The question must be asked, *"What can we do to allow patients to live until they die?"*[7] notes Nessa Coyle, M.S., R.N., A.N.P., the Director of Supportive Care, Department of Neurology, Pain Service, Memorial Sloan-Kettering Cancer Center.

Patients need doctors and nurses who are not going to "treat them to death." A recent article in the *Journal of the American Medical Association* noted that in many instances that is what is taking place with cancer patients, who spend time in intensive care units being treated to death and/or returning home, where the average length of survival is three months. The cost often bankrupts the family emotionally and financially.

Patients need doctors who care about the complete human being and not just relentless treatment that offers neither hope of cure nor hope of any improved quality of life.

Howard Silverman, M.D., and Nancy Croker, R.N., M.D., of Good Samaritan Medical Center in Phoenix, notes three attributes of physicians that are essential for the care of dying patients. They are:

Temperament
Refers to values and beliefs. Specifically, the practitioner must view palliation (to relieve pain of disease, but not to cure it) as a worthy and attainable outcome that is balanced with efforts toward a cure. Adequate treatment of pain and other terminal symptoms requires a careful combination of technology and compassion. The unit of care becomes "the whole person" plus the family, rather than the sum of affected organ systems.

Skill in Terminal Care

Temperament alone is not sufficient in treating these patients; technique is also essential. Unfortunately, few physicians have specific training in caring for dying patients and therefore may avoid doing so. This accentuates the sense of loss and abandonment experienced by the patients.

Time

Time is the least available commodity for most practitioners, and care of the dying patient can consume large quantities of time. To remedy this, a multidisciplinary approach that coordinates a variety of personalities and professional services is important.[8]

ASSESSMENT AND CARE

Many of the measurement tools found in other chapters can be used for pain assessment. However, some cannot be used with certain patients near the end of life because they may *not* be able to respond to questions regarding the level of comfort. The *0–10 Numeric Pain Intensity Scale* can often be used as effectively.

0–10 Numeric Pain Intensity Scale

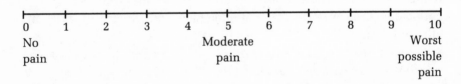

| 0 | 1 | 2 | 3 | 4 | 5 | 6 | 7 | 8 | 9 | 10 |

No pain   Moderate pain   Worst possible pain

It is important to take the time to find out what kind of pain is being experienced by the patient. A helpful assessment tool is the *Short-Form McGill Pain Questionnaire.*

The more that is known about a patient's pain, the more specific and successful the treatment plan will be.

All of the drugs and their methods of administration mentioned in other chapters are an option for these patients.

Many patients can take oral medication. Morphine is the drug of choice, because of the flexibility of dosage, method of delivery, and, if taken orally, low cost of use. There is an oral timed-release morphine that will provide pain relief for up to twelve hours. One of

Short-Form McGill Pain Questionnaire

PATIENT'S NAME: _____ DATE: _____

	NONE	MILD	MODERATE	SEVERE
THROBBING	0)_____	1)_____	2)_____	3)_____
SHOOTING	0)_____	1)_____	2)_____	3)_____
STABBING	0)_____	1)_____	2)_____	3)_____
SHARP	0)_____	1)_____	2)_____	3)_____
CRAMPING	0)_____	1)_____	2)_____	3)_____
GNAWING	0)_____	1)_____	2)_____	3)_____
HOT–BURNING	0)_____	1)_____	2)_____	3)_____
ACHING	0)_____	1)_____	2)_____	3)_____
HEAVY	0)_____	1)_____	2)_____	3)_____
TENDER	0)_____	1)_____	2)_____	3)_____
SPLITTING	0)_____	1)_____	2)_____	3)_____
TIRING–EXHAUSTING	0)_____	1)_____	2)_____	3)_____
SICKENING	0)_____	1)_____	2)_____	3)_____
FEARFUL	0)_____	1)_____	2)_____	3)_____
PUNISHING–CRUEL	0)_____	1)_____	2)_____	3)_____

NO PAIN |_____| WORST POSSIBLE PAIN

PPI [Present Pain Intensity]

0 NO PAIN _____
1 MILD _____
2 DISCOMFORTING _____
3 DISTRESSING _____
4 HORRIBLE _____
5 EXCRUCIATING _____

© R. Melzack. Reprinted by permission, 1993.

the longest-acting is MS Contin. It should be remembered there is no set dose or ceiling of dose for these patients. The right dose is the dose that relieves pain.

Pain patches, known as transdermal patches, can provide forty-eight hours or more of pain relief to patients who cannot take oral medication and cannot tolerate intravenous doses. One patch is known as Duragesic, which is Fentanyl. In addition, continuous infusions can significantly improve the quality of life for patients in the home care setting who cannot take oral medications. PCA or PCA-plus is an option which allows patients to self-administer the dose of morphine or other drugs through a preset computer. The WHO ladder can also be used as a guideline for patients to a certain point, and then the measurement of doses must be guided by the level of relief achieved. Doctors and nurses need to learn not to fear high doses of opioids.

Some patients may be depressed. As discussed, relief of pain may relieve the depression. Antidepressants can be used as an enhancer for pain relief and/or to help lift depression.

To counteract sedation, some patients can benefit from amphetamines, which can also enhance pain relief. In addition, some patients may experience anxiety. Tranquilizers can often offset anxiety and reduce the total pain experience. Tranquilizers should not be withheld from a patient in need, for fear of respiratory depression. If used properly, they are not lethal.

Nessa Coyle, R.N., notes that many times doctors and nurses are reluctant to give large doses of morphine to a patient for fear of hastening death. Sometimes they panic and think, " 'Is this pain medication helping the patient's pain or is it euthanasia?' It is important to realize that these patients may need huge doses of pain medications to manage pain."[9]

Dame Cicely Saunders, considered the founder of the hospice movement, writes, "Every time a patient dies within a short time of an injection, many families—and indeed many nurses—need reassurance that this was not the cause of death."[10]

Rosette Poletti, Ed.D., of the School of Nursing of the Swiss Red Cross in Lausanne, writes that nurses who are concerned about administering drugs should remember that *"constant pain is also a factor in abbreviating a patient's life, probably much more than morphine when it is knowledgeably administered."*[11]

It should also be remembered that if one drug does not provide pain relief, the dose may not be high enough and/or another drug should be tried.

A knowledgeable pharmacologist can help select proper doses when the patient is being switched over to a new drug. It is important to monitor a patient after switching, to watch for side effects and also for the success or failure of pain relief.

Family Care

The role of the family as caregiver, and all that it implies, has been discussed in Chapter 5. Doctors, nurses, and health care professionals need to consider the role of the family. They also need to consider the toll that is taken on the family when pain management is inadequate. It is not all that uncommon for family members to be put in the "begging," "pleading," or "screaming" role as they attempt to convince doctors, nurses, and others that their loved one needs more pain medication. It is a sorry state in which to place the family. The caregiver, already burdened with the reality of losing a loved one, suffers horribly, watching unrelieved pain hour after hour, day after day. All too often the pleas fall on deaf ears.

Dr. Betty Ferrell points out that the way a person dies has a lasting impact on the family. If a person dies "well," with pain controlled, the memory is "At least he died without suffering." If a person dies "badly" and in pain, that memory is etched indelibly in the survivors' minds.[12] To allow a person to die in pain without aggressively attempting to control pain is inexcusable. As a researcher once pointed out, the guidelines for protecting research animals from pain are often more compassionate than those for humans.

Hospice

Hospice represents a supportive philosophy of care to those whose life expectancy is measured in weeks or months. In the hospice, the emphasis is changed from the disease to the patient. Twycross notes that

> . . . [the] major goals of hospice care are to provide the patient with the following:
>
> (a) relief from pain and other distressing symptoms
> (b) psychologic care
> (c) A support system to help the patient live as actively as possible in the face of impending death
> (d) psychologic care for the family during the period of illness and bereavement

Patients with terminal diseases often need more care than those whose sickness is curable. Hospice offers intensive care for the terminally ill. Hospice philosophy is not limited by "the tyranny of cure." The National Organization of the United States states that:

> *The purpose of hospice is to provide support and care for persons in the last phases of disease so that they can live as fully as possible. Hospice affirms life and regards dying as a normal process. Hospice neither hastens nor postpones death. Hospice believes that through personalized services and a caring community, patients and families can attain the necessary preparation for a death that is satisfactory to them.*
>
> Hospice care is distinct from geriatric medicine or the care of the chronically ill, two specialites with which it is frequently compared.[13]

Hospice care is made up of an interdisciplinary team composed of professionals and volunteers who provide individual care for patients and family, usually in the home. Some hospitals have hospice care, and there are also freestanding hospices. There is no age limit for hospice care. Adults and children can receive the support of hospice programs.

In 1989 there were 1,529 operating hospices in this country. Of these, 41% were independent, 30% were operated by or directly affiliated with hospitals, 23% were operated by home health agencies, and 5% were run by other organizations. The average length of stay for patients in Medicare-certified hospice programs was 58 days.[14]

The Hospice care team usually is made up of the following:

- *Physician:* Approves plan of care.
- *Nursing:* Registered nurses provide direct patient care, check symptoms, and monitor medication.
- *Social services:* A social worker counsels the patient and family members and helps to access community resources.
- *Spiritual:* Clergy provide support for the patient and family.
- *Home services:* Homemakers and/or home health aides provide personal care for the patient and may do light housekeeping.
- *Continuous care:* Round-the-clock staffing if needed.
- *Physical therapy and occupational therapy:* Can help with daily living tasks—dressing, feeding, range of motion, etc.
- *Meals:* At-home delivery of meals and/or preparation of meals.
- *Volunteers:* Trained volunteers provide companionship and help with daily tasks, such as shopping, baby-sitting, driving, and support for patient or family.

- *Twenty-four-hour availability:* Can address emergency problems on the phone or by visit.
- *Respite care:* To relieve family members and give them some time off.
- *Bereavement counselor:* To assist the patient and family with issues on dying and death.

Guidelines for Home Hospice Care

- A life expectancy of six months or less
- Need for palliative care rather than curative treatment
- A family member or friend who can provide support
- Request to be cared for at home

Paying for Hospice Care

Medicare or Medicaid and some private insurance companies pay for hospice care. As mentioned, it is less expensive to be cared for in the home than in the hospital. In addition, it is possible to be in familiar surroundings with family and friends.

Of note and concern: At this time Medicare will pay only for intravenous medication in home hospice. Thus, a patient who needs oral morphine for pain control will have to go back to the hospital. It does not make sense, and certainly is not cost-effective. Not only does this policy cause human suffering, it costs a great deal of money to keep a patient in a hospital.

The Foundation for Hospice and Homecare, located in Washington, D.C., provides a *Hospice Patients' Bill of Rights.*

Hospice Patients' Bill of Rights

The Hospice Association of America has developed the following Hospice Patients' Bill of Rights.

Patients have a right to be notified in writing of their rights and obligations before hospice care begins. Consistent with state laws, the patient's family or guardian may exercise the patient's rights when the patient is unable to do so. Hospice organizations have an obligation to protect and promote the rights of their patients, including the following:

DIGNITY AND RESPECT

Patients and their hospice caregivers have a right to mutual respect and dignity. Caregivers are prohibited from accepting personal gifts and borrowing from patients/families/primary caregivers.

. *Patients have the right:*

- to have relationships with hospice organizations that are based on honesty and ethical standards of conduct;
- to be informed of the procedures they can follow to lodge complaints with the hospice organization about the care that is (or fails to be) furnished and regarding a lack of respect for property (to lodge complaints call the Foundation for Hospice and Homecare at 202-547-6586);
- to know about the disposition of such complaints;
- to voice their grievances without fear of discrimination or reprisal for having done so.

DECISION MAKING

Patients have the right:

- to be notified in writing of the care that is to be furnished, the types (disciplines) of caregivers who will furnish the care, and the frequency of the services that are proposed to be furnished;
- to be advised of any change in the plan of care before the change is made;
- to participate in the planning of the care and in planning changes in the care, and to be advised that they have the right to do so;
- to refuse services and to be advised of the consequences of refusing care;
- to request a change in caregiver without fear of reprisal or discrimination.

The hospice organization or the patient's physician may be forced to refer the patient to another source of care if the client's refusal to comply with the plan of care threatens to compromise the provider's commitment to quality care.

PRIVACY

Patients have the right:

- to confidentiality with regard to information about their health, social, and financial circumstances and about what takes place in the home;
- to expect the hospice organization to release information only as consistent with its internal policy, required by law, or authorized by the client.

FINANCIAL

Patients have the right:

- to be informed of the extent to which payment may be expected from Medicare, Medicaid or any other payor known to the hospice organization;
- to be informed of any charges that will not be covered by Medicare;
- to be informed of the charges for which the patient may be liable;
- to receive this information, orally and in writing, within fifteen working

days of the date the hospice organization becomes aware of any changes in charges;

- to have access, upon request, to all bills for service received, regardless of whether they are paid out-of-pocket or by another party;
- to be informed of the hospice's ownership status and its affiliation with any entities to which the patient is referred.

QUALITY OF CARE

Patients have the right:

- to receive care of the highest quality;
- to be admitted by a hospice organization only if it is assured that all necessary palliative and supportive services will be provided to promote the physical, psychological, social, and spiritual well-being of the dying patient. An organization with less than optimal resources may, however, admit the patient if a more appropriate hospice organization is not available—but only after fully informing the client of its limitations and the lack of suitable alternative arrangements; and
- to be told what to do in the case of an emergency.

The hospice organization shall assure that:

- all medically-related hospice care is provided in accordance with physician's orders and that a plan of care, which is developed by the patient's physician and the hospice interdisciplinary group in conjunction with the patient, specifies the services to be provided and their frequency and duration; and
- all medically-related personal care is provided by an appropriately trained homemaker–home health aide who is supervised by a nurse or other qualified hospice professional.

Reprinted with permission of the Foundation for Hospice and Homecare, 1993.

SUMMARY

Patients who are incurably ill and are near the end of life need to have their pain controlled. Not to attempt to control a patient's pain is morally, ethically, medically, and legally wrong. It is also cruel and inhumane.

With the state-of-the-art pain management tools available to doctors, nurses, and health care professionals, there is no excuse for inadequate pain management.

Medical directives can help patients die with control and dignity. The inclusion of a proxy or proxies who can make health care decisions if the patient cannot act for himself/herself can help to ensure that the patient's wishes will be carried out.

Hospice at home or in the hospital can provide the patient with a caring and supportive team near the end of life.

The following are national resources for hospices.

HOSPICE RESOURCES

Choice in Dying
200 Varick Street
New York, NY 10014
(212) 366-5540

A not-for-profit organization advocating the recognition and protection of individual rights at the end of life. It can provide information on life-sustaining technology, the laws of every state on advanced directives like living wills, the medical and ethical issues that arise for people at the very end of their lives, as well as booklets on such matters as pain management. Copies of living wills and health-care proxies (appropriate to each state) are free. People in difficult situations who need advice and counsel, or those who would like to request a speaker, may call Mary Meyer, associate director of education.

Children's Hospice International
901 North Washington Street, Suite 700
Alexandria, VA 22314
(800) 2-4-CHILD
In VA (703) 684-0330

Promotes pediatric hospice care through an information clearinghouse, symposia, projects, fellowships, annual conference, membership newsletter, and publications.

National Hospice Organization
1901 North Moore Street, Suite 901
Arlington, VA 22209
(800) 658-8898
In VA (703) 243-5900

An organization representing independent hospice providers. Provides referrals, advocacy, educational programs, and publications. Newsletter *NHO Hospice News.*

Good Grief Program
Judge Baker Guidance Center
295 Longwood Avenue
Boston, MA 02115
(617) 232-8390

Provides crisis intervention to schools and community groups to help children when a friend is terminally ill or dies. Resource materials. Fee.

Compassionate Friends
P.O. Box 3696
Oak Brook, IL 60522-3696
(708) 990-0010

Self-help organization for bereaved parents to assist in the positive resolution of grief experienced on death of their child and to foster physical and emotional health of bereaved families. No professional counseling. Local chapters. Publishes newsletter and other written, audio, and video materials on parent and sibling bereavement.

American Association of Retired
  Persons
601 East Street, N.W.
Washington, DC 20049
(202) 434-2277

Purdue Frederick Company
100 Connecticut Avenue
Norwalk, CT 06850-3590

Offers "Home Care of the Hospice Patient," an information/instructional booklet for caregivers in the home.

Elisabeth Kübler-Ross offers her famous "Life, Death, and Transition Workshops" at various locations around the country. Call (703) 396-3441.

NOTES

[1]Ferrell, B., personal communication, 1993.

[2]Twycross, R. G., "Terminal Care of Cancer Patients: Hospice and Home Care," *The Management of Pain*, second edition, ed. Bonica, J. (Philadelphia: Lea & Febiger, 1990), vol. 1, 446.

[3]Solomon, M., O'Donnell, L., Jennings, B., et al., "Decisions Near the End of Life: Professional Views on Life-Sustaining Treatments," *American Journal of Public Health*, vol. 83, no. 1 (January 1993), 14–25.

[4]Solomon, M., O'Donnell, L., Jennings, B., et al., "Decisions Near the End of Life: Professional Views on Life-Sustaining Treatments," *American Journal of Public Health*, vol. 83, no. 1 (January 1993), 14–25.

[5]Charap, A. D., "The Knowledge, Attitudes and Experience of Medical Personnel Treating Pain in the Terminally Ill," *Mount Sinai Journal of Medicine*, vol. 45, no. 4 (July–August 1978), 561–77.

[6]Lamers, W. M., "Hospice: Enhancing the Quality of life," *Oncology*, May 1990.

[7]Coyle, N., "The Nature of Terminal Illness in the Cancer Patient: Pain and Other Symptoms in the Last Four Weeks of Life," Innovations in Cancer Pain: Assessment and Treatment, First International Nursing Research Symposium on Cancer Pain, University of Washington, Seattle, July 22, 1992.

[8]Silverman, H. D., Criker, N. A., "Pain in Management in Terminally Ill Patients," *Pain Management, Postgraduate Med.*, vol. 83, no. 8 (June 1988) 181.

[9]Coyle, N., "The Nature of Terminal Illness in the Cancer Patient: Pain and Other Symptoms in the Last Four Weeks of Life," Innovations in Cancer Pain: Assessment and Treatment, First International Nursing Research Symposium on Cancer Pain, University of Washington, Seattle, July 22, 1992.

[10]Saunders, C., "Pain and Impending Death," *Textbook of Pain*, ed. Wall and Melzack (New York: Churchill Livingstone, 1984), 474.

[11]Poletti, R., "Ethics of Death and Dying," *International Journal of Nursing Studies*, vol. 22, no. 4 (1985), 329–34.

[12]Ferrell, B., personal communication, 1993.

[13]Twycross, R. G., "Terminal Care of Cancer Patients: Hospice and Home Care," *The Management of Pain*, second edition, ed. Bonica, J. (Philadelphia: Lea & Febiger, 1990), vol. 1, 446.

[14]Rogarz, P., Schwartz, F., Dennis, J., "A Community Based Hospice Program," *New York State Journal of Medicine*, vol. 91, November 1992, 500.

11

PAIN CENTERS

When all other measures fail to control pain, it may be helpful for the patient to enter an outpatient or inpatient pain center.

Not all pain centers are equal, and investigation should be thorough when a patient is looking for one. Caution is advisable.

The International Association for the Study of Pain Task Force has published "Desirable Characteristics for Pain Treatment Facilities," guidelines on pain centers. The task force does not address the issues of pain management in the postoperative or post-trauma setting; rather, the emphasis is on the quality of the pain center's assessment and treatment of chronic pain. The following describes the characteristics of each type of facility:

Pain Treatment Facility:
- A generic term used to describe all forms of pain treatment facilities.

Multidisciplinary Pain Center:
- An organization of health care professionals and basic scientists which includes research, teaching, and patient care related to acute and chronic pain. Ideally, the center is part of a teaching hospital or medical school.
- Care is provided by a team made up of physicians, psychologists, nurses, physical therapists, occupational therapists, vocational counselors, social workers, and other specialized health care providers.
- Inpatient and outpatient programs are available.

Multidisciplinary Pain Clinic:
- A health care delivery facility staffed by physicians of different specialties and other nonphysician health care providers who spe-

cialize in the diagnosis and management of patients with chronic pain. This facility does not have research and teaching activities in its regular programs.
- It may be inpatient and/or outpatient.

Pain Clinic:
- A health care delivery facility focusing upon the diagnosis and management of patients' chronic pain. A pain clinic may specialize in specific diagnoses or in pain related to a specific region of the body.
- A pain clinic may be large or small, but it should never be a label for an isolated solo practitioner. A single physician functioning within a complex health care institution that offers appropriate consultative and therapeutic services could qualify as a pain clinic.

Modality-Oriented Clinic:
- This is a health care facility which offers a specific type of treatment and does not provide comprehensive assessment or management. Examples include nerve block clinic, transcutaneous nerve stimulation clinic, acupuncture clinic, biofeedback clinic, etc. Because of its limited treatment options and the lack of an integrated, comprehensive approach, it does not qualify for the term "multidisciplinary."

The following is a list of resources and pain centers.*

PAIN CENTER RESOURCES

COMMISSION ON ACCREDITATION OF REHABILITATION FACILITIES: COMPREHENSIVE PAIN MANAGEMENT

Advanced Rehabilitative Medical Arts
Indianapolis, IN

Alberta Society for the Study and
Management of Pain
Edmonton, AB, Canada

Alvarado Rehabilitation and Pain Clinic
San Diego, CA

Anaheim Hills Pain and Stress
Management Center
Anaheim, CA

Anesthesia Center for Pain
Fitchburg, MA

Anesthesia Pain Clinic/Diagnostic and
Therapeutic Nerve Block Clinic
Chapel Hill, NC

Anesthesia Pain Therapy Center
San Diego, CA

Anesthesiology Pain Clinic
Milwaukee, WI

Arthritis and Back Pain Center—
Swezey Institute
Santa Monica, CA

*Courtesy of Commission on Accreditation of Rehabilitation Facilities.

Thomas L. Ashcraft, M.D., and
Associates
Tulsa, OK

Auburn Pain Rehabilitation Medical
Clinic
Auburn, CA

Betty Bacharach Rehabilitation Hospital
Chronic Pain Management Program
Pomona, NJ

Baptist Hospital of Miami Pain
Treatment Center
Miami, FL

Baylor College Pain Control and
Functional Restoration Clinic
Houston, TX

Behavioral Medicine Clinic
Olympia, WA

Behavioral Medicine Clinic and Stress
Disorders Research Laboratory
Norfolk, VA

Behavioural Health Clinic
Toronto, ON, Canada

Beth Israel Hospital Pain Management
Center
Boston, MA

Beverly Hills Orthopedic Neurological
Group
Beverly Hills, CA

Jacob and Hilda Blaustein Pain
Treatment Center
Baltimore, MD

Booth Memorial Medical Center
Flushing, NY

Boston Pain Management Team
Boston, MA

Boulder Memorial Hospital Pain
Rehabilitation Program
Boulder, CO

Bowyer Cancer Pain Clinic
Los Angeles, CA

Brookwood Pain and Rehabilitation
Center
Birmingham, AL

Buffalo General Hospital Pain
Management Center
Buffalo, NY

Burns Clinic—Department of
Preventive and Rehabilitative
Medicine
Petoskey, MI

Butterworth Hospital Pain Management
Center
Grand Rapids, MI

Capron Pain Rehabilitation Program
Colorado Springs, CO

Cardinal Hill Hospital Comprehensive
Pain Management Program
Lexington, KY

Casa Colina Hospital Comprehensive
Back Services and Pain Disorders
Program
Pomona, CA

Center for Behavioral Medicine
Radford, VA

Center for Pain and Stress Management
West Hills, CA

Center for Pain Control and
Rehabilitation
Cape Coral, FL

Center for Pain Management at St.
Francis Hospital
Pittsburgh, PA

Center for Pain Studies
Chicago, IL

Chapman General Hospital Chronic
Pain Control Program
Orange, CA

Charter Suburban Hospital Drug-Free
Pain Management Center
Paramount, CA

Chedoke-McMaster Pain Program
Hamilton, ON, Canada

Chicago Osteopathic Medical Centers
Chicago, IL

Child Health Research Institute
London, ON, Canada

Children's Hospital and Medical Center
Seattle, WA

Children's Hospital of Philadelphia Pain
Management Program
Philadelphia, PA

Chronic Pain Assessment and
Management Service
Vancouver, BC, Canada

Cleveland Clinic Foundation Pain
Management Unit
Cleveland, OH

Clinic for Pain Management
Clearwater, FL

Columbia Centre for Integrated Health
Services
Vancouver, BC, Canada

Columbia-Presbyterian Medical Center
Pain Treatment Service
New York, NY

Columbia University School of Dental
and Oral Surgery, TMJ and Facial
Pain Clinic
New York, NY

Comprehensive Back, Pain, and Work
Center
Knoxville, TN

Comprehensive Medical Rehabilitation
Center
Lexington, KY

Comprehensive Medical Rehabilitation
Center
Fort Lauderdale, FL

Comprehensive Pain Management
Center
Sarasota, FL

Comprehensive Pain Therapy Center
Plainview, NY

Controlling Our Pain Effectively Center
Vestal, NY

Cranio-Facial Pain Center of Boston
Boston, MA

Craniofacial Pain TMJ Clinic
San Francisco, CA

Dartmouth Hitchcock Medical Center
Pain Management Service
Hanover, NH

Day Surgery of Independence—Pain
Management
Independence, MO

Dekalb Pain Management and
Rehabilitation Center
Decatur, GA

Delaware Pain Clinic
Newark, DE

Diamond Headache Clinic
Chicago, IL

Doctors Pain Clinic
Youngstown, OH

Downstate Headache Center
Brooklyn, NY

Duke Pain Clinic
Durham, NC

Durango Pain Rehabilitation Center
Durango, CO

Eastern Maine Medical Center Pain
Program
Bangor, ME

Elmbrook Memorial Hospital
Brookfield, WI

Elyria Pain Clinic
Elyria, OH

Emanuel Pain Center
Portland, OR

Englewood Pain Clinic
Englewood, NJ

Essex County Pain Management Center
Orange, NJ

Facial Pain Research Center
San Francisco, CA

Fair Oaks Hospital Pain Program
Fairfax, VA

Fairview General Hospital Pain
Management Center
Cleveland, OH

Farmbrook Pain Control Center
Southfield, MI

Ellis Fischel Cancer Center
Columbia, MO

Fort Worth Back Institute
Fort Worth, TX

Gastrointestinal Pain Center
Baltimore, MD

Gateway Institute
Bethlehem, PA

Gateway Pain Center
Bridgeton, MO

General Health Science Centre Pain
Clinic
Winnipeg, MB, Canada

General Hospital Pain Clinic
Winnipeg, MB, Canada

Georgia Baptist Medical Center Pain
Management Program
Atlanta, GA

Good Samaritan Hospital and Medical
Center Pain Clinic
Portland, OR

Good Samaritan Medical Center Pain
Management Program
Zanesville, OH

John R. Graham Headache Centre
Boston, MA

Great Jersey Pain Management Center
Voorhees, NJ

Great Lakes Regional Rehabilitation
Center Pain Program
Lorain, OH

Greensboro Rehabilitation Center
Greensboro, NC

Hahnemann University Pain Treatment
Program
Philadelphia, PA

Harmarville Rehabilitation Center—
Chronic Pain Program
Pittsburgh, PA

Harvard Medical School Children's
Hospital Pain Treatment Service
Boston, MA

HCA Lewis-Gale Hospital Pain Control
Center
Salem, VA

HCA Portsmouth Hospital Pain Center
Portsmouth, NH

Headache Management and Neurology
Pensacola, FL

Headache Management Center
Winter Park, FL

Headache Treatment Center of Orange
County
Tustin, CA

Healing Resources
Walnut Creek, CA

Hennepin Pain Clinic and Research
Center
Minneapolis, MN

Hillside Rehabilitation Hospital Chronic
Pain Treatment Program
Warren, OH

Hopital Hotel-Dieu de Montreal
Clinique Anti-douleur
Montreal, PQ, Canada

Hotel Dieu Hospital Pain Treatment
Center
New Orleans, LA

Houston Pain Center
Houston, TX

Humana Hospital Pain Management
Center
Baytown, TX

Fred Hutchinson Cancer Research
Center Pain and Toxicity Research
Program
Seattle, WA

Illinois Masonic Medical Center Pain
Treatment Center
Chicago, IL

Incentives
York, PA

Indiana Center for Rehabilitation
Medicine
Indianapolis, IN

Indiana University Pain Clinic
Indianapolis, IN

Industrial Rehabilitation Center
Baltimore, MD

Ingham Medical Center Pain Clinic
Lansing, MI

Institute for Behavioral Medicine
Providence, RI

Institute for Complementary Medicine
Victoria, BC, Canada

Institute of Pain Management
Ceres, CA

Institution for Functional and
Occupational Restoration
Walla Walla, WA

Interdisciplinary Chronic Pain
Management Center
Augusta, GA

Iowa Methodist Pain Management
Center
Des Moines, IA

Thomas Jefferson Pain Center
Philadelphia, PA

Jewish Hospital of Cincinnati Pain
Center
Cincinnati, OH

Joliet Headache and Neurology Center
Joliet, IL

Kansas City Pain Consortium
Leawood, KS

Kansas University Medical Center Pain
Clinic
Kansas City, KS

Sister Kenny Institute Chronic Pain
Rehabilitation Program
Minneapolis, MN

Kessler Institute for Rehabilitation
East Orange, NJ

Kim Rehabilitation Institute
West Orange, NJ

Kingston General Hospital
Kingston, ON, Canada

Kingwood Hospital Pain Management
Center
Michigan City, IN

Klein Clinic
Gainesville, FL

Lafayette General Pain Management
Center
Lafayette, LA

Lahey Clinic Out-Patient Pain
Management Program
Burlington, MA

Lake Forest Hospital Pain Treatment
Center
Lake Forest, IL

Lakes Area Human Services
Lindstrom, MN

Lakeshore Pain Management Center
Birmingham, AL

Lansing Pain Management Services
Lansing, MI

Laval University Hospital Pain Control
Center
Sainte-Foy, PQ, Canada

Ronald M. Lawrence, M.D., Ph.D.
Agoura, CA

Lenox Hill Hospital Pain Evaluation
and Treatment Service
New York, NY

Gertrude Levin Pain Clinic
Detroit, MI

Jeffrey H. Levy Center for Pain Control
Walnut Creek, CA

Litchfield Rehabilitation Center Chronic
Pain Treatment Program
Akron, OH

Lourdes Regional Rehabilitation Center
Camden, NJ

Loyola University Medical Center Pain
Treatment Center
Maywood, IL

Magee Rehabilitation Hospital Pain
Management/Rehabilitation Services
Philadelphia, PA

Maimonides Medical Center
Brooklyn, NY

Michael Margoles, M.D.
San Jose, CA

Clorinda G. Margolis and Associates PC
Philadelphia, PA

Marianjoy Rehabilitation Center
Wheaton, IL

Marquette General Hospital Pain
Management Center
Marquette, MI

Mayo Clinic
Rochester, MN

McGill Pain Management Centre
Montreal, PQ, Canada

McMaster University Health Science
Centre Acupuncture Clinic
Hamilton, ON, Canada

Medical Center for Pain Control
Houston, TX

Medical College of Virginia Facial Pain
Management Program
Richmond, VA

Medical College of Virginia Pain
Management Center
Richmond, VA

Medical Ergonomic and Therapeutic
Services
San Rafael, CA

Medical Illness Counseling Center Pain
Program
Chevy Chase, MD

Medical University of South Carolina
Chronic Pain Rehabilitation Program
Charleston, SC

Memorial Pain Management Program
Long Beach, CA

Mercy Center for Health Care Services
Pain Treatment Center
Aurora, IL

Mercy Hospital Nerve Block Center
Des Moines, IA

Mercy Hospital Pain Center
Des Moines, IA

Methodist Hospital Pain Management
Program
Houston, TX

Methodist Medical Center of Illinois
Pain Management Clinic
Peoria, IL

Metropolitan Hospital Center for Pain
Control
Richmond, VA

Michigan Headache and Neurological
Institute
Ann Arbor, MI

Midcities Headache and Pain Clinic
Hunt, TX

Mid-Hudson Pain Management
Physicians
Kingston, NY

Mills-Peninsula Hospitals Injured
Workers Program
Burlingame, CA

Milwaukee County Medical Complex
Pain Clinic
Milwaukee, WI

Minnesota Head and Neck Pain Clinic
Minneapolis, MN

Misericordia Hospital Palliative Case
Service
Edmonton, AB, Canada

H. Lee Moffitt Cancer Center and
Research Institute
Tampa, FL

Monmouth Medical Center Pain
Treatment Center
Long Branch, NJ

Montefiore Medical Center Headache
Unit
Bronx, NY

Mt. Diablo Hospital Pain Management
Center
Concord, CA

Mt. Sinai Medical Center Pain
Management Center
New York, NY

Mt. Sinai Pain Management Center
Bloomfield, CT

Musculoskeletal Injury Rehabilitation
Program
Mechanicsburg, PA

Nassau Pain and Stress Center
Mineola, NY

Neurological Rehabilitation Center
Tamarac, FL

Neuropsychiatric Pain Rehabilitation
Clinic
New Port Richey, FL

New Directions Rehabilitation Center
Pain Management Program
Inglewood, CA

New Jersey Dental School Center for
TMJ and Orofacial Pain Management
Newark, NJ

New Mexico Pain and Rehabilitation
Clinic
Albuquerque, NM

New York Pain Treatment Program
New York, NY

New York University Medical Center
Comprehensive Pain Center
New York, NY

New York University Medical Center
Pain Management Center
New York, NY

Newport Hospital Pain Management
Center
Newport, RI

Newport Pain and Neurodiagnostic
Center
Newport Beach, CA

North Carolina Memorial Hospital Pain
Management Program
Chapel Hill, NC

North Coast Center
Eureka, CA

North County Pain Management Center
Carlsbad, CA

North Fullerton Regional Hospital
Disability Medicine Program
Roswell, GA

Northern California Pain and
Rehabilitation Program
Redding, CA

Northwest Pain Center Associates
Portland, OR

Northwestern Memorial Hospital
Department of Anesthesia Pain
Control Unit
Chicago, IL

Norton Hospital Pain Management
Program
Louisville, KY

Oklahoma Spine Pain Management
Clinic—Working Back Clinic
Oklahoma City, OK

Oregon Health Sciences University Pain
Management Center
Portland, OR

Oregon Pain Center
Springfield, OR

Orthopaedic-Arthritis Pain Center
New York, NY

Osteopathic Hospital of Maine Pain
Control Center
Portland, ME

Outpatient Pain Management Center
Billings, MT

Pacific Spine and Pain Center
Ashland, OR

Pain Alleviation Center
Roslyn, NY

Pain and Rehabilitation Center
New Orleans, LA

Pain and Stress Management Clinic
San Leandro, CA

Pain Clinic of Colorado Springs PC
Colorado Springs, CO

Pain Clinic of the Group Health Centre
Sault Sainte Marie, ON, Canada

Pain Control and Rehabilitation Institute
of Georgia
Decatur, GA

Pain Control Center
Winston-Salem, NC

Pain Control Center of America
Lauderdale Lakes, FL

Pain Control Center of Beverly Hills
Beverly Hills, CA

Pain Control Clinic
Saginaw, MI

Pain, Headache and Rehabilitation
Clinic
Port Orange, FL

Pain Institute of Nevada
Las Vegas, NV

Pain Management and Behavioral
Medicine Center
Farmington, CT

Pain Management Associates
Beverly Hills, CA

Pain Management Center
San Clemente, CA

Pain Management Center of New
England
Hamden, CT

Pain Management Clinic
Monterey, CA

Pain Management Consultants
Chicago, IL

Pain Management Consultants
Whittier, CA

Pain Management Foundation of Dallas
Dallas, TX

Pain Management Group
Tempe, AZ

Pain Management Program at
Behavioral Health and Rehabilitation
Orlando, FL

Pain Rehabilitation and Biofeedback
Center of West Georgia
Austell, GA

Pain Rehabilitation and Thermography
Center of Westchester
White Plains, NY

Pain Therapy Center of Greenville
Greenville, SC

Pain Therapy Medical Clinic
Hemet, CA

Pain Treatment Center of Central
Pennsylvania
Mechanicsburg, PA

Pain Treatment Center of Psychological
Services
Annapolis, MD

Pain Treatment Centers
San Diego, CA

Paincare Centers of America
Big Bear Lake, CA

PAINWAY
Pekin, IL

Y. S. Palchick, D.D.S.
Akron, OH

Pathways Medical Center
Richmond, VA

Pennsylvania Pain Rehabilitation Center
Doylestown, PA

Physicians and Surgeons Hospital
Center for Pain Management
Shreveport, LA

Piedmont Physical Medicine and
Rehabilitation
Greenville, SC

Pilling Pain Clinic
Minneapolis, MN

Pipp Community Hospital Center for
Pain Management
Plainwell, MI

Pocatello Regional Medical Center Pain
Management Programme
Pocatello, ID

Presbyterian University Hospital Pain
Control Center
Pittsburgh, PA

Providence Hospital Pain Control
Center
Everett, WA

Providence Hospital Pain Control
Center
Southfield, MI

Providence Hospital Pain Rehabilitation
Center
Cincinnati, OH

REACT Center
Marietta, GA

Redwood Center Medical Clinic
Santa Rosa, CA

Rehabilitation Center for Pain
Indianapolis, IN

Rehabilitation Centre
Ottawa, ON, Canada

Rehabilitation Institute
Glendale, CA

Rehabilitation Institute of Chicago
Center for Pain Studies
Chicago, IL

Rehabilitation Institute of Sarasota
Sarasota, FL

Rehabilitation Medicine Center of New
Jersey
Wayne, NJ

Jack Richman Acupuncture Therapy
Oakville, ON

Richmond Pain Clinic
Richmond, VA

Rio Grande Health Center
El Paso, TX

Robb Pain Management Group
Los Angeles, CA

Royal Victoria Hospital Pain
Management Centre,
Montreal, PQ, Canada

Rush Pain Center
Chicago, IL

Rusk Rehabilitation Center and Pain
Management Program
Columbia, MO

Sacre-Coeur Hospital
Montreal, PQ, Canada

Sacred Heart Medical Center Pain Clinic
Spokane, WA

St. Alphonsus Regional Medical Center
Pain Management Clinic
Boise, ID

St. Boniface Hospital Pain Clinic
Winnipeg, MB, Canada

St. Charles Hospital Pain Management
Center
Toledo, OH

St. Cloud Hospital Pain Management
Center
Saint Cloud, MN

St. David's Hospital Pain Management
Program
Austin, TX

St. Helena Hospital Pain Rehabilitation
Center
Deer Park, CA

St. Johns Hospital Pain Management
Center
Santa Monica, CA

St. Joseph Hospital Pain Management
Program
Baltimore, MD

St. Joseph Hospital Palliative Care
Program
Nashua, NH

St. Joseph's Health Centre Chronic Pain
Unit
London, ON, Canada

St. Joseph's Hospital and Medical
Center Pain Program
Phoenix, AZ

St. Joseph's Hospital Pain Therapy
Center
Asheville, NC

St. Joseph's Medical Center Pain
Rehabilitation Unit
South Bend, IN

St. Jude Hospital Pain Center
Fullerton, CA

St. Louis University Pain Management
Program
St. Louis, MO

St. Luke's Hospital Pain Management
Center
Kansas City, MO

St. Luke's Hospital Pain Management
Program
Cleveland, OH

St. Mary's Pain and Rehabilitation
Center
West Palm Beach, FL

St. Vincent Hospital Pain Control
Center
Worcester, MA

San Francisco Center for
Comprehensive Pain Management
San Francisco, CA

Richard A. Sandler, M.D.
San Diego, CA

Santa Barbara Pain Center at St. Francis
Santa Barbara, CA

Santa Fe Pain Center
Santa Fe, NM

Scott and White Chronic Pain Center
Temple, TX

Scripps Memorial Hospital—Pain
Center
La Jolla, CA

Sequoia Hospital Pain Treatment Center
Redwood City, CA

Shadyside Hospital Pain Clinic
Pittsburgh, PA

Shealy Institute for Comprehensive Pain
and Health Care
Springfield, MO

Sierra Pain Institute
Reno, NV

Irene Eleanor Smythe Pain Clinic
Toronto, ON, Canada

South Side Physical Medicine Center
Chicago, IL

South Sound Oral Medicine
Federal Way, WA

Southeast Pain Management Center
Charlotte, NC

Southwest Medical Pain Management
Program
Dallas, TX

Southwest Pain Control and Sports
Therapy Center
Palm Desert, CA

Southwest Pain Control Center
Albuquerque, NM

Spalding Rehabilitation Hospital Pain
Program
Denver, CO

Spaulding Rehabilitation Hospital
Boston Pain Center
Boston, MA

Spectrum Wellness Center
Schenectady, NY

State University of New York at
Syracuse Pain Treatment Service
Syracuse, NY

State University of New York Pain
Management Service
Brooklyn, NY

Charles E. Still Hospital Jefferson City
Rehabilitation Center
Jefferson City, MO

Sunnyview Hospital and Rehabilitation
Center Chronic Pain Management
Program
Schenectady, NY

Swedish Covenant Hospital TMJ and
Facial Pain Center
Chicago, IL

Tampa General Hospital Pain
Management Program
Tampa, FL

Arthur Taub, M.D., Ph.D., PC
New Haven, CT

Temple University Pain Control Center
Philadelphia, PA

Texas Tech University Health Sciences
Center Pain Clinic
Lubbock, TX

Texas Tech University Pain Treatment
Center
El Paso, TX

Theda Pain Center
Neenah, WI

Touro Infirmary Center for Chronic Pain
and Disability Rehabilitation
New Orleans, LA

Tri-State Headache and Pain
Management Associates
Evansville, IN

Unified Pain Service
Bronx, NY

Unite de Traitement de Douleur de
L'Hopital St. Luc
Montreal, PQ, Canada

University Hospital Pain Management
Service
Saskatoon, SK, Canada

University Hospitals of Cleveland Pain
Center
Cleveland, OH

University of Alabama Birmingham
Pain Treatment Center
Birmingham, AL

University of Alabama Medical Center
Pain Control Program
Birmingham, AL

University of Arizona Pain Clinic
Tucson, AZ

University of Calgary Foothills Hospital
Pain Relief Clinic
Calgary, AB, Canada

University of California Irvine Medical
Center
Orange, CA

University of California Los Angeles
Pain Management Center
Los Angeles, CA

University of California Los Angeles
Temporomandibular and Facial Pain
Clinic
Los Angeles, CA

University of California San Francisco
Pain Clinic
San Francisco, CA

University of Illinois Hospital Pain
  Control Center
Chicago, IL

University of Massachusetts Medical
  Center Pain Control Center
Worcester, MA

University of Medicine and Dentistry,
  New Jersey Medical School, Pain
  Management Center
Newark, NJ

University of Miami Comprehensive
  Pain and Rehabilitation Center
Miami Beach, FL

University of Michigan Medical Center
  Coordinated Chronic Pain Program
Ann Arbor, MI

University of Minnesota TMJ and
  Craniofacial Pain Clinic
Minneapolis, MN

University of Nebraska Medical
  Center/Pain Management Center
Omaha, NE

University of New Mexico Pelvic Pain
  Clinic
Albuquerque, NN

University of Pennsylvania Hospital
  Anesthesia Pain Service
Philadelphia, PA

University of Pittsburgh Center for Pain
  Evaluation and Treatment
Pittsburgh, PA

University of Southern California Pain
  Management Center
Los Angeles, CA

University of Tennessee Center for
  Comprehensive Pain Control
Memphis, TN

University of Texas Center for Pain
  Medicine at Hermann
Houston, TX

University of Texas Health Science
  Center
San Antonio, TX

U.S. DEPARTMENT OF HEALTH AND HUMAN SERVICES, AGENCY FOR HEALTH CARE POLICY AND RESEARCH: ACUTE PAIN MANAGEMENT GUIDELINE PEER REVIEWERS, CONSULTANTS, AND CONTRIBUTORS

Robert G. Addison, M.D.
Director, Medical Planning
Rehabilitation Institute of Chicago

Gerald M. Aronoff, M.D.
Director, Boston Pain Center
Assistant Clinical Professor
Tufts Medical School

Charles Berde, M.D., Ph.D.
Director, Pain Treatment Service
Associate in Anesthesia
Children's Hospital, Boston
Associate Professor of Anesthesia
Harvard Medical School

Kenneth Blazier, M.D.
Department of Anesthesia
Mercy Hospital, Portland, ME

Alan Jeffry Breslau
Executive Director
Phoenix Society for Burn Survivors,
  Levittown, PA

Dorothy Y. Brockopp, R.N., Ph.D.
Clinical Nurse Researcher
Associate Professor of Nursing
University of Kentucky

Marion E. Broome, R.N., Ph.D.
Associate Professor, Assistant
  Chairperson, Maternal-Child Nursing
Rush-Presbyterian–St. Lukes Medical
  Center, Chicago

James N. Campbell, M.D.
Associate Director, Department of
  Neurosurgery
Professor of Neurosurgery
Johns Hopkins Medical School

Daniel B. Carr, M.D.
Director, Division of Pain Management,
  Department of Anesthesia
Massachusetts General Hospital

C. Richard Chapman, Ph.D.
Professor of Anesthesiology
School of Medicine, University of
  Washington

Charles Samuel Cleeland, Ph.D.
Director, World Health Organization
  Collaborating Center for Symptom
  Evaluation
Director, Pain Research Group
Professor of Neurology
University of Wisconsin Medical School

David E. Cohen, M.D.
Director, Pain Management Program
Department of Anesthesiology and
  Critical Care Medicine
Assistant Professor of Anesthesia
University of Pennsylvania

Judy M. Diekmann, R.N., Ed.D., O.C.N.
Associate Professor of Nursing
University of Wisconsin

Seymour Diamond, M.D.
Executive Director
National Headache Foundation, Chicago

Marion B. Dolan
Executive Director and President
Heritage Home Health and Heritage
  Hospice, Bristol, NH

Marilee Donovan, R.N., Ph.D.
Associate Hospital Director
Oregon Health Sciences Center

JoAnn Eland, R.N., Ph.D., F.A.A.N.
Associate Professor of Nursing
University of Iowa

Joyce Marie Engel, O.T.R., Ph.D.
Assistant Professor of Occupational
  Therapy
University of Wisconsin

Margaret Faut-Callahan, C.R.N.A.,
  DNSc, F.A.A.N.
American Association of Nurse
  Anesthetists
Associate Chairperson
Operating Room and Surgical Nursing
Rush-Presbyterian–St. Luke's Medical
  Center, Chicago

Michael Ferrante, M.D.
Director, Pain Treatment Services
Brigham and Women's Hospital
Assistant Professor of Anesthesia
Harvard Medical School

Howard L. Fields, M.D., Ph.D.
Professor, Departments of Neurology
  and Physiology
University of California, San Francisco

Roxie Foster, R.N., Ph.D.
Coordinator, Pain Management Service
Children's Hospital
Assistant Research Professor
School of Nursing, University of
  Colorado Health Sciences Center

Rollin M. Gallagher, M.D.
Director, Pain Center
Stony Brook Health Science Center
State University of New York

Randall D. Gaz, M.D.
Associate Visiting Surgeon
Massachusetts General Hospital
Assistant Professor
Harvard Medical School

Stuart A. Grossman, M.D.
Director, Neuro-Oncology
Associate Professor of Oncology and
  Medicine
Johns Hopkins Oncology Center

Kenneth M. Hargreaves, D.D.S., Ph.D.
Associate Professor of Endodontics and
  Pharmacology
University of Minnesota School of
  Dentistry

George Heidrich III, R.N., M.A.
Instructor, Department of Neurology,
  University of Wisconsin Medical
  School
Clinical Nurse Specialist Affiliate
University of Wisconsin School of
  Nursing

Ada K. Jacox, R.N., Ph.D. F.A.A.N.
Independence Foundation Chair in
  Health Policy
School of Nursing, Johns Hopkins
  University

C. Celeste Johnson, R.N., DEd
Director, Pain Group
Montreal Children's Hospital
Associate Professor
McGill University

Maryalice Jordan-Marsh, R.N., Ph.D.
American Nurses Association
Director, Nursing Research Division
Harbor-UCLA Medical Center

Steven A. King, M.D., M.S.
Director, Pain Service
Department of Psychiatry
Maine Medical Center

Arthur G. Lipman, Pharm.D.
Professor of Clinical Pharmacy
College of Pharmacy, University of Utah

Rev. Jerry L. Loch, C.R.N.A., Ph.D.
American Association of Nurse
Anesthetists

John D. Loeser, M.D.
President-Elect, International
Association for the Study of Pain
Director and Chief, Pain Service and
Multidisciplinary Pain Center
Professor of Neurological Surgery and
Anesthesia
University of Washington

Mitchell Max, M.D.
Secretary, American Pain Society
Clinical Coordinator, Pain Research
Clinic
National Institute of Dental Research,
National Institutes of Health

Margo McCaffery, R.N., M.S., F.A.A.N.
Pain Consultant, Los Angeles, CA

Ruth McCorkle, R.N., Ph.D.
Professor and Chairperson, Adult
Health and Illness
University of Pennsylvania

Charles L. McGarvey III, M.S.
Chief, Physical Therapy Service
Department of Rehabilitation Medicine,
National Institutes of Health

Patricia A. McGrath, Ph.D.
Director, Child Health Research
Institute
Associate Professor, Department of
Pediatrics,
Western Ontario University

Deborah B. McGuire, R.N., Ph.D.
Director of Nursing Research
Johns Hopkins Oncology Center
Assistant Professor of Nursing
Johns Hopkins University

Christine A. Miaskowski, R.N., Ph.D.
Associate Professor
Department of Physiological Nursing,
University of California, San
Francisco

David Stevenson Mulder, M.D.
Professor of Surgery
McGill University
Surgeon-in-Chief, Montreal General
Hospital

Paul M. Paris, M.D., F.A.C.E.P.
Associate Professor
Chief, Division of Emergency Medicine
University of Pittsburgh School of
Medicine

Richard Payne, M.D.
Associate Professor of Neurology
University of Texas, M. D. Anderson
Cancer Center

L. Brian Ready, M.D., F.R.C.P.(C)
Director, Acute Pain Service
University of Washington Medical
Center
Professor of Anesthesiology
University of Washington

Patrick M. Renfro, R.N., M.S., C.R.C.
National Rehabilitation Consultants
Denver, CO

Linda Jo Rice, M.D.
Associate Professor of Anesthesiology
and Pediatrics, Children's National
Medical Center
Catholic University of America

Anthony J. Richtsmeier, M.D.
Director, Section of Behavioral
Pediatrics, Department of Pediatrics
Rush-Presbyterian–St. Luke's Medical
Center, Chicago

Marilyn Savedra, R.N., Ph.D., F.A.A.N.
Professor and Acting Chair, Department
of Family Health Care Nursing
University of California School of
Nursing

Vivian R. Sheidler, M.S., R.N.
Research Associate and Nursing Clinical
   Specialist
Johns Hopkins Hospital

George Shorten, M.D.
Clinical Research Fellow, Department of
   Anesthesia
Massachusetts General Hospital

Robert S. Smith, Ph.D.
Director, Institute for Medicine in
   Contemporary Society
State University of New York Medical
   Center at Stony Brook

Judith Spross, R.N., M.S., O.C.N.
Assistant Professor
Institute of Health Professions
Massachusetts General Hospital

Earl Steinberg, M.D., M.P.H.
Director, Medical Technology and
   Practice Assessment Program
Associate Professor of Health Policy and
   Management
Johns Hopkins University

Carole V. Tsou, M.D.
Division of Family Medicine, Center for
   the Health Sciences
University of California, Los Angeles

Dennis C. Turk, Ph.D.
Director, Pain Evaluation and Treatment
   Institute
Center for Sports Medicine and
   Rehabilitation
Professor of Psychiatry and
   Anesthesiology
University of Pittsburgh School of
   Medicine

Gail Ulshafer, C.R.N.A.
American Association of Nurse
   Anesthetists, Park Ridge, IL
Anesthesia Care Associates, Yucca
   Valley, CA

Sridhar V. Vasudevan, M.D.
President-Elect, American Academy of
   Pain Medicine
Chairman, Department of Physical
   Medicine and Rehabilitation
St. Joseph's Hospital, Milwaukee, WI

Loretta Vecchiarelli, M.S.
Rehabilitation Hospital of Western New
   England

Andrew L. Warshaw, M.D.
Associate Chief of Surgery
Massachusetts General Hospital
Harold and Ellen Danser Professor of
   Surgery
Harvard Medical School

Steven Woolf, M.D.
Consultant, Oakton, VA

Donald M. Yealy, M.D.
Assistant Professor
Director of Research, Division of
   Emergency Medicine
Texas A & M University Medical Center
   and Scott and White Memorial
   Hospital

Lonnie Zeltzer, M.D.
Professor of Pediatrics
Head, Pediatric Pain Program
UCLA School of Medicine

J. M. Zimmerman, M.D.
Chief of Surgery, Church Hospital
Associate Professor of Surgery
Johns Hopkins University

12

ALTERNATIVE HEALTH CARE

Because many patients throughout the country are dissatisfied with traditional medicine, it is not unusual for them to turn to alternative approaches to health care. The National Institutes of Health and Congress are currently investigating this $27-billion-a-year industry.

There is substantial public pressure to address alternative care for arthritis, AIDS, low back pain, autoimmune disorders, advanced-stage cancer, and other chronic illnesses which do not respond to standard medical treatment.

The *New England Journal of Medicine* recently reported that Americans turn to alternative medicine with surprising frequency, spend vast sums of money on alternative care, and rarely tell their doctors that they are seeking it.

Based on a survey by researchers at Harvard Medical School, *it is estimated that 34% of Americans visited alternative therapists in 1990 on an average of 19 times a year, accounting for 425 million visits altogether. Those visits surpassed the 388 million visits by patients to all mainstream medical practitioners, who include internists, pediatricians, and family doctors.*

Patients sought alternative care for anxiety, back pain, allergies, and chronic pain. The patients feel that there is something missing in a more traditional medical care model. Some patients also visit alternative care practitioners as a life-style choice, out of curiosity, or for other non-chronic-disease reasons.

Seventy-two percent of the patients who visited alternative care practitioners did not tell their medical doctor about those visits and/or therapies.

Scientific evidence seems to indicate that there is an ongoing communication between the nervous, immune, and endocrine systems. The concept that negative emotions depress the immune system, and, conversely, that positive emotions bolster the immune system, continues to be the object of intensive investigation.

Some of the health care alternatives, such as chiropractic, acupuncture, osteopathy, biofeedback, hypnosis, guided imagery, and the Alexander technique, are well known.

Homeopathy, color therapy, and crystal healing are some of the less-well-known forms of healing.

A 1991 poll conducted by *Time* magazine and CNN asked five hundred American adults whether they would consider seeking medical help from an alternative doctor if conventional medicine failed to help them. Sixty-two percent said "yes"; 29% said "no." When asked if they would go back to an alternative doctor, 84% said "yes" and 10% said "no."

Although the majority of medical doctors still embrace traditional medicine, a growing number are now more open to some of these alternative approaches as they become more aware of the interaction between the mind and body.

A word of caution: One should always be concerned about any health care decision, most particularly about alternative health care. If you are considering this avenue, always check the references or accreditation of the therapist.

As Bill Moyers notes in his book *Healing and the Mind*, "People are taking a new look at the meaning of sickness and health." Moyers quotes Eric J. Cassell in *The Nature of Suffering and the Goals of Medicine*: "Without system and training, being responsive in the face of suffering remains the attribute of individual physicians who have come to this mastery alone or gained it from a few inspirational teachers." Cassell adds, "Healing powers consist only in and no more than in allowing, causing, or bringing to bear those things or forces for getting better (whatever they may be) that already exist in the patient." Moyers acknowledges the importance of the mind/body medicine as an integral part of the healing process.

The following is a list of the most popular alternative medical options.

ALTERNATIVE MEDICINE AND HEALTH CARE

Acupressure—A variation of acupuncture in which the fingers are used instead of needles.

Acupuncture—A system for pain alleviation in which small solid needles are inserted into the skin at varying depths to penetrate and relieve underlying musculature pain.

Alexander technique—Therapeutic training to improve poor posture and thereby alleviate pain.

Aromatherapy—Use of essential oils from plants and flowers, massaged into the skin or inhaled.

Ayurvedic medicine—Indian system of medicine in which diet and therapy utilize herbs and massage.

Bioenergetics—A purported exchange of energy between the therapist and the patient.

Biofeedback—Conditioning technique devised to observe, control, and modify emotional, nervous, and muscular responses, including blood pressure and pulse.

Chiropractic—An ancient Chinese technique now employed by Western practitioners, in which manual manipulation of the spine is employed to alleviate back pain and other ailments.

Color therapy—Use of colored light on the body to alter a patient's aura.

Cryotherapy—The localized use of cold on the body to relieve pain there or in other parts of the body.

Crystal healing—New Age therapy purportedly utilizing healing energy from quartz and other minerals.

Faith/religious healing—A method of attempting to cure disease by prayer and religious faith.

Guided imagery—Therapy in which patients are encouraged to envision their immune system battling disease.

Heat therapy—The localized use of heat on the body to relieve pain there or in other parts of the body.

Herbal healing—Promoting health and and treating illness with botanically derived potions.

Holistic medicine—A variation of medicine emphasizing life-style and psychological factors by treating the "whole" person.

Homeopathy—Treatment for disease using small amounts of natural substances which in larger amounts would cause the same symptoms as the ailment.

Hypnosis/hypnotherapy—Making therapeutic suggestions to patients who are induced into a state of semiconsciousness, to relieve pain, decrease anxiety, or speed the healing process.

Macrobiotics—Use of grains and vegetables to form a healthy and life-expanding diet.

Meditation—The use of soothing thought, reflection, and contemplation to alleviate pain.

Music/distraction—Use of music to alter the focus from pain or illness.

Naturopathy—A method of treating disease using diet, exercise, and heat to assist the natural healing process.

Osteopathy—A therapeutic system of medicine based upon the premise that restoring or preserving health can best be accomplished by manipulation of the skeleton and muscles.

Reflexology—Manipulation of areas of the feet to alleviate pain in other parts of the body.

Rolfing—A deep and sometimes painful massage to realign the body.

Shiatsu—Therapeutic Japanese massage using the manipulation of pressure points.

Tactile strategies—Strategies that provide comfort through the sense of touch, such as stroking or massage.

TENS—Transcutaneous electrical nerve stimulation, a variation of acupuncture in which electrical impulses are passed through the needles into muscle.

Postscript

You have read about the complexities of pain. You now know that pain is as individual as your fingerprint. No two people's pain is experienced in the same way, nor should it be treated the same by doctors, nurses, and health care professionals. When you say you are in pain, you should be believed.

You need to become an advocate for yourself.

Always discuss your pain history with your doctor, and never enter into any diagnostic, medical, or surgical procedure without first discussing pain control, how pain will be assessed, what pain treatment is planned, who will be accountable for your pain management, and who will respond to you if your pain is not managed.

Using the *0–10 Numeric Pain Intensity Scale* should become as familiar as taking a temperature. Use the scale whenever you discuss your pain level with your doctor or other health care professionals. Also learn how to describe your pain. Is it stabbing, hot, dull, pulsing? Does it stay in one place? Does it radiate? How long have you had it? Does anything make it better? Did you injure yourself? What have you taken to relieve the pain?

It you call your doctor and say, "My elbow hurts," he or she will be in the dark. If you say, "I have a stabbing, continuous pain located in my right elbow that began twenty-four hours ago; there is no position that relieves the pain; I have taken three aspirins every four hours, with no reduction in pain; the pain is a 7 on the 0–10 pain scale; I did not fall or injure myself," then you have immediately given your doctor a great deal of information. Write down what you want to tell the doctor. Be as specific as possible.

Insist that your pain be measured on the 0–10 scale. Keep track of your pain before, during, and after treatment. If a health care professional says he or she is not familiar with the scale, respond that it is simple to use and it is how you will be communicating about your level of pain.

Don't get intimidated.

If your doctor refuses to discuss pain management plans, including the drugs or treatments he will use with you, he has denied you your right to informed consent. It is federal law that doctors must discuss any medical or surgical treatment with their patients and obtain their consent beforehand. Not to do so is seen as an assault on the patient. Patients must participate in decisions about their care. The same principles apply to nurses and other health care professionals.

You can change the way pain is managed. Learn the language of pain and the use of pain assessment tools, and understand that the way your pain is managed is an important part of your medical or surgical care. Help yourself by becoming an active partner with your doctor and other health care professionals. You can achieve pain relief!

Guide for the Consumer

PHARMACEUTICAL COMPANIES AND THE SPECIFIC PAIN-RELIEVING DRUGS THEY MANUFACTURE*

Abbott Laboratories
Butesin® Picrate (butamben picrate), Nembutal® Sodium Capsules (pentobarbital sodium capsules, USP)

A.H. Robins Co.
Phenaphen, Robaxin, Robaxisal

Astra Pharmaceutical Products, Inc.
Astramorph/PF℠ (morphine sulfate injection, USP), Cocaine Hydrochloride, Dalgan® (dezocine), Duranest® (etidocaine hydrochloride), Dyclone® (dyclonine HCl), Fentanyl citrate and droperidol injection, morphine sulfate injection, USP, Nesacaine® (chloroprocaine HCl), Sensorcaine® (bupivacaine HCl injection), Xylocaine® (lidocaine hydrochloride)

Burroughs Wellcome
Anectine, Empirin, Nuromax, Retrovir, Tracrium, Vasoxyl, Zovirax

Central Pharmaceuticals, Inc.
Azdone® (hydrocodone bitartrate), Mono-Gesic® (salsalate)

Dista Products Company
Prozac® (fluoxetine hydrochloride)

DuPont Pharmaceuticals
Moban, Narcan, Nubain, Numorphan, Percocet, Percodan, Sublimaze, Sufenta

Eli Lilly and Company
Bevital sodium, Darvon, Dolophine hydrochloride, Methadone hydochloride, Phenobarbitol

Elkins-Sinn, Inc.
Duramorph® (morphine sulfate injection), Infumorph℠ (morphine sulfate solution for continuous microinfusion devices)

Gebauer Company
Ethyl Chloride (chloroethane), Fluori-Methane® (dichlorodifluoromethane 15%, trichloromonofluoromethane 85%), Fluro-Ethyl® (ethyl chloride, U.S.P., 25%, dichlorotetrafluoroethane, N.F., 75%)

GenDerm Corporation
Zostrix® (capsaicin 0.025% and 0.075%)

Hoffmann–La Roche
Levo-Dromoran, Noludar, Pantopon, Valrelease, Versed

---

*© *Physicians' Desk Reference,* 46th edition (Montvale, N.J.: Medical Economics Data, 1992). Reprinted by permission. All rights reserved.

Janssen
Alfenta, Inapsine, Innovar, Duragesic
transdermal system

Knoll Pharmaceuticals
Dilaudid, Vicodin

Mason Pharmaceuticals, Inc.
Damuson-P (hydrocodone bitastrate 5
mg., and aspirin 500 mg.), Duocet™
(hydrocodone bitartrate and
acetaminophen tablets 5 mg/500 mg)

McNeil Consumer Products Company
Medipren, Maximum Strength Sine-Aid,
Tylenol, Trexan, Zydone

McNeil Pharmaceutical
Haldol, Paraflex, Parafon Forte,
Tolectin, Tylenol with Codeine,
Tylox

Parke-Davis
Centrax, Easprin, Ergostat, Ketalar,
Meclomen, Ponstel, Pyridium, Surital,
Vira-A

Purdue Frederick
DHC Plus™ (dihydrocodeine), MS
Contin, MSIR Norzine
(thiethylperazine), Torecan
(thiethylperazine), Trilisate

Roche Products, Inc.
Dalmane, Librium, Limbitrol, Valium

*Rhône-Poulenc Rorer Pharmaceuticals
Inc.*
Ascriptin® (Aspirin buffered with
Maalox®), Ascriptin® A/D for
arthritis pain

Richwood Pharmaceutical Co. Inc.
Acuprin®, Hydrostat (hydromorphone
hydrochloride), MS/S Suppositories
(rectal morphine sulfate)

Roxane Laboratories, Inc.
Methadone Hydrochloride, Morphine
Sulfate, Oramorph SR™, Roxanol™
(100 UD, Rescudose) morphine
sulfate, Roxicet™ (oxycodone and
acetaminophen)

Sanofi–Winthrop
Carbacaine, Demerol, Marcaine,
Mebarol, Novocain, Pontocaine,
Talacen, Talwin

Schering Corporation
Etrafon, Solganal

SmithKline Beecham
Anexsia, Ecotrin, Ridaura, Thorazine

Upjohn Company
Ansaid, Motrin, Xanax

Upsher-Smith Laboratories, Inc.
Feverall® (acetaminophen rectal
suppositories), OMS® (immediate
release morphine sulfate) oral, RMS®
(rectal morphine sulfate)

Wallace Laboratories
Butisol Sodium® (butabarbital sodium),
Soma® (carisoprodol tablets, USP)

Webcon Pharmaceuticals
Anestacon® (2% lidocaine
hydrochloride viscous solution for
topical use), B & O Supprettes®
(belladonna and opium suppositories)

Whitby Pharmaceuticals, Inc.
Lortab® tablets and liquid
(hydrocodone bitartrate and
acetaminophen)

Whitehall Laboratories
Advil, Anacin, Anbesol, Dermoplast

Wyeth-Ayerst Laboratories
Children's Advil® Suspension
(ibuprofen), Ativan® (lorazepam),
Fluothane® (halothane, USP),
Lodine™ (etodolac), Orudis®
(ketoprofen), Serax® (oxazepam),
Synalgos-DC® (dihydrocodeine
bitartrate, aspirin and caffeine),
Wygesic® (propoxyphene HCl and
acetaminophen)

SPECIFIC TYPES OF ANXIETY AND PAIN, AND TARGET DRUGS:*

Anxiety disorders, management of
Ativan Tablets (Lorazepam)
  Wyeth-Ayerst
BuSpar (Buspirone Hydrochloride)
  Mead Johnson Pharmaceuticals
Centrax (Prazepam) Parke-Davis
Etrafon (Perphenazine, Amitriptyline
  Hydrochloride) Schering
Libritabs Tablets (Chlordiazepoxide
  Hydrochloride) Roche Products
Librium Capsules (Chlordiazepoxide)
  Roche Products
Librium Injectable (Chlordiazepoxide
  Hydrochloride) Roche Products
Mebaral Tablets (Mephobarbital) Sanofi
  Winthrop Pharmaceuticals
Miltown Tablets (Meprobamate) Wallace
Phenergan Injection (Promethazine
  Hydrochloride) Wyeth-Ayerst
Phenergan Suppositories (Promethazine
  Hydrochloride) Wyeth-Ayerst
Phenergan Syrup (Promethazine
  Hydrochloride) Wyeth-Ayerst
Phenergan Tablets (Promethazine
  Hydrochloride) Wyeth-Ayerst
Serax Capsules (Oxazepam)
  Wyeth-Ayerst
Serax Tablets (Oxazepam) Wyeth-Ayerst
Trancopal Caplets (Chlormezanone)
  Sanofi Winthrop Pharmaceuticals
Tranxene (Clorazepate Dipotassium)
  Abbott
Valium Injectable (Diazepam) Roche
  Products
Valium Tablets (Diazepam) Roche
  Products
Valrelease Capsules (Diazepam) Roche
  Laboratories
Vistaril Intramuscular Solution
  (Hydroxyzine Hydrochloride) Roerig
Xanax Tablets (Alprazolam) Upjohn

Anxiety, generalized nonpsychotic,
short term treatment of
Compazine (Prochlorperazine)
  SmithKline Beecham Pharmaceuticals

Stelazine (Trifluoperazine
  Hydrochloride) SmithKline Beecham
  Pharmaceuticals

Anxiety, mental depression–induced
Ativan Tablets (Lorazepam)
  Wyeth-Ayerst
Etrafon (Perphenazine, Amitriptyline
  Hydrochloride) Schering
Limbitrol (Chlordiazepoxide,
  Amitriptyline Hydrochloride) Roche
  Products
Ludiomil Tablets (Maprotiline
  Hydrochloride) CIBA Pharmaceutical
Serax Capsules (Oxazepam)
  Wyeth-Ayerst
Serax Tablets (Oxazepam) Wyeth-Ayerst
Sinequan (Doxepin Hydrochloride)
  Roerig
Triavil Tablets (Perphenazine,
  Amitriptyline Hydrochloride) Merck
  Sharp & Dohme
Vistaril Intramuscular Solution
  (Hydroxyzine Hydrochloride) Roerig
Xanax Tablets (Alprazolam) Upjohn

Anxiety, preoperative
Ativan Injection (Lorazepam)
  Wyeth-Ayerst
Inapsine Injection (Droperidol) Janssen
Innovar Injection (Fentanyl Citrate,
  Droperidol) Janssen
Libritabs Tablets (Chlordiazepoxide
  Hydrochloride) Roche Products
Librium Capsules (Chlordiazepoxide)
  Roche Products
Librium Injectable (Chlordiazepoxide
  Hydrochloride) Roche Products
Thorazine (Chlorpromazine) SmithKline
  Beecham Pharmaceuticals
Valium Injectable (Diazepam) Roche
  Products
Vistaril Capsules (Hydroxyzine
  Pamoate) Pfizer Labs Division
Vistaril Intramuscular Solution
  (Hydroxyzine Hydrochloride) Roerig
Vistaril Oral Suspension (Hydroxyzine
  Pamoate) Pfizer Labs Division

Anxiety, short-term symptomatic relief of

Atarax Tablets & Syrup (Hydroxyzine Hydrochloride) Roerig

Ativan Tablets (Lorazepam) Wyeth-Ayerst

BuSpar (Buspirone Hydrochloride) Mead Johnson Pharmaceuticals

Centrax (Prazepam) Parke-Davis

Libritabs Tablets (Chlordiazepoxide Hydrochloride) Roche Products

Librium Capsules (Chlordiazepoxide) Roche Products

Librium Injectable (Chlordiazepoxide Hydrochloride) Roche Products

Miltown Tablets (Meprobamate) Wallace

Numorphan Hydrochloride Injection (Oxymorphone Hydrochloride) Du Pont Multi-Source Products

Serax Capsules (Oxazepam) Wyeth-Ayerst

Serax Tablets (Oxazepam) Wyeth-Ayerst

Tranxene (Clorazepate Dipotassium) Abbott

Valium Injectable (Diazepam) Roche Products

Valium Tablets (Diazepam) Roche Products

Valrelease Capsules (Diazepam) Roche Laboratories

Vistaril Capsules (Hydroxyzine Pamoate) Pfizer Labs Division

Vistaril Intramuscular Solution (Hydroxyzine Hydrochloride) Roerig

Vistaril Oral Suspension (Hydroxyzine Pamoate) Pfizer Labs Division

Xanax Tablets (Alprazolam) Upjohn

Headache

Acetaminophen Uniserts Suppositories (Acetaminophen) Upsher-Smith

Advil Ibuprofen Tablets and Caplets (Ibuprofen) Whitehall

Alka-Seltzer Effervescent Antacid and Pain Reliever (Aspirin, Sodium Bicarbonate, Citric Acid) Miles Consumer

Alka-Seltzer Extra Strength Effervescent Antacid and Pain Reliever (Aspirin, Sodium Bicarbonate, Citric Acid) Miles Consumer

Alka-Seltzer (Flavored) Effervescent Antacid and Pain Reliever (Aspirin, Sodium Bicarbonate, Citric Acid) Miles Consumer

Anacin (Aspirin, Caffeine) Whitehall

Anacin Maximum Strength Analgesic Coated Tablets (Aspirin, Caffeine) Whitehall

Aspirin Free Anacin Maximum Strength Acetaminophen Film Coated Caplets (Acetaminophen) Whitehall

Aspirin Free Anacin Maximum Strength Acetaminophen Film Coated Tablets (Acetaminophen) Whitehall

Maximum Strength Arthritis Pain Formula By the Makers of Anacin Analgesic Tablets and Caplets (Aspirin, Aluminum Hydroxide, Magnesium Hydroxide) Whitehall

Regular Strength Ascriptin Tablets (Aluminum Hydroxide Gel, Dried, Aspirin, Magnesium Hydroxide, Calcium Carbonate) Rhone-Poulenc Rorer Consumer

BC Powder (Aspirin, Salicylamide, Caffeine) Block

Children's Bayer Chewable Aspirin (Aspirin) Glenbrook

Genuine Bayer Aspirin Tablets & Caplets (Aspirin) Glenbrook

Maximum Bayer Aspirin Tablets & Caplets (Aspirin) Glenbrook

8 Hour Bayer Timed-Release Aspirin (Aspirin) Glenbrook

Extra Strength Bufferin Analgesic Tablets (Aspirin) Bristol-Myers Products

Bufferin Analgesic Tablets and Caplets (Aspirin) Bristol-Myers Products

Datril Extra-Strength Analgesic Tablets (Acetaminophen) Bristol-Myers Products

Dimetapp Plus Caplets (Acetaminophen, Brompheniramine Maleate, Phenylpropanolamine Hydrochloride) Robins

Dorcol Children's Fever & Pain Reducer (Acetaminophen) Sandoz Consumer

Ecotrin (Aspirin, Enteric Coated) SmithKline Beecham Consumer Brands

Empirin Aspirin (Aspirin) Burroughs Wellcome

Aspirin Free Excedrin Analgesic Caplets (Acetaminophen, Caffeine) Bristol-Myers Products

Excedrin Extra-Strength Analgesic Tablets & Caplets (Acetaminophen, Aspirin, Caffeine) Bristol-Myers Products

Excedrin P.M. Analgesic/Sleeping Aid Tablets, Caplets and Liquid (Acetaminophen, Diphenhydramine Citrate) Bristol-Myers Products

Fiorinal with Codeine Capsules (Codeine Phosphate, Butalbital, Caffeine, Aspirin) Sandoz Pharmaceuticals

Haltran Tablets (Ibuprofen) Roberts

Ibuprofen (Ibuprofen) Ohm Laboratories

Liquiprin (Acetaminophen) Menley & James

Medipren Ibuprofen Caplets and Tablets (Ibuprofen) McNeil Consumer

Mobigesic Analgesic Tablets (Magnesium Salicylate, Phenyltoloxamine Citrate) Ascher

Headache with upset stomach
Alka-Seltzer Advanced Formula Antacid & Non-Aspirin Pain Reliever (Acetaminophen, Calcium Carbonate, Citric Acid, Sodium Bicarbonate, Potassium Bicarbonate) Miles Consumer

Alka-Seltzer Effervescent Antacid and Pain Reliever (Aspirin, Sodium Bicarbonate, Citric Acid) Miles Consumer

Alka-Seltzer Extra Strength Effervescent Antacid and Pain Reliever (Aspirin, Sodium Bicarbonate, Citric Acid) Miles Consumer

Alka-Seltzer (Flavored) Effervescent Antacid and Pain Reliever (Aspirin, Sodium Bicarbonate, Citric Acid) Miles Consumer

Headache, migraine
Cafergot/Cafergot P-B (Ergotamine Tartrate, Caffeine) Sandoz Pharmaceuticals

D.H.E. 45 Injection (Dihydroergotamine Mesylate) Sandoz Pharmaceuticals

Ergostat (Ergotamine Tartrate) Parke-Davis

Inderal LA Long Acting Capsules (Propranolol Hydrochloride) Wyeth-Ayerst

Medihaler Ergotamine Aerosol (Ergotamine Tartrate) 3M Pharmaceuticals

Wigraine Tablets & Suppositories (Ergotamine Tartrate, Caffeine) Organon

Headache, migraine, "possibly" effective in
Isocom Capsules (Acetaminophen, Isometheptene Mucate, Dichloralphenazone) Nutripharm

Midrin Capsules (Isometheptene Mucate, Dichloralphenazone, Acetaminophen) Carnrick

Headache, migraine, prevention or reduction of intensity and frequency of
Cafergot/Cafergot P-B (Ergotamine Tartrate, Caffeine) Sandoz Pharmaceuticals

D.H.E. 45 Injection (Dihydroergotamine Mesylate) Sandoz Pharmaceuticals

Ergostat (Ergotamine Tartrate) Parke-Davis

Sansert Tablets (Methysergide Maleate) Sandoz Pharmaceuticals

Headache, migraine, prophylaxis of (see also under Headache, migraine, prevention or reduction of intensity and frequency of)
Blocadren Tablets (Timolol Maleate) Merck Sharp & Dohme

Inderal (Propranolol Hydrochloride) Wyeth-Ayerst

Headache, tension (see also under Pain, unspecified; Pain with anxiety and tension)
Esgic-Plus Tablets (Butalbital, Acetaminophen, Caffeine) Forest Pharmaceuticals

Esgic Tablets & Capsules (Butalbital, Acetaminophen) Forest Pharmaceuticals

Fioricet Tablets (Butalbital, Acetaminophen, Caffeine) Sandoz Pharmaceuticals

Fiorinal Capsules (Butalbital, Aspirin) Sandoz Pharmaceuticals

Fiorinal with Codeine Capsules (Codeine Phosphate, Butalbital, Caffeine, Aspirin) Sandoz Pharmaceuticals

Fiorinal Tablets (Butalbital, Aspirin) Sandoz Pharmaceuticals

Phrenilin (Butalbital, Acetaminophen) Carnick

Sedapap Tablets 50 mg/650 mg (Acetaminophen, Butalbital) Mayrand Pharmaceuticals

Norwich Extra-Strength Aspirin (Aspirin) Chattem

Norwich Regular Strength Aspirin (Aspirin) Chattem

Nuprin Ibuprofen/Analgesic Tablets & Caplets (Ibuprofen) Bristol-Myers Products

P-A-C Analgesic Tablets (Aspirin, Caffeine Anhydrous) Roberts

Children's Panadol Chewable Tablets, Liquid, Infants' Drops (Acetaminophen) Glenbrook

Junior Strength Panadol (Acetaminophen) Glenbrook

Maximum Strength Panadol Tablets and Caplets (Acetaminophen) Glenbrook

St. Joseph Adult Chewable Aspirin (81 mg.) (Aspirin) Schering-Plough HealthCare

Trendar Ibuprofen Tablets (Ibuprofen) Whitehall

Tylenol, Extra Strength, acetaminophen Adult Liquid Pain Reliever (Acetaminophen) McNeil Consumer

Tylenol, Extra Strength, acetaminophen Gelcaps, Caplets, Tablets (Acetaminophen) McNeil Consumer

Tylenol, Junior Strength, acetaminophen Coated Caplets, Grape and Fruit Chewable Tablets (Acetaminophen) McNeil Consumer

Tylenol, Regular Strength, acetaminophen Tablets and Caplets (Acetaminophen) McNeil Consumer

Vanquish Analgesic Caplets (Acetaminophen, Aspirin, Caffeine) Glenbrook

Headache accompanied by insomnia

Bufferin AF Nite Time Analgesic/Sleeping Aid Caplets (Acetaminophen, Diphenhydramine Citrate) Bristol-Myers Products

Excedrin P.M. Analgesic/Sleeping Aid Tablets, Caplets and Liquid (Acetaminophen, Diphenhydramine Citrate) Bristol-Myers Products

Mobigesic Analgesic Tablets (Magnesium Salicylate, Phenyltoloxamine Citrate) Ascher

Sominex Pain Relief Formula (Acetaminophen, Diphenhydramine Hydrochloride) SmithKline Beecham

Tylenol PM, Extra Strength Caplets and Tablets (Acetaminophen, Diphenhydramine Hydrochloride) McNeil Consumer

Unisom Dual Relief Nighttime Sleep Aid/Analgesic (Diphenhydramine Hydrochloride, Acetaminophen) Pfizer Consumer Health

Headache associated with common cold

Advil Cold & Sinus Caplets (formerly CoAdvil) (Ibuprofen, Pseudoephedrine Hydrochloride) Whitehall

Day-Night Comtrex (Acetaminophen, Chlorpheniramine Maleate, Dextromethorphan Hydrobromide, Pseudoephedrine Hydrochloride) Bristol-Myers Products

Dristan Cold Nasal Decongestant/ Antihistamine/Analgesic Coated Tablets (Phenylephrine Hydrochloride, Chlorpheniramine Maleate, Acetaminophen) Whitehall

Sinus Excedrin Analgesic, Decongestant Tablets & Caplets (Acetaminophen, Pseudoephedrine Hydrochloride) Bristol-Myers Products

Children's Tylenol Cold Liquid Formula and Chewable Tablets (Acetaminophen, Chlorpheniramine Maleate, Pseudoephedrine Hydrochloride) McNeil Consumer

Headache with gastric hyperacidity
Alka-Seltzer Advanced Formula
Antacid & Non-Aspirin Pain Reliever
(Acetaminophen, Calcium Carbonate,
Citric Acid, Sodium Bicarbonate,
Potassium Bicarbonate) Miles
Consumer
Alka-Seltzer Effervescent Antacid and
Pain Reliever (Aspirin, Sodium
Bicarbonate, Citric Acid) Miles
Consumer
Alka-Seltzer Extra Strength Effervescent
Antacid and Pain Reliever (Aspirin,
Sodium Bicarbonate, Citric Acid)
Miles Consumer
Alka-Seltzer (Flavored) Effervescent
Antacid and Pain Reliever (Aspirin,
Sodium Bicarbonate, Citric Acid)
Miles Consumer

*Pain associated with upper respiratory
infection*
Actifed Plus Caplets (Acetaminophen,
Pseudoephedrine Hydrochloride,
Triprolidine Hydrochloride)
Burroughs Wellcome
Actifed Plus Tablets (Acetaminophen,
Pseudoephedrine Hydrochloride,
Triprolidine Hydrochloride)
Burroughs Wellcome
Advil Cold & Sinus Caplets (formerly
CoAdvil) (Ibuprofen,
Pseudoephedrine Hydrochloride)
Whitehall
Advil Ibuprofen Tablets and Caplets
(Ibuprofen) Whitehall
BC Cold Powder (Aspirin,
Phenylpropanolamine Hydrochloride,
Chlorpheniramine Maleate) Block
Benadryl Plus (Acetaminophen,
Diphenhydramine Hydrochloride,
Pseudoephedrine Hydrochloride)
Parke-Davis
Benadryl Plus Nighttime
(Acetaminophen, Diphenhydramine
Hydrochloride, Pseudoephedrine
Hydrochloride) Parke-Davis
Extra Strength Bufferin Analgesic
Tablets (Aspirin) Bristol-Myers
Products
Bufferin Analgesic Tablets and Caplets
(Aspirin) Bristol-Myers Products

Cough Formula Comtrex
(Pseudoephedrine Hydrochloride,
Acetaminophen, Guaifenesin,
Dextromethorphan Hydrobromide)
Bristol-Myers Products
Comtrex Multi-Symptom Cold Reliever
Tablets/Caplets/Liqui-Gels/Liquid
(Pseudoephedrine Hydrochloride,
Phenylpropanolamine Hydrochloride,
Dextromethorphan Hydrobromide,
Acetaminophen, Chlorpheniramine
Maleate) Bristol-Myers Products
Day-Night Comtrex (Acetaminophen,
Chlorpheniramine Maleate,
Dextromethorphan Hydrobromide,
Pseudoephedrine Hydrochloride)
Bristol-Myers Products
Non-Drowsy Comtrex (Acetaminophen,
Dextromethorphan Hydrobromide,
Pseudoephedrine Hydrochloride)
Bristol-Myers Products
Congespirin For Children Aspirin Free
Chewable Cold Tablets
(Acetaminophen, Phenylephrine
Hydrochloride) Bristol-Myers
Products
Contac Cough & Sore Throat Formula
(Acetaminophen, Dextromethorphan
Hydrobromide, Guaifenesin)
SmithKline Beecham
Contac Jr. Children's Cold Medicine
(Acetaminophen, Dextromethorphan
Hydrobromide, Pseudoephedrine
Hydrochloride) SmithKline Beecham
Contac Nighttime Cold Medicine
(Acetaminophen, Dextromethorphan
Hydrobromide, Doxylamine
Succinate, Pseudoephedrine
Hydrochloride) SmithKline Beecham
Contac Severe Cold and Flu Formula
Caplets (Acetaminophen,
Chlorpheniramine Maleate,
Dextromethorphan Hydrobromide,
Phenylpropanolamine Hydrochloride)
SmithKline Beecham
Contac Sinus Caplets Maximum
Strength Non-Drowsy Formula
(Acetaminophen, Pseudoephedrine
Hydrochloride) SmithKline Beecham
Contac Sinus Tablets Maximum
Strength Non-Drowsy Formula
(Acetaminophen, Pseudoephedrine
Hydrochloride) SmithKline Beecham

Dimetapp Plus Caplets (Acetaminophen, Brompheniramine Maleate, Phenylpropanolamine Hydrochloride) Robins

Dristan Cold Nasal Decongestant/Antihistamine/Analgesic Coated Tablets (Phenylephrine Hydrochloride, Chlorpheniramine Maleate, Acetaminophen) Whitehall

No Drowsiness Dristan Cold Nasal Decongestant/Analgesic Coated Caplets (Acetaminophen, Pseudoephedrine Hydrochloride) Whitehall

Dristan Sinus Caplets (Ibuprofen, Pseudoephedrine Hydrochloride) Whitehall

Drixoral Plus Extended-Release Tablets (Acetaminophen, Dexbrompheniramine Maleate, Pseudoephedrine Sulfate) Schering-Plough HealthCare

Excedrin Extra-Strength Analgesic Tablets & Caplets (Acetaminophen, Aspirin, Caffeine) Bristol-Myers Products

4-Way Cold Tablets (Acetaminophen, Chlorpheniramine Maleate, Phenylpropanolamine Hydrochloride) Bristol-Myers Products

Liquiprin (Acetaminophen) Menley & James

Medi-Flu Caplet, Liquid (Acetaminophen, Chlorpheniramine Maleate, Dextromethorphan Hydrobromide, Pseudoephedrine Hydrochloride) Parke-Davis

Ornex Caplets (Acetaminophen, Pseudoephedrine Hydrochloride) Menley & James

Pyrroxate Capsules (Acetaminophen, Chlorpheniramine Maleate, Phenylpropanolamine Hydrochloride) Roberts

Robitussin Night Relief (Acetaminophen, Dextromethorphan Hydrobromide, Phenylephrine Hydrochloride, Pyrilamine Maleate) Robins

Sine-Off Maximum Strength Allergy/Sinus Formula Caplets (Acetaminophen, Chlorpheniramine Maleate, Pseudoephedrine Hydrochloride) SmithKline Beecham

Sine-Off Maximum Strength No Drowsiness Formula Caplets (Acetaminophen, Pseudoephedrine Hydrochloride) SmithKline Beecham

Sine-Off Sinus Medicine Tablets-Aspirin Formula (Aspirin, Chlorpheniramine Maleate, Phenylpropanolamine Hydrochloride) SmithKline Beecham

Sinulin (Acetaminophen, Phenylpropanolamine Hydrochloride, Chlorpheniramine Maleate) Carnrick

Sinutab Maximum Strength (Acetaminophen, Chlorpheniramine Maleate, Pseudoephedrine Hydrochloride) Parke-Davis

Sinutab Maximum Strength Without Drowsiness Tablets & Caplets (Acetaminophen, Pseudoephedrine Hydrochloride) Parke-Davis

Sinutab Regular Strength Without Drowsiness Formula (Acetaminophen, Pseudoephedrine Hydrochloride) Parke-Davis

St. Joseph Nighttime Cold Medicine (Chlorpheniramine Maleate, Pseudoephedrine Hydrochloride, Dextromethorphan Hydrobromide, Acetaminophen) Schering-Plough HealthCare

Tempra, Acetaminophen (Acetaminophen) Mead Johnson Nutritionals

TheraFlu Flu and Cold Medicine (Acetaminophen, Chlorpheniramine Maleate, Pseudoephedrine Hydrochloride) Sandoz Consumer

Triaminicin Tablets (Acetaminophen, Chlorpheniramine Maleate, Phenylpropanolamine Hydrochloride) Sandoz Consumer

Children's Tylenol Cold Liquid Formula and Chewable Tablets (Acetaminophen, Chlorpheniramine Maleate, Pseudoephedrine Hydrochloride) McNeil Consumer

Tylenol Cold & Flu No Drowsiness Hot Medication, Packets (Acetaminophen, Dextromethorphan Hydrobromide, Pseudoephedrine Hydrochloride) McNeil Consumer

Tylenol Cold Medication Caplets and Tablets (Acetaminophen, Chlorpheniramine Maleate, Pseudoephedrine Hydrochloride, Dextromethorphan Hydrobromide) McNeil Consumer

Tylenol Cold Medication, Effervescent Tablets (Acetaminophen, Phenylpropanolamine Hydrochloride, Chlorpheniramine Maleate) McNeil Consumer

Tylenol Cold Medication No Drowsiness Formula Caplets (Acetaminophen, Pseudoephedrine Hydrochloride, Dextromethorphan Hydrobromide) McNeil Consumer

Tylenol Cold Night Time Medication Liquid (Acetaminophen, Chlorpheniramine Maleate, Pseudoephedrine Hydrochloride, Dextromethorphan Hydrobromide) McNeil Consumer

Tylenol Cough Medication Liquid, Maximum Strength (Dextromethorphan Hydrobromide, Acetaminophen) McNeil Consumer

Tylenol Cough Medication Liquid with Decongestant, Maximum Strength (Dextromethorphan Hydrobromide, Acetaminophen, Pseudoephedrine Hydrochloride) McNeil Consumer

Vicks Daycare (Acetaminophen, Dextromethorphan Hydrobromide, Pseudoephedrine Hydrochloride, Guaifenesin) Richardson-Vicks Inc.

Vicks Formula 44M Multi-Symptom Cough Medicine (Acetaminophen, Dextromethorphan Hydrobromide, Chlorpheniramine Maleate, Pseudoephedrine Hydrochloride) Richardson-Vicks Inc.

Vicks NyQuil Nighttime Colds Medicine—Original & Cherry Flavor (Acetaminophen, Dextromethorphan Hydrobromide, Doxylamine Succinate, Pseudoephedrine Hydrochloride) Richardson-Vicks Inc.

Pain due to common cold
(see under Pain associated with upper respiratory infection)

Pain due to urinary tract infections, symptomatic relief of
Azo Gantanol Tablets (Sulfamethoxazole, Phenazopyridine Hydrochloride) Roche Laboratories
Azo Gantrisin Tablets (Sulfisoxazole, Phenazopyridine Hydrochloride) Roche Laboratories

Pain with anxiety and tension
Equagesic Tablets (Meprobamate, Aspirin) Wyeth-Ayerst
Fiorinal with Codeine Capsules (Codeine Phosphate, Butalbital, Caffeine, Aspirin) Sandoz Pharmaceuticals

Pain with gastric hyperacidity
Alka-Seltzer Effervescent Antacid and Pain Reliever (Aspirin, Sodium Bicarbonate, Citric Acid) Miles Consumer
Alka-Seltzer Extra Strength Effervescent Antacid and Pain Reliever (Aspirin, Sodium Bicarbonate, Citric Acid) Miles Consumer
Alka-Seltzer (Flavored) Effervescent Antacid and Pain Reliever (Aspirin, Sodium Bicarbonate, Citric Acid) Miles Consumer

Pain, anogenital
Americaine Hemorrhoidal Ointment (Benzocaine) Fisons Consumer Health
Dermoplast Anesthetic Pain Relief Spray (Benzocaine, Menthol) Whitehall
Dyclone 0.5% and 1% Topical Solutions, USP (Dyclonine Hydrochloride) Astra
Pazo Hemorrhoid Ointment & Suppositories (Ephedrine Sulfate, Zinc Oxide) Bristol-Myers Products
Preparation H (Yeast Cell Derivative, Live) Whitehall
Tronothane Hydrochloride Cream (Pramoxine Hydrochloride) Abbott

Pain, anorectal
Fleet Relief (Zinc Oxide, Mineral Oil, Petrolatum, White) Fleet

Nupercainal Cream and Ointment
(Dibucaine) CIBA Pharmaceutical
Nupercainal Suppositories (Zinc Oxide)
CIBA Pharmaceutical
proctoFoam/non-steroid (Pramoxine
Hydrochloride) Reed & Carnrick
Tronolane Anesthetic Cream for
Hemorrhoids (Pramoxine
Hydrochloride) Ross
Tronothane Hydrochloride Cream
(Pramoxine Hydrochloride) Abbott

Pain, arthritic, minor
Advil Ibuprofen Tablets and Caplets
(Ibuprofen) Whitehall
Anacin (Aspirin, Caffeine) Whitehall
Anacin Maximum Strength Analgesic
Coated Tablets (Aspirin, Caffeine)
Whitehall
Aspirin Free Anacin Maximum Strength
Acetaminophen Film Coated Caplets
(Acetaminophen) Whitehall
Aspirin Free Anacin Maximum Strength
Acetaminophen Film Coated Tablets
(Acetaminophen) Whitehall
Maximum Strength Arthritis Pain
Formula By the Makers of Anacin
Analgesic Tablets and Caplets
(Aspirin, Aluminum Hydroxide,
Magnesium Hydroxide) Whitehall
Arthritis Strength BC Powder (Aspirin,
Salicylamide, Caffeine) Block
BC Powder (Aspirin, Salicylamide,
Caffeine) Block
Genuine Bayer Aspirin Tablets &
Caplets (Aspirin) Glenbrook
Maximum Bayer Aspirin Tablets &
Caplets (Aspirin) Glenbrook
Bayer Plus Aspirin Tablets (Aspirin)
Glenbrook
Therapy Bayer Aspirin Caplets (Aspirin,
Enteric Coated) Glenbrook
8 Hour Bayer Timed-Release Aspirin
(Aspirin) Glenbrook
Arthritis Strength Bufferin Analgesic
Caplets (Aspirin) Bristol-Myers
Products
Extra Strength Bufferin Analgesic
Tablets (Aspirin) Bristol-Myers
Products
Bufferin Analgesic Tablets and Caplets
(Aspirin) Bristol-Myers Products

Ecotrin (Aspirin, Enteric Coated)
SmithKline Beecham Consumer
Brands
Empirin Aspirin (Aspirin) Burroughs
Wellcome
Aspirin Free Excedrin Analgesic Caplets
(Acetaminophen, Caffeine)
Bristol-Myers Products
Excedrin Extra-Strength Analgesic
Tablets & Caplets (Acetaminophen,
Aspirin, Caffeine) Bristol-Myers
Products
Haltran Tablets (Ibuprofen) Roberts
Ibuprofen (Ibuprofen) Ohm Laboratories
Medipren Ibuprofen Caplets and Tablets
(Ibuprofen) McNeil Consumer
Motrin IB Caplets and Tablets
(Ibuprofen) Upjohn
Norwich Extra-Strength Aspirin
(Aspirin) Chattem
Norwich Regular Strength Aspirin
(Aspirin) Chattem
Nuprin Ibuprofen/Analgesic Tablets &
Caplets (Ibuprofen) Bristol-Myers
Products
Maximum Strength Panadol Tablets and
Caplets (Acetaminophen) Glenbrook
Tylenol, Regular Strength,
acetaminophen Tablets and Caplets
(Acetaminophen) McNeil Consumer
Vanquish Analgesic Caplets
(Acetaminophen, Aspirin, Caffeine)
Glenbrook

Pain, breast, postpartum
Metandren Linguets and Tablets
(Methyltestosterone) CIBA
Pharmaceutical

Pain, dental
Advil Ibuprofen Tablets and Caplets
(Ibuprofen) Whitehall
Anacin (Aspirin, Caffeine) Whitehall
Anacin Maximum Strength Analgesic
Coated Tablets (Aspirin, Caffeine)
Whitehall
Aspirin Free Anacin Maximum Strength
Acetaminophen Film Coated Caplets
(Acetaminophen) Whitehall
Aspirin Free Anacin Maximum Strength
Acetaminophen Film Coated Tablets
(Acetaminophen) Whitehall

Baby Anbesol Teething Gel Anesthetic (Benzocaine) Whitehall

Anbesol (Benzocaine) Whitehall

Maximum Strength Arthritis Pain Formula By the Makers of Anacin Analgesic Tablets and Caplets (Aspirin, Aluminum Hydroxide, Magnesium Hydroxide) Whitehall

Arthritis Strength BC Powder (Aspirin, Salicylamide, Caffeine) Block

BC Powder (Aspirin, Salicylamide, Caffeine) Block

Children's Bayer Chewable Aspirin (Aspirin) Glenbrook

Genuine Bayer Aspirin Tablets & Caplets (Aspirin) Glenbrook

Maximum Bayer Aspirin Tablets & Caplets (Aspirin) Glenbrook

8 Hour Bayer Timed-Release Aspirin (Aspirin) Glenbrook

Extra Strength Bufferin Analgesic Tablets (Aspirin) Bristol-Myers Products

Bufferin Analgesic Tablets and Caplets (Aspirin) Bristol-Myers Products

Cēpacol Anesthetic Lozenges (Troches) (Benzocaine, Cetylpyridinium Chloride) Marion Merrell Dow

Dyclone 0.5% and 1% Topical Solutions, USP (Dyclonine Hydrochloride) Astra

Empirin Aspirin (Aspirin) Burroughs Wellcome

Aspirin Free Excedrin Analgesic Caplets (Acetaminophen, Caffeine) Bristol-Myers Products

Gly-Oxide Liquid (Carbamide Peroxide) Marion Merrell Dow

Haltran Tablets (Ibuprofen) Roberts

Hyland's Teething Tablets (Calcium Phosphate, Homeopathic Medications) Standard Homeopathic

Ibuprofen (Ibuprofen) Ohm Laboratories

Medipren Ibuprofen Caplets and Tablets (Ibuprofen) McNeil Consumer

Mobigesic Analgesic Tablets (Magnesium Salicylate, Phenyltoloxamine Citrate) Ascher

Norwich Extra-Strength Aspirin (Aspirin) Chattem

Norwich Regular Strength Aspirin (Aspirin) Chattem

Nuprin Ibuprofen/Analgesic Tablets & Caplets (Ibuprofen) Bristol-Myers Products

Children's Panadol Chewable Tablets, Liquid, Infants' Drops (Acetaminophen) Glenbrook

Junior Strength Panadol (Acetaminophen) Glenbrook

Tylenol, Children's (Acetaminophen) McNeil Consumer

Vanquish Analgesic Caplets (Acetaminophen, Aspirin, Caffeine) Glenbrook

ZilaDent/ZilaBrace/Zilactin (Benzocaine) Zila Pharmaceuticals

Pain, ear

Americaine Otic Topical Anesthetic Ear Drops (Benzocaine) Fisons Pharmaceuticals

Children's Panadol Chewable Tablets, Liquid, Infants' Drops (Acetaminophen) Glenbrook

Junior Strength Panadol (Acetaminophen) Glenbrook

Pain, general

Acetaminophen Uniserts Suppositories (Acetaminophen) Upsher-Smith

Alka-Seltzer Advanced Formula Antacid & Non-Aspirin Pain Reliever (Acetaminophen, Calcium Carbonate, Citric Acid, Sodium Bicarbonate, Potassium Bicarbonate) Miles Consumer

Alka-Seltzer Effervescent Antacid and Pain Reliever (Aspirin, Sodium Bicarbonate, Citric Acid) Miles Consumer

Alka-Seltzer Extra Strength Effervescent Antacid and Pain Reliever (Aspirin, Sodium Bicarbonate, Citric Acid) Miles Consumer

Alka-Seltzer (Flavored) Effervescent Antacid and Pain Reliever (Aspirin, Sodium Bicarbonate, Citric Acid) Miles Consumer

Aspirin Free Anacin Maximum Strength Acetaminophen Film Coated Caplets (Acetaminophen) Whitehall

Maximum Strength Arthritis Pain Formula By the Makers of Anacin Analgesic Tablets and Caplets (Aspirin, Aluminum Hydroxide, Magnesium Hydroxide) Whitehall

Children's Bayer Chewable Aspirin (Aspirin) Glenbrook

Genuine Bayer Aspirin Tablets & Caplets (Aspirin) Glenbrook

Maximum Bayer Aspirin Tablets & Caplets (Aspirin) Glenbrook

Bayer Plus Aspirin Tablets (Aspirin) Glenbrook

Therapy Bayer Aspirin Caplets (Aspirin, Enteric Coated) Glenbrook

8 Hour Bayer Timed-Release Aspirin (Aspirin) Glenbrook

Campho-Phenique Liquid (Phenol, Camphor) Winthrop Consumer Products

Dorcol Children's Fever & Pain Reducer (Acetaminophen) Sandoz Consumer

Aspirin Free Excedrin Analgesic Caplets (Acetaminophen, Caffeine) Bristol-Myers Products

Feverall Sprinkle Caps (Acetaminophen) Upsher-Smith

Feverall Suppositories (Acetaminophen) Upsher-Smith

Haltran Tablets (Ibuprofen) Roberts

Ibuprofen (Ibuprofen) Ohm Laboratories

Liquiprin (Acetaminophen) Menley & James

Medipren Ibuprofen Caplets and Tablets (Ibuprofen) McNeil Consumer

Motrin IB Caplets and Tablets (Ibuprofen) Upjohn

Norwich Extra-Strength Aspirin (Aspirin) Chattem

Norwich Regular Strength Aspirin (Aspirin) Chattem

P-A-C Analgesic Tablets (Aspirin, Caffeine Anhydrous) Roberts

Children's Panadol Chewable Tablets, Liquid, Infants' Drops (Acetaminophen) Glenbrook

Junior Strength Panadol (Acetaminophen) Glenbrook

Maximum Strength Panadol Tablets and Caplets (Acetaminophen) Glenbrook

St. Joseph Adult Chewable Aspirin (81 mg.) (Aspirin) Schering-Plough HealthCare

St. Joseph Aspirin-Free Fever Reducer for Children Chewable Tablets, Liquid & Infant Drops (Acetaminophen) Schering-Plough HealthCare

Tempra, Acetaminophen (Acetaminophen) Mead Johnson Nutritionals

Trendar Ibuprofen Tablets (Ibuprofen) Whitehall

Trilisate (Choline Magnesium Trisalicylate) Purdue Frederick

Tylenol acetaminophen Children's Chewable Tablets & Elixir (Acetaminophen) McNeil Consumer

Tylenol Cold & Flu No Drowsiness Hot Medication, Packets (Acetaminophen, Dextromethorphan Hydrobromide, Pseudoephedrine Hydrochloride) McNeil Consumer

Tylenol, Extra Strength, acetaminophen Adult Liquid Pain Reliever (Acetaminophen) McNeil Consumer

Tylenol, Extra Strength, acetaminophen Gelcaps, Caplets, Tablets (Acetaminophen) McNeil Consumer

Tylenol, Infants' Drops (Acetaminophen) McNeil Consumer

Tylenol, Junior Strength, acetaminophen Coated Caplets, Grape and Fruit Chewable Tablets (Acetaminophen) McNeil Consumer

Tylenol, Regular Strength, acetaminophen Tablets and Caplets (Acetaminophen) McNeil Consumer

Tylenol PM, Extra Strength Caplets and Tablets (Acetaminophen, Diphenhydramine Hydrochloride) McNeil Consumer

Vanquish Analgesic Caplets (Acetaminophen, Aspirin, Caffeine) Glenbrook

Pain, hemorrhoidal
(see under Pain, anorectal)

Pain, intractable chronic
(see also under Pain, severe)
Infumorph 200 and Infumorph 500 Sterile Solutions (Morphine Sulfate) Elkins-Sinn

Pain, menstrual
Advil Ibuprofen Tablets and Caplets (Ibuprofen) Whitehall

Anacin (Aspirin, Caffeine) Whitehall

Anacin Maximum Strength Analgesic Coated Tablets (Aspirin, Caffeine) Whitehall

Aspirin Free Anacin Maximum Strength Acetaminophen Film Coated Caplets (Acetaminophen) Whitehall

Aspirin Free Anacin Maximum Strength Acetaminophen Film Coated Tablets (Acetaminophen) Whitehall

Maximum Strength Arthritis Pain Formula By the Makers of Anacin Analgesic Tablets and Caplets (Aspirin, Aluminum Hydroxide, Magnesium Hydroxide) Whitehall

Regular Strength Ascriptin Tablets (Aluminum Hydroxide Gel, Dried, Aspirin, Magnesium Hydroxide, Calcium Carbonate) Rhone-Poulenc Rorer Consumer

BC Powder (Aspirin, Salicylamide, Caffeine) Block

Genuine Bayer Aspirin Tablets & Caplets (Aspirin) Glenbrook

Maximum Bayer Aspirin Tablets & Caplets (Aspirin) Glenbrook

Extra Strength Bufferin Analgesic Tablets (Aspirin) Bristol-Myers Products

Bufferin Analgesic Tablets and Caplets (Aspirin) Bristol-Myers Products

Datril Extra-Strength Analgesic Tablets (Acetaminophen) Bristol-Myers Products

Empirin Aspirin (Aspirin) Burroughs Wellcome

Aspirin Free Excedrin Analgesic Caplets (Acetaminophen, Caffeine) Bristol-Myers Products

Excedrin Extra-Strength Analgesic Tablets & Caplets (Acetaminophen, Aspirin, Caffeine) Bristol-Myers Products

Feminine Gold (Camphor, Menthol) Au Pharmaceuticals

Haltran Tablets (Ibuprofen) Roberts

Ibuprofen (Ibuprofen) Ohm Laboratories

Medipren Ibuprofen Caplets and Tablets (Ibuprofen) McNeil Consumer

Midol 200 Cramp Relief Formula (Ibuprofen) Glenbrook

Maximum Strength Midol Multi-Symptom Menstrual Formula (Cinnamedrine Hydrochloride, Acetaminophen) Glenbrook

Maximum Strength Midol PMS Premenstrual Syndrome Formula (Acetaminophen, Pamabrom, Pyrilamine Maleate) Glenbrook

Regular Strength Midol Multi-Symptom Menstrual Formula (Cinnamedrine Hydrochloride, Acetaminophen) Glenbrook

Mobigesic Analgesic Tablets (Magnesium Salicylate, Phenyltoloxamine Citrate) Ascher

Motrin IB Caplets and Tablets (Ibuprofen) Upjohn

Norwich Extra-Strength Aspirin (Aspirin) Chattem

Norwich Regular Strength Aspirin (Aspirin) Chattem

Nuprin Ibuprofen/Analgesic Tablets & Caplets (Ibuprofen) Bristol-Myers Products

Junior Strength Panadol (Acetaminophen) Glenbrook

Maximum Strength Panadol Tablets and Caplets (Acetaminophen) Glenbrook

Premsyn PMS Capsules & Caplets (Acetaminophen, Pamabrom, Pyrilamine Maleate) Chattem

St. Joseph Adult Chewable Aspirin (81 mg.) (Aspirin) Schering-Plough HealthCare

Trendar Ibuprofen Tablets (Ibuprofen) Whitehall

Tylenol, Regular Strength, acetaminophen Tablets and Caplets (Acetaminophen) McNeil Consumer

Vanquish Analgesic Caplets (Acetaminophen, Aspirin, Caffeine) Glenbrook

Pain, mild

Regular Strength Ascriptin Tablets (Aluminum Hydroxide Gel, Dried, Aspirin, Magnesium Hydroxide, Calcium Carbonate) Rhone-Poulenc Rorer Consumer

Arthritis Strength Bufferin Analgesic Caplets (Aspirin) Bristol-Myers Products

Cama Arthritis Pain Reliever (Aspirin, Aluminum Hydroxide Gel, Dried, Magnesium Oxide) Sandoz Consumer

Datril Extra-Strength Analgesic Tablets (Acetaminophen) Bristol-Myers Products

Ecotrin (Aspirin, Enteric Coated) SmithKline Beecham Consumer Brands

Empirin with Codeine Phosphate Nos. 2, 3 & 4 (Aspirin, Codeine Phosphate) Burroughs Wellcome

Excedrin Extra-Strength Analgesic Tablets & Caplets (Acetaminophen, Aspirin, Caffeine) Bristol-Myers Products

Norwich Extra-Strength Aspirin (Aspirin) Chattem

Norwich Regular Strength Aspirin (Aspirin) Chattem

Tylenol, Extra Strength, acetaminophen Adult Liquid Pain Reliever (Acetaminophen) McNeil Consumer

Tylenol, Extra Strength, acetaminophen Gelcaps, Caplets, Tablets (Acetaminophen) McNeil Consumer

Tylenol, Junior Strength, acetaminophen Coated Caplets, Grape and Fruit Chewable Tablets (Acetaminophen) McNeil Consumer

Tylenol, Regular Strength, acetaminophen Tablets and Caplets (Acetaminophen) McNeil Consumer

Pain, mild to moderate

Anaprox and Anaprox DS Tablets (Naproxen Sodium) Syntex

Children's Advil Suspension (Ibuprofen) Wyeth-Ayerst

Darvon-N/Darvocet-N (Propoxyphene Napsylate, Acetaminophen) Lilly

Darvon (Propoxyphene Hydrochloride, Aspirin, Caffeine) Lilly

Darvon-N Suspension & Tablets (Propoxyphene Napsylate) Lilly

Dolobid Tablets (Diflunisal) Merck Sharp & Dohme

Easprin (Aspirin, Enteric Coated) Parke-Davis

Meclomen Capsules (Meclofenamate Sodium) Parke-Davis

Motrin Tablets (Ibuprofen) Upjohn

Nalfon Pulvules & Tablets (Fenoprofen Calcium) Dista

Naprosyn (Naproxen) Syntex

Orudis Capsules (Ketoprofen) Wyeth-Ayerst

PediaProfen Suspension (Ibuprofen) McNeil Consumer

Phenaphen with Codeine Capsules (Codeine Phosphate, Acetaminophen) A.H. Robins

Phenaphen-650 with Codeine Tablets (Acetaminophen, Codeine Phosphate) A.H. Robins

Rufen Tablets (Ibuprofen) Boots Pharmaceuticals

Talacen (Pentazocine Hydrochloride) Sanofi Winthrop Pharmaceuticals

Trilisate (Choline Magnesium Trisalicylate) Purdue Frederick

Wygesic Tablets (Propoxyphene Hydrochloride, Acetaminophen) Wyeth-Ayerst

Pain, mild to moderate, acute musculo-skeletal

Norgesic (Orphenadrine Citrate, Aspirin) 3M Pharmaceuticals

Paraflex Caplets (Chlorzoxazone) McNeil Pharmaceutical

Parafon Forte DSC Caplets (Chlorzoxazone) McNeil Pharmaceutical

Soma Compound w/Codeine Tablets (Carisoprodol, Aspirin, Codeine Phosphate) Wallace

Soma Compound Tablets (Carisoprodol, Aspirin) Wallace

Soma Tablets (Carisoprodol) Wallace

Pain, moderate

Empirin with Codeine Phosphate Nos. 2, 3 & 4 (Aspirin, Codeine Phosphate) Burroughs Wellcome

Levo-Dromoran (Levorphanol Tartrate) Roche Laboratories

Ponstel (Mefenamic Acid) Parke-Davis

Talwin Compound (Pentazocine Hydrochloride, Aspirin) Sanofi Winthrop Pharmaceuticals

Pain, moderate to moderately severe

Anexsia 5/500 Tablets (Hydrocodone Bitartrate, Acetaminophen) SmithKline Beecham Pharmaceuticals

Anexsia 7.5/650 Tablets (Hydrocodone Bitartrate, Acetaminophen) SmithKline Beecham Pharmaceuticals

Azdōne Tablets (Hydrocodone Bitartrate, Aspirin) Central Pharmaceuticals

Damason-P (Hydrocodone Bitartrate, Aspirin) Mason

DHC Plus (dihydrocodeine, acetaminophen, caffeine) Purdue Frederick

Lortab ASA Tablets (Hydrocodone Bitartrate, Aspirin) Whitby

Lortab (Hydrocodone Bitartrate, Acetaminophen) Whitby

Roxicodone Tablets, Oral Solution & Intensol (Oxycodone) (Oxycodone Hydrochloride) Roxane

Synalgos-DC Capsules (Dihydrocodeine Bitartrate, Aspirin) Wyeth-Ayerst

Tylenol with Codeine (Acetaminophen, Codeine Phosphate) McNeil Pharmaceutical

Tylox Capsules (Oxycodone Hydrochloride, Acetaminophen) McNeil Pharmaceutical

Vicodin Tablets (Hydrocodone Bitartrate, Acetaminophen) Knoll

Vicodin ES Tablets (Hydrocodone Bitartrate, Acetaminophen) Knoll

Pain, moderate to severe

Astramorph/PF Injection, USP (Preservative-Free) (Morphine Sulfate) Astra

B & O No. 15A & No. 16A Supprettes (Belladonna Extract, Opium Preparations) Webcon

Dalgan Injection (Dezocine) Astra

Demerol (Meperidine Hydrochloride) Sanofi Winthrop Pharmaceuticals

Dilaudid (Hydromorphone Hydrochloride) Knoll

Dilaudid-HP Injection (Hydromorphone Hydrochloride) Knoll

Duragesic Transdermal System (Fentanyl) Janssen

Duramorph (Morphine Sulfate) Elkins-Sinn

Empirin with Codeine Phosphate Nos. 2, 3 & 4 (Aspirin, Codeine Phosphate) Burroughs Wellcome

Hydrocet Capsules (Acetaminophen, Hydrocodone Bitartrate) Carnrick

Levo-Dromoran (Levorphanol Tartrate) Roche Laboratories

MS Contin Tablets (Morphine Sulfate) Purdue Frederick

MSIR (Morphine Sulfate) Purdue Frederick

Nubain Injection (Nalbuphine Hydrochloride) Du Pont Multi-Source Products

Numorphan Hydrochloride Injection (Oxymorphone Hydrochloride) Du Pont Multi-Source Products

Numorphan Suppositories (Oxymorphone Hydrochloride) Du Pont Multi-Source Products

Percocet Tablets (Oxycodone Hydrochloride, Acetaminophen) Du Pont Pharmaceuticals

Percodan (Oxycodone Hydrochloride, Oxycodone Terephthalate, Aspirin) Du Pont Pharmaceuticals

Stadol (Butorphanol Tartrate) Bristol Laboratories

Talwin Injection (Pentazocine Lactate) Sanofi Winthrop Pharmaceuticals

Talwin Nx (Pentazocine Hydrochloride, Naloxone Hydrochloride) Sanofi Winthrop Pharmaceuticals

Zydone Capsules (Acetaminophen, Hydrocodone Bitartrate) Du Pont Multi-Source Products

Pain, muscular, temporary relief of

Advil Ibuprofen Tablets and Caplets (Ibuprofen) Whitehall

Alka-Seltzer Effervescent Antacid and Pain Reliever (Aspirin, Sodium Bicarbonate, Citric Acid) Miles Consumer

Alka-Seltzer Extra Strength Effervescent Antacid and Pain Reliever (Aspirin, Sodium Bicarbonate, Citric Acid) Miles Consumer

Alka-Seltzer (Flavored) Effervescent Antacid and Pain Reliever (Aspirin, Sodium Bicarbonate, Citric Acid) Miles Consumer

Aspirin Free Anacin Maximum Strength Acetaminophen Film Coated Caplets (Acetaminophen) Whitehall

Aspirin Free Anacin Maximum Strength Acetaminophen Film Coated Tablets (Acetaminophen) Whitehall

Aspercreme Creme & Lotion Analgesic Rub (Trolamine Salicylate) Thompson Medical

Maximum Bayer Aspirin Tablets & Caplets (Aspirin) Glenbrook

Bayer Plus Aspirin Tablets (Aspirin) Glenbrook

Therapy Bayer Aspirin Caplets (Aspirin, Enteric Coated) Glenbrook

8 Hour Bayer Timed-Release Aspirin (Aspirin) Glenbrook

Extra Strength Bufferin Analgesic Tablets (Aspirin) Bristol-Myers Products

Bufferin Analgesic Tablets and Caplets (Aspirin) Bristol-Myers Products

Empirin Aspirin (Aspirin) Burroughs Wellcome

Aspirin Free Excedrin Analgesic Caplets (Acetaminophen, Caffeine) Bristol-Myers Products

Excedrin Extra-Strength Analgesic Tablets & Caplets (Acetaminophen, Aspirin, Caffeine) Bristol-Myers Products

Fluori-Methane (Dichlorodifluoromethane, Trichloromonofluoromethane) Gebauer

Haltran Tablets (Ibuprofen) Roberts

Ibuprofen (Ibuprofen) Ohm Laboratories

Icy Hot Balm (Menthol, Methyl Salicylate) Richardson-Vicks Inc.

Medipren Ibuprofen Caplets and Tablets (Ibuprofen) McNeil Consumer

Momentum Muscular Backache Formula (Aspirin, Phenyltoloxamine Citrate) Whitehall

Nuprin Ibuprofen/Analgesic Tablets & Caplets (Ibuprofen) Bristol-Myers Products

Maximum Strength Panadol Tablets and Caplets (Acetaminophen) Glenbrook

St. Joseph Adult Chewable Aspirin (81 mg.) (Aspirin) Schering-Plough HealthCare

Therapeutic Mineral Ice Pain Relieving Gel (Menthol) Bristol-Myers Products

Trendar Ibuprofen Tablets (Ibuprofen) Whitehall

Tylenol, Junior Strength, acetaminophen Coated Caplets, Grape and Fruit Chewable Tablets (Acetaminophen) McNeil Consumer

Tylenol, Regular Strength, acetaminophen Tablets and Caplets (Acetaminophen) McNeil Consumer

Vanquish Analgesic Caplets (Acetaminophen, Aspirin, Caffeine) Glenbrook

Pain, neurogenic

Anacin (Aspirin, Caffeine) Whitehall

Anacin Maximum Strength Analgesic Coated Tablets (Aspirin, Caffeine) Whitehall

Maximum Strength Arthritis Pain Formula By the Makers of Anacin Analgesic Tablets and Caplets (Aspirin, Aluminum Hydroxide, Magnesium Hydroxide) Whitehall

Arthritis Strength BC Powder (Aspirin, Salicylamide, Caffeine) Block

Regular Strength Ascriptin Tablets (Aluminum Hydroxide Gel, Dried, Aspirin, Magnesium Hydroxide, Calcium Carbonate) Rhone-Poulenc Rorer Consumer

BC Powder (Aspirin, Salicylamide, Caffeine) Block

Genuine Bayer Aspirin Tablets & Caplets (Aspirin) Glenbrook

Maximum Bayer Aspirin Tablets & Caplets (Aspirin) Glenbrook

Mobigesic Analgesic Tablets (Magnesium Salicylate, Phenyltoloxamine Citrate) Ascher

Sarapin (Sarracenia purpurea) High Chemical

St. Joseph Adult Chewable Aspirin (81 mg.) (Aspirin) Schering-Plough HealthCare

Tegretol Chewable Tablets (Carbamazepine) Basel

Tegretol Suspension (Carbamazepine) Basel

Tegretol Tablets (Carbamazepine) Basel

Tylenol, Regular Strength, acetaminophen Tablets and Caplets (Acetaminophen) McNeil Consumer

Vanquish Analgesic Caplets (Acetaminophen, Aspirin, Caffeine) Glenbrook

Zostrix/Zostrix-HP (Capsaicin) GenDerm

Pain, neurogenic, post-herpes zoster
infections, topical relief of
Zostrix/Zostrix-HP (Capsaicin) GenDerm

Pain, obstetrical
Demerol (Meperidine Hydrochloride)
Sanofi Winthrop Pharmaceuticals
Ethrane (Enflurane) Anaquest
Nubain Injection (Nalbuphine
Hydrochloride) Du Pont Multi-Source
Products
Numorphan Hydrochloride Injection
(Oxymorphone Hydrochloride) Du
Pont Multi-Source Products
Stadol (Butorphanol Tartrate) Bristol
Laboratories

Pain, oral mucosal and gingival
Cetacaine Topical Anesthetic
(Benzocaine) Cetylite

Pain, pre- and postoperative, adjunct to
Levo-Dromoran (Levorphanol Tartrate)
Roche Laboratories
Phenergan Injection (Promethazine
Hydrochloride) Wyeth-Ayerst
Sublimaze Injection (Fentanyl Citrate)
Janssen

Pain, pre- and postoperative, relief of
Alfenta Injection (Alfentanil
Hydrochloride) Janssen
Demerol (Meperidine Hydrochloride)
Sanofi Winthrop Pharmaceuticals
Ethyl Chloride, U.S.P. (Chloroethane,
Ethyl Chloride) Gebauer
Fluro-Ethyl (Dichlorotetrafluoroethane,
Ethyl Chloride) Gebauer
Levo-Dromoran (Levorphanol Tartrate)
Roche Laboratories
Mepergan Injection (Meperidine
Hydrochloride, Promethazine
Hydrochloride) Wyeth-Ayerst
Nubain Injection (Nalbuphine
Hydrochloride) Du Pont Multi-Source
Products
Sufenta Injection (Sufentanil Citrate)
Janssen
Talwin Injection (Pentazocine Lactate)
Sanofi Winthrop Pharmaceuticals
Toradol IM Injection (Ketorolac
Tromethamine) Syntex

Pain, severe
Astramorph/PF Injection, USP
(Preservative-Free) (Morphine Sulfate)
Astra

Dolophine Hydrochloride Ampoules &
Vials (Methadone Hydrochloride)
Lilly
Dolophine Hydrochloride Tablets
(Methadone Hydrochloride) Lilly
Duramorph (Morphine Sulfate)
Elkins-Sinn
Levo-Dromoran (Levorphanol Tartrate)
Roche Laboratories
Methadone Hydrochloride Oral Solution
& Tablets (Methadone Hydrochloride)
Roxane
MS Contin Tablets (morphine sulphate)
Purdue Frederick
MSIR (morphine sulphate) Purdue
Frederick
Oramorph SR (Morphine Sulfate
Sustained Release Tablets) (Morphine
Sulfate) Roxane
Pantopon Injectable (Opium
Preparations) Roche Laboratories
Roxanol (Morphine Sulfate) Roxane

Pain, suprapubic, symptomatic relief of
Urispas Tablets (Flavoxate
Hydrochloride) SmithKline Beecham
Pharmaceuticals

Pain, topical relief of
Americaine (Benzocaine) Fisons
Consumer Health
Aspercreme Creme & Lotion Analgesic
Rub (Trolamine Salicylate) Thompson
Medical
Aurum—The Gold Lotion (Methyl
Salicylate, Menthol, Camphor) Au
Pharmaceuticals
Aveeno Anti-Itch Concentrated Lotion
(Calamine, Pramoxine Hydrochloride)
Rydelle
Aveeno Anti-Itch Cream (Calamine,
Pramoxine Hydrochloride) Rydelle
Bactine Antiseptic/Anesthetic First Aid
Spray (Benzalkonium Chloride,
Lidocaine Hydrochloride) Miles
Consumer
Benadryl Anti-Itch Cream
(Diphenhydramine Hydrochloride)
Parke-Davis
Benadryl Spray, Maximum Strength
(Diphenhydramine Hydrochloride)
Parke-Davis

Ben-Gay External Analgesic Products (Menthol, Methyl Salicylate) Pfizer Consumer

BiCozene Creme (Benzocaine, Resorcinol) Sandoz Consumer

Butesin Picrate Ointment (Butamben Picrate) Abbott

Caladryl Cream, Lotion, Spray (Calamine, Diphenhydramine Hydrochloride) Parke-Davis

Campho-Phenique Triple Antibiotic Ointment Plus Pain Reliever (Bacitracin, Neomycin Sulfate, Polymyxin B Sulfate) Winthrop Consumer Products

Chloresium (Chlorophyllin Copper Complex) Rystan

Dermoplast Anesthetic Pain Relief Lotion (Benzocaine) Whitehall

Dermoplast Anesthetic Pain Relief Spray (Benzocaine, Menthol) Whitehall

Ethyl Chloride, U.S.P. (Chloroethane, Ethyl Chloride) Gebauer

Eucalyptamint 100% All Natural Ointment (Menthol) CIBA Consumer

Flex-all 454 Pain Relieving Gel (Menthol) Chattem

Fluori-Methane (Dichlorodifluoromethane, Trichloromonofluoromethane) Gebauer

Fluro-Ethyl (Dichlorotetrafluoroethane, Ethyl Chloride) Gebauer

Gold Plus—The Gold Lotion (Methyl Salicylate, Menthol, Camphor) Au Pharmaceuticals

Icy Hot (Menthol, Methyl Salicylate) Richardson-Vicks Inc.

Itch-X Gel (Pramoxine Hydrochloride, Benzyl Alcohol) Ascher

Lanacane Spray (Benzocaine) Combe

Mantadil Cream (Chlorcyclizine Hydrochloride) Burroughs Wellcome

Mobisyl Analgesic Creme (Trolamine Salicylate) Ascher

Mycitracin Plus Pain Reliever (Bacitracin, Neomycin Sulfate, Lidocaine, Polymyxin B Sulfate) Upjohn

Nupercainal Cream and Ointment (Dibucaine) CIBA Pharmaceutical

PRID Salve (Ichthammol) Walker Pharmacal

Rhulicream (Benzocaine, Calamine) Rydelle

Rhuligel (Benzyl Alcohol, Camphor, Menthol) Rydelle

Rhulispray (Benzocaine, Calamine, Camphor, Isopropyl Alcohol, Menthol) Rydelle

Solarcaine (Lidocaine, Benzocaine) Schering-Plough HealthCare

Thera-Gesic (Methyl Salicylate, Menthol) Mission

Aurum/Gold Plus/Theragold (Methyl Salicylate, Menthol, Camphor) Au Pharmaceuticals

Therapeutic Mineral Ice Pain Relieving Gel (Menthol) Bristol-Myers Products

Therapeutic Mineral Ice Exercise Formula, Pain Relieving Gel (Menthol) Bristol-Myers Products

Tronothane Hydrochloride Cream (Pramoxine Hydrochloride) Abbott

Xylocaine Ointment 2.5% (Lidocaine Base) Astra

Xylocaine 5% Ointment (Lidocaine) Astra

Ziradryl Lotion (Diphenhydramine Hydrochloride, Zinc Oxide) Parke-Davis

Zostrix-HP Topical Analgesic Cream (Capsaicin) GenDerm

Pain, unguis aduncus, temporary relief of

Outgro Solution (Chlorobutanol, Tannic Acid) Whitehall

Pain, unspecified

Ascriptin A/D Caplets (Aluminum Hydroxide Gel, Dried, Aspirin, Magnesium Hydroxide, Calcium Carbonate) Rhone-Poulenc Rorer Consumer

Regular Strength Ascriptin Tablets (Aluminum Hydroxide Gel, Dried, Aspirin, Magnesium Hydroxide, Calcium Carbonate) Rhone-Poulenc Rorer Consumer

Ecotrin (Aspirin, Enteric Coated) SmithKline Beecham Consumer Brands

Lodine Capsules (Etodolac)
Wyeth-Ayerst

Pain, urethritis-induced
Anestacon Solution (Lidocaine
Hydrochloride) Webcon
Xylocaine 2% Jelly (Lidocaine
Hydrochloride) Astra

Pain, urinary tract
Pyridium (Phenazopyridine
Hydrochloride) Parke-Davis
Pyridium Plus (Phenazopyridine
Hydrochloride, Hyoscyamine
Hydrobromide, Butabarbital)
Parke-Davis

General Pain Resources

SUPPORT CENTERS

American Pain Society
5700 Old Orchard Road, 1st floor
Skokie, IL 60077-1057
(708) 966-5595

National Hospice Organization
1901 North Monroe Street, Suite 901
Arlington, VA 22209
(800) 658-8898

Patient Advocates for Advanced
  Treatments
1143 Parmelee, N.W.
Grand Rapids, MI 49504
(616) 453-1477

Vital Options
4419 Coldwater Canyon Avenue,
  Suite A
Studio City, CA 91604
(818) 508-5687

International Association for the Study
  of Pain
909 N.E. 43d Street, Suite 306
Seattle, WA 98105-6020
(206) 547-6409
Fax (206) 547 1703

Collaborating Center for Symptom
  Evaluation
610 Walnut Street
Madison, WI 53705

National Institute of Health
9000 Rockville Pike
Bethesda, MD 20892
(301) 496-4000

American Self-Help Clearing House
St. Clare's–Riverside Medical Center
Pocono Road
Denville, NJ 07834
(201) 625-7101

American Occupational Therapy
  Association
1383 Piccard Drive
Rockville, MD 20850

Mayday Fund
30 Rockefeller Plaza
New York, NY 10112
(212) 649-5800
  The Mayday Fund provides public education, helping individuals to seek and receive effective treatment for pain.

Department of Health and Human
  Services
Social and Rehabilitation Services
Rehabilitation Service Administration
Washington, DC 20014

National Institute of Mental Health
5600 Fishers Lane
Rockville, MD 20852

National Rehabilitation Association
633 South Washington Street
Alexandria, VA 22314

National Organization for Rare
  Disorders
P.O. Box 8923
New Fairfield, CT 06812

National Rehabilitation Information
Center
4407 Eighth Street, N.E.
Catholic University of America
Washington, DC 20017
(800) 34-NARIC

American Medical Association
535 North Dearborn Street
Chicago, IL 60610

National Association of the Physically
Handicapped
2810 Terrace Road, S.E.
Washington, DC 20020

American Physical Therapy Association
1156 15th Street, N.W.
Washington, DC 20005

American Psychiatric Association
1700 18th Street, N.W.
Washington, DC 20009

American Psychological Association
1200 17th Street, N.W.
Washington, DC 20036

National Association of Social Workers
1425 H Street, N.W., Suite 600
Washington, DC 20005

National Mental Health Association
1021 Prince Street
Alexandria, VA 22314-2971

Handicapped Organized Women
P.O. Box 35481
Charlotte, NC 28235
    A newly formed organization acting as
a support group and outreach organization for handicapped women. State chapters now forming.

Vocational Guidance and Rehabilitation
Services
2289 East 55th Street
Cleveland, OH 44103

American Association of Marriage and
Family Counselors
225 Yale Avenue
Claremont, CA 91711

PUBLICATIONS

*Acute Pain Management: Operative or Medical Procedures and Trauma. Clinical
    Practice Guideline* (AHCPR Pub. #92-0032). U.S. Department of Health and Human
    Services, 1992.
Complete Guide to Prescription and Non-Prescription Drugs by Winter Griffith. The
    Body Press, 1993.
Disability and Chronic Disease Quarterly (newsletter), Irving K. Zola, Brandeis Univer-
    sity, Department of Sociology, Waltham, MA 02254.
Mainstream, Magazine of the Able-Disabled, P.O. Box 2781, Escondido, CA 92025.
The Management of Pain by John J. Bonica. Lea & Febiger, 1990.
Pain: A Sourcebook for Nurses and Other Health Professionals by Ada K. Jacox. Little,
    Brown & Co., 1977.
Pain: Clinical Manual for Nursing Practice by M. McCaffery and A. Beebe. C. V. Mosby
    Co., 1989.
Pain Erasure: The Bonnie Prudden Way by Bonnie Prudden. Ballantine Books, 1982.
The Prevention How-To Dictionary of Healing Remedies and Techniques, edited by
    John Feltman. Rodale Press, 1992.

Professional Journals

American Journal of Pain Management.
    University of the Pacific, Stockton,
    CA 95211, (209) 946-3145.
American Pain Society Journal.
    Churchill Livingstone Fulfillment
    Center, 5 South 250 Frontenac Road,
    Naperville, IL 60563, (800) 553-5426.

The Clinical Journal of Pain. Raven
    Press, 1185 Avenue of the Americas,
    New York, NY 10036.
*Journal of Pain and Symptom
    Management.* Elsevier Science
    Publishing Co., 655 Avenue of the
    Americas, New York, NY 10010.

Pain. Elsevier Science Publishing Co., 655 Avenue of the Americas, New York, NY 10010.

Pain Digest. Springer-Verlag, Journal Promotions, 175 Fifth Avenue, New York, NY 10010.

MAIL ORDER

Abbey Medical Catalog Sales
13782 Crenshaw Boulevard
Gardena, CA 90249
(800) 421-5126
In CA (800) 262-1294

ABLE DATA
National Rehabilitation Information
Center
4407 Eighth Street, N.E.
Washington, DC 20017
(202) 635-6090
TTD (202) 635-5884
This is a computerized national database for rehabilitation products.

Accent on Living Magazine
Gillum Road and High Drive,
P.O. Box 700
Bloomington, IL 61702
Supplier to the disabled and chronically ill; write for catalogue.

Access Travel: A Guide to Accessibility
of Airport Terminals
U.S. General Services Administration
Washington, DC 20405

Accurate Medical Service
8004 West Chester Pike
Upper Darby, PA 19082

Air Travel for the Handicapped
TWA
605 Third Avenue
New York, NY 10016

Air Travelers Fly Rights
Office of Consumer Affairs, Civil
Aeronautics Board
Washington, DC 20428

Alda Industries
214 Harvard Avenue
Boston, MA 02134
E-Z up chair to help people who have difficulty with sitting or getting out of a chair.

All Ways Medical
786 East 7th Street
St. Paul, MN 55106
(612) 771-0046
Can call collect. Three- and four-wheel scooters, electric and manual wheelchairs, and other adaptive equipment.

Appliance Information Service
Whirlpool Corporation
Administrative Center
Benton Harbor, MI 49022
Ask for "Designs for Independent Living" and other booklets.

Clearinghouse on the Handicapped,
Office of Special Education and
Rehabilitative Services
Department of Education
330 C Street, S.W.
Switzer Building, Room 3106
Washington, DC 20202

Comfortably Yours
52 West Hunter Avenue
Maywood, NJ 07607
Write for catalogue on aids for easier living.

Consumer Product Information Service
Public Documents Distribution Center
Pueblo, CO 81009

Coping Catalogue
2019 North Carothers
Franklin, TN 37064
(615) 790-2400

Cosco Home Products
2525 State Street
Columbus, IN 47201

Elder Ensembles
7400 Metro Boulevard, Suite 410
Edina, MN 55435
Adapted clothing and shoe service, catalogue, convenience items.

Enrichments: Helping Hands for Special Needs
P.O. Box 579
145 Tower Drive
Hinsdale, IL 60921

Everest and Jennings
3233 E. Mission Oaks Boulevard
Camarillo, CA 93010
Wheelchairs, home and hospital medical supplies.

Helping Hand for Independent Living
P.O. Box 19083
Washington, DC 20036-9083
Write for a $3 catalogue of products for people with special needs.

Mainstream
1200 15th Street, N.W., Suite 403
Washington, DC 20005
(202) 833-1160
A nonprofit organization seeking to provide better employment for the disabled.

Medic Alert Foundation International
P.O. Box 1009
Turlock, CA 95380
(209) 634-4917

Can call collect. A confidential, 24-hour medical information service providing emergency information related to members' medical conditions; free medical information bracelet or necklace provided with membership fee.

New Jersey Self-Help Clearing House
St. Clares–Riverside Medical Center
Pocono Road
Denville, NJ 07834
(201) 625-9565
Will put you in touch with your state's clearinghouse.

The Self-Help Source Book
St. Clares–Riverside Medical Center
Denville, NJ 07834
For help finding and forming mutual aid self-help groups—$8 and well worth it.

Ways and Means
28001 Citrin Drive
Romulus, MI 48174
Write for catalogue for access to over 1,000 adaptive aids and general-use products for daily living.

COMPUTER DATABASES

BRS Information Systems
Maxwell Online Limited
8000 Westpark Drive
McLean, VA 22102
(800) 468-0908

Data Star
485 Devon Park Drive, Suite 10
Wayne, PA 19087
(800) 221-7754

DIALOG Information Services
3460 Hillview Avenue
Palo Alto, CA 94304
(800) 3-DIALOG

The Health Resource
209 Katherine Drive
Conway, AZ 72032
(501) 329-5272
Excellent computer research on medical topics and alternative treatment.

Medlars Management Section
National Library of Medicine
8600 Rockville Pike, Building 38,
Room 4N421
Bethesda, MD 20894
(301) 496-4000

Glossary

Acetaminophen—An analgesic used to treat mild pain and reduce fever (for example, Tylenol).

Acupressure—A variation of acupuncture in which finger pressure is applied instead of needles.

Acupuncture—A therapeutic practice of Chinese origin consisting of the introduction of fine needles at certain points in the skin along vital "lines of force," sometimes far removed from the point where the pain is suffered.

Acute pain—Severe pain usually of short duration, the cause of which is usually known and which may or may not be the result of an acute condition.

Addiction—Overwhelming involvement with obtaining and using a drug for its psychic effects, not for approved medical or social reasons.

Adrenaline—A hormone that increases heart and breathing rates and blood pressure. Its release in the body can be triggered by stress, exercise, or fear. Also called epinephrine.

Affective—Expressing emotion or feeling.

Alexander technique—Therapeutic training to improve poor posture and thereby alleviate pain.

Alternative medicine—Types of health care that use unconventional means with the objective of relieving symptoms.

Amnesiac—A drug administered to block the patient's memory of a painful procedure or operation.

Amphetamine—A group of stimulant drugs that increase nerve activity in the brain, making the user more wakeful and alert.

Analgesia—Loss of pain sensation without sedation.

Analgesic drug—Pain medication used in the treatment of mild to moderate pain.

Anesthesiologist—A physician who specializes in "putting the patient to sleep" in preparation for an operation and monitors body functions during the procedure.

Anesthetic—A drug that causes insensibility to pain and other sensations.

387

Angiography—A procedure that enables blood vessels to be seen on film after the film has been filled with a contrast medium. Used to detect diseases that alter the appearance of the blood vessel channel.

Anticoagulant—A drug given to treat the blood to prevent it from clotting.

Anticonvulsant—Drug that reduces the frequency and severity of seizures.

Antidepressant—A medicine used to treat depression.

Aromatherapy—The use of essential oils from plants and flowers, either massaged into skin or inhaled, in the treatment of psychosomatic and stress-related disorders.

Ayurvedic medicine—Indian system of medicine in which diet and therapy use herbs and massage.

Axillary block—A regional block to treat pain generated from the shoulder, forearm, or hand.

Benign tumor—An abnormal growth that is nonmalignant and does not spread to other parts of the body.

Bioenergetics—A purported exchange of energy between the therapist and the patient.

Biopsy—A diagnostic test in which tissue or cells are excised for microscopic examination.

Biofeedback—A behavioral technique to control and modify emotional, nervous, and muscle responses by altering blood pressure and pulse. Must be taught by a professional.

Breakthrough pain—A sudden flare-up of pain.

Carcinoma—Any malignant (cancerous) tumor that develops in tissues covering or lining organs of the body, such as the skin, the uterus, the lung, or the breast.

Chemotherapy—Treatment of infections or malignant disease that acts selectively on the cause of the disorder.

Chiropractic—A theory of healing that relies on manual manipulation and adjustment of the spine. It is based on the belief that disease results from lack of normal nerve function.

Chronic pain—Prolonged pain, usually lasting for more than six months, for which the cause may or may not be known. Intensity may range from mild to severe.

Codeine—A weak opiate used for pain relief, often with other drugs in tablet or liquid mixtures.

Color therapy—Use of colored light on the body to alter a patient's "aura."

Combination chemotherapy—Combines two or more chemicals to achieve the most effective results in the treatment of malignant disease.

Combined modality therapy—Two or more types of treatment—surgery, radiation, chemotherapy, or immunotherapy—used alternatively or together for maximum effectiveness in the treatment of cancer.

Coping strategies—Varying methods patients use to deal with a particular disease or diagnosis.

Cordotomy—Surgery to divide bundles of nerve fibers of the spinal cord. Used to relieve persistent pain which has not responded to more conservative treatment.

Counterirritant—An agent that is used to produce irritation at one site in order to decrease the perception of pain there or at a distant site.

Cryotherapy—The localized use of cold on the body to relieve pain there or in another part of the body.

Crystal healing—New Age therapy that uses healing energy from quartz and other minerals.

Cutaneous pain—Pain generated from the skin.

Cystic fibrosis—A chronic hereditary disease of the pancreas and lungs that interferes with the absorption of fats and other nutrients from food. The disorder manifests itself in infancy.

Cytodestructive—Having a damaging effect on cells.

Distraction—A method to relieve pain by taking the sufferer's attention away from it.

Dose—The amount of medication prescribed.

Drug tolerance—The loss of effectiveness of a drug prescribed for the relief of pain after repeated administration.

Dura mater—The tough membrane surrounding the spinal cord.

Duration—The length of time the effect of a medication lasts.

EKG—Electrocardiagram, a device that records the electrical impulses that immediately precede contraction of the heart muscle. It is used to detect disorders of the heart.

Embolism—Blockage of an artery by a clump of material traveling in the bloodstream. It may be a blood clot, bubble of air or other gas, piece of tissue or tumor, etc.

EMLA—A topical anesthetic applied to the skin to diminish pain from injections, punctures, or sutures.

Enhancers—Drugs that are given in combination with other drugs to increase their effectiveness.

Epidural anesthesia—A method of pain relief from surgery in which a local anesthetic is injected into the epidural space in the middle and lower back to numb the nerves leading to the chest and lower half of the body.

Equianalgesic—Having equal painkilling effect. (For example, morphine sulfate 10 mg injected intramuscularly is generally used for opioid analgesic comparisons.)

Esophagitis—Painful swelling of the esophagus, making swallowing difficult.

Etiology—Study of the causes of disease, many of which are multifactorial in origin. Many diseases are of unknown etiology.

Faith/religious healing—A method of trying to cure disease by prayer and religious faith.

Femoral nerve block—A regional pain block in the area of the thigh.

Fentanyl—An opioid analgesic used as a supplementary analgesic in anesthesia. Also used in the transdermal pain patch.

Field block—Injection of anesthetic to numb a large treatment area.

Frequency—How often a medication is taken.

General anesthetic—Loss of sensation and conciousness induced by an anesthesiologist, most often to prevent pain and discomfort during surgery.

Guided imagery—Therapy in which patients are encouraged to imagine a real or imaginary setting.

Heat therapy—The use of heat to relieve pain in parts of the body.

Herbal healing—A method of promoting health and treating illness with botanically derived potions.

Herpes, oral—Small painful blisters on the lips and mouth.

Herpes zoster—Medical term for shingles: an infection of the nerves that supply certain areas of the skin, causing a rash of painful small blisters.

Holistic medicine—An alternative therapy aimed at treating the whole person, both body and mind.

Homeopathy—Treatment for disease using small amounts of natural substances which in larger amounts would cause the same symptoms as the ailment.

Hormones—A group of chemical compounds released into the bloodstream by a particular gland or tissue. Hormones control body functions such as the metabolism of cells, growth, sexual development, and the body's response to illness or stress. Glands that primarily produce hormones make up the endocrine system.

Hospice—A hospital or part of a hospital devoted to the care of patients who are dying. Hospice care can take place in the home.

Hypersensitivity—Heightened sensitivity from illness or an adverse allergic reaction.

Hypnosis/hypnotherapy—A technique by which therapeutic suggestions are made to patients in a state of semiconciousness to relieve pain, decrease anxiety, or speed healing.

Imagery—A pain-relief technique that uses mental images produced by memory or imagination.

Immunosuppression—A lowering of the body's immune system.

Immunotherapy—A treatment that stimulates the body's own defense mechanisms to combat disease.

Informed Consent—A discussion between patient and physician that explains exactly what procedure the physician will perform and its risks and benefits.

Intercostal nerve block—A regional block used in the area of the rib cage to block the nerves leading to the chest and abdominal walls.

Interpleura—An area situated between the membrane surrounding the lungs and the membrane lining in the thoracic cavity.

Intramuscular (IM)—Injection into a muscle.

Intrathecal (IC)—Injection into the spinal cord.

Intravenous (IV)—Injection into a vein.

Invasive procedure—A procedure in which body tissues are penetrated by an instrument that may could cause pain or discomfort.

Local nerve block—An injection of local anesthetic around a peripheral nerve to numb the area supplied by the nerve.

Lumbar puncture—A procedure in which a hollow needle is inserted into the lower part of the spinal canal to withdraw cerebrospinal fluid.

Lymphangiogram—A procedure in which dye is injected into lymph vessels so they can be studied on x-ray film.

Malignant—A term primarily used to refer to cancer that spreads from its original site to affect other parts of the body, with potentially life-threatening results.

Meditation—A technique using soothing thought, reflection, and contemplation to alleviate pain.

Metabolism—The chemical and physical processes of the body—for example, the use of glucose in body cells, by which energy is made available.

Metastasis—The spread of cancer from one part of the body to another by way of the lymph system or bloodstream.

Migraine—A severe headache lasting from a few hours to a few days, accompanied by disturbances of vision and/or nausea and vomiting.

Morbidity—The state of being diseased.

Mortality—The death rate, or the number of deaths per 100,000 of the population per year.

Mucosal—Referring to the mucous membranes which line the respiratory tract, alimentary canal, urinary and genital passages, and eyelids. The membranes secrete a fluid that contains mucus to keep them moist and lubricated.

Music distraction—The use of music to alter the focus from pain or illness.

Narcotic—A drug derived from opium or opium-like compounds, with potent analgesic effects, and with the potential for dependence and tolerance after repeated administration.

Naturopathy—A method of treating disease using diet, exercise, and heat to assist the healing process.

Neoplasm—Any new abnormal growth, whether benign or malignant.

Neuron—A nerve cell.

Neuropathic pain—Pain that arises from a damaged nerve.

Neuropeptide—A neural secretion that transmits a chemical message from one neuron to another.

Nociception—The process of pain transmission, usually related to a receptive neuron for painful sensation.

Noxious—Harmful, causing injury to health or well-being.

NSAID—Nonsteroidal anti-inflammatory drug, an aspirin-like drug that alleviates pain and inflammation arising from injured tissue.

Oncology—The medical specialty which deals with the physical, chemical, and biological properties and features of cancer, including causes, disease process, and treatment.

Onset of action—The time at which medicine begins to work.

Opioid—A morphine-like drug that produces pain relief.

Osteopathy—A therapeutic system of medicine based upon the premise that the human body is a unified organism that can be treated by restoring or preserving health by manipulation of the musculoskeletal system.

Oxymorphone—A synthetic opioid with analgesic actions similar to those of morphine but more potent.

Pain—A localized sensation that ranges from mild discomfort to unbearable. Pain is the result of stimulation of special sensory nerve endings following injury or disease.

Pain assessment—The determination of a patient's pain through one or more predetermined modalities.

Pain diary—A daily journal used to chart a patient's pain.

Pain history—Information taken by a physician from a patient about past pain treatments and medications.

Pain patch—A patch worn on the skin that delivers pain-relieving medication on a continuous basis.

Pain team—A diverse group of health care providers in a hospital or other facility who work together in providing pain relief to patients.

Pain threshold—The point at which increasing stimuli are perceived as pain.

Pain tolerance—The level of pain, in intensity and/or duration, that a patient is able to endure.

Palliative treatment—Therapy that relieves symptoms, such as pain, but does not alter the course of disease. Its primary purpose is to improve the quality of life.

Patient-controlled analgesia (PCA)—Self-administration of an analgesic by a patient. PCA is available either from a programmed pump that delivers the drug though an intravenous line or taken orally.

PCA-plus—Continuous infusion of pain medication coupled with the patient's self-administration.

Patient education—Provision of information to the patient on preoperative procedures and expected postoperative sensations, plus instruction to help decrease mobility-related discomfort.

Penile nerve block—A pain block given to dull the pain of circumcision.

Phantom limb pain—The persistence of pain from a limb that was amputated.

Pharmacology—The science dealing with the discovery and development of drugs, their chemical structure, the ways in which they act in the body, their use in prevention or treatment of disease, and their toxicity and side effects.

Phenothiazines—Drugs used to treat psychotic illness, and also used as antihistamines and antiemetics.

Physical dependence—A state in which, after repeated administration of an opiate, a patient may suffer withdrawal symptoms if suddenly deprived of the drug.

Physical therapy—The health profession that treats pain in muscles, nerves, joints, and bones with exercise, electrical stimulation, hydrotherapy, and the use of massage, heat, cold, and electrical devices.

Physiology—The foundation of medical science: the study of body functions, the physical and chemical processes of its cells, tissues, organs, and systems, including their interactions.

Prognosis—A medical appraisal of the course of disease and the prospects for recovery.

PRN (pro re nata)—Instruction for giving a medication "as needed."

Radiation therapy—Treatment with high energy from x-ray or other sources to kill cancer cells.

Referred pain—Pain that is generated from one area but felt in another.

Reflexology—Manipulation of areas of the feet to alleviate pain in other parts of the body.

Regional nerve block—Nerve block that cuts off the pain message to an entire area. Types include axillary, intercostal, and femoral.

Relaxation—A variety of techniques used to decrease anxiety and muscle tension, such as imagery, distraction, and progressive muscle relaxation.

Rhizotomy—Incision of nerve roots within the spinal canal.

Rolfing—A deep and sometimes painful massage to realign the body.

Sedation—The use of a drug to reduce excessive anxiety, often used as premedication to produce relaxation before an uncomfortable procedure.

Sedative—A drug used to produce calmness. Sedatives include sleep medications, antianxiety drugs, antipsychotic drugs, and antidepressant drugs.

Serotonin—A neurotransmitter released by the brain which is thought to be involved in controlling states of conciousness and mood.

Shiatsu—Therapeutic Japanese massage using the manipulation of pressure points.

Sickle cell anemia—A hereditary disease characterized by the presence of abnormally shaped red blood cells, resulting in a very severe form of anemia.

Side effect—Usually describes a secondary consequence of medication or therapy, usually an unwanted or adverse effect.

Somatic pain—Pain associated with the body.

Subcutaneous—The area just beneath the skin.

Subcutaneous anesthetic—A substance injected under the skin to numb the area just beneath the site.

Suffer—To feel pain or distress; to sustain harm, injury, pain, or death; to tolerate or endure pain, evil, injury, or death.

TAC—A topical anesthetic that can be dripped into wounds to numb the area to be sutured.

Tactile strategies—Techniques that provide comfort through the sense of touch, such as stroking or massage.

TENS—(Transcutaneous electrical nerve stimulation, a variation of acupuncture in which a battery-powered generator transmits electrical impulses through electrodes on the skin.

Thrombembolism—The blockage of a blood vessel by a fragment that has broken off and been carried from a blood clot elsewhere in the circulatory system.

Topical anesthesia—An anesthetic applied locally on the skin to produce temporary numbness.

Ultrasound—The use of high-frequency sound waves as a diagnostic tool to detect abnormalities in the body. The procedure is considered painless and safe, and is particularly useful for examining fluid-filled organs and soft organs.

Visceral pain—Pain associated with the abdominal cavity.

Visual Analogue Scale—A pain assessment tool in which the patient is asked to rate his or her pain on a scale of zero (no pain) to ten (severe pain).

WHO—World Health Organization.

WPI—Wisconsin Pain Initiative, dedicated to treating and relieving cancer pain statewide.

Index

abdominal surgery, 52–53
Abrass, I., 302
acetaminophen, 47–48, 100, 123,
    233
  for children, 154
activities of daily living
    (ADL), 306–7
acupressure, 359
acupuncture, 93, 359
acute pain, 7–8
  from cancer, 204–6
  in children, 151
  chronic pain as consequence
    of, 10–11
  treatment of, 8–10
  unrelieved, effects of, 209
addiction, fears of, 11, 31–32, 71,
    201
  in adolescents, 194–96
  in children, 143
  physical dependence
    distinguished from, 234–35
adjuvant (enhancing)
    medications, 34, 50, 233,
    235–37
administration of
    medications, 46–47, 237–38
Adolescent Daily Pain Charts, 194,
    195
Adolescent Pediatric Pain
    Tool, 191–93
adolescents, 186–87

assessment of pain in, 191–94
  pain control in, 194–97
  stages of adolescence, 187–91
Agency for Health Care Policy and
    Research, 144
aging, 302
AIDS (acquired immune deficiency
    syndrome), 284–85
  assessment of pain with, 286–87
  drug-abusing patients
    with, 288–89
  nondrug pain management
    for, 289
  prevalence of pain with, 285–86
  resources for, 290
  treatments for pain with,
    287–89
Alexander technique, 359
alternative health care, 357–60
Altman, Arnold, 160, 162
American Association of Retired
    Persons (AARP), 295–96, 319
American Cancer Society, 20
American Pain Society, 8
  chronic pain defined by, 61–62
American Pain Society Task
    Force, 20
American Society of
    Anesthesiologists, 29
amnesics (medications), 27
amphetamines, 50, 237, 334
amputations, 27

analgesics
  for children, 149, 154–55
  opioids, 48–50
  patient-controlled analgesia
    (PCA), 35–36, 151–54, 194,
    334
  World Health Organization
    (WHO) "ladder" of, 231–33
  see also medications
Anand, K. J., 142
Andrasik, Frank, 94, 97
anesthesiologists, 29–30
anesthetics, 25
  choosing anesthesiologists, 29–30
  for circumcision, 141
  epidural, 26–28
  general, 28–29
  patient-controlled analgesia (PCA)
    for, 35–36, 151–54, 194, 287,
    334
  spinal, 28
  for surgery on infants, 142
anger, 243–44
antianxiety medications, 101, 150
anticonvulsants, 101, 236
antidepressants, 50, 101, 236, 287,
    334
antihistamines, 50, 101
anti-inflammatory medications, 130
antinausea medications, 101–2
anti-rheumatic
    medications, 130–31
anxiety, 243
anxiolytics, 236
aqua-therapy, 92
aromatherapy, 359
Aronoff, Gerald, 64
arthritis, 125
  assessment of, 128–30
  osteoarthritis, 125–26
  physical therapy for, 126–27
  rheumatoid arthritis, 127–28
  self-management of, 131–32
  treatment of, 130–31

Arthritis Self-Efficacy
    Scale, 128–29
Arthritis Society of Canada, 134–35
art therapy, 246
aspirin, 47, 100, 233
assessment of pain, 37–41
  in adolescents, 191–94
  with AIDS, 286–87
  of arthritis, 128–30
  Biobehavioral Pain Profile for, 41,
    44–45, 218–22
  Brief Pain Inventory for, 212–18
  of cancer pain, 210
  in children, 156–59
  communications in, 211–12
  Daily Pain Diaries for, 24, 88–90
  in dying patients, 332–34
  among elderly people, 304–7
  McGill Pain Questionnaire
    for, 42–44
  Memorial Pain Assessment Card
    for, 222, 223
  see also evaluation of pain
at-home care, see home care
Ativan (anxiolytic), 236
aura symptoms, 97–99
axillary blocks, 26
Ayurvedic medicine, 359

back pain, low, 108, 117–25
back surgery, 53
Barcus, Carol, 145
Beck, Susan, 217
Beebe, A.
  on attitudes communicated by
    nurses, 45
  on children in health care
    settings, 148
  on misidentification of "drug
    abuse," 70–71
  on physician-patient conflicts, 65
  on rights of parents of children in
    pain, 144
Bennett, Gary, 63

Berde, Charles, 144, 146, 160
beta blockers, 100
Bills of Rights
  Children's, 161
  Hospice Patients', 337–39
  Pain Patient's, 57
Biobehavioral Pain Profile, 41–44,
    218–22
bioenergetics, 359
biofeedback, 55, 90, 359
Bond, M. B., 62
Bonica, John
  on acute cancer pain, 204
  on assessment of cancer
    pain, 210
  on cancer pain, 200
  on headache histories, 95
  on lack of medical education on
    pain, 2
  on multimodal treatment of
    pain, 13
  on work lost because of chronic
    pain, 61
books, for pain control, 55
boys, see men
breakthrough pain, 32
breast cancer, 21
breathing, 54–55
Breitbart, William S., 284, 285,
    288–89
Brief Pain Inventory (BPI), 212–17
Brin, Edward, 74, 75, 76–78
Brown, Gregory, 71–72
Bruera, Eduardo, 225

calcium-channel blockers, 101,
    103
cancer care centers, 257–59
cancer pain, 199–200, 251–52
  with AIDS and, 284–87
  assessment of, 210–24
  cancer centers for, 257–59
  in children, 160–61
  chronic, 13–15

community resources and
    support groups for, 276–79
  costs of, 21
  ethical issues involving, 208–9
  family caregivers and, 247–51
  individual responses to, 206–7
  management of, 231–41
  multidisciplinary teams for, 246
  poor control of, 207–8
  psychological aspects of, 241–46
  quality of life and, 225–31
  resources for, 252–56
  resources for, in
    children, 260–76
  types of, 204–6
  undertreated, 200–203
  unrelieved, effects of, 209–10
capsaicin (Zostrix), 103, 131
capsules, 46, 237
cardiac surgery, 52
caregivers, family as, 247–51, 335
Cassell, Eric J., 358
Cats-Baril, William, 108, 117, 124
ceiling effects, 233
Chapman, C. Richard
  on assessment of cancer
    pain, 212, 217
  on cancer pain, 199–200, 225
  on descriptions of pain, 211
  on evaluation of chronic
    pain, 75–76
  on problems in assessment of
    pain, 78–79
  on psychological aspects of
    cancer pain, 243–44
Charap, Arthur David, 324–25
chemotherapy, 204
chest and chest-wall surgery,
    51–52
childbirth, 28
children, 140–42
  adolescents distinguished
    from, 190
  cancer pain in, 160–62

children (*continued*)
  cancer resources for, 260–76
  control-coping measures
    for, 159–60
  of disabled parents, 73
  elderly people compared
    with, 303
  evaluation of pain in, 144–47
  hospitals for, 167–83
  insufficient pain medication given
    to, 142–43
  pain assessment in, 156–59
  Pain Plans for, 147–56
  pain professionals for, 163–67
  patient-controlled analgesia (PCA)
    used by, 36
  publications on pain in, 162
  undertreated postoperative pain
    in, 143–44
Children's Pain Bill of Rights, 161
chiropractic, 359
chronic cancer pain, 13–15, 204,
  206
chronic headaches, 94
  see also headaches
chronic pain, 11–13, 60–61
  arthritis, 125–32
  from cancer, 204, 206
  cancer pain, 13–15
  in children, 160
  complexity of, 67–73
  as consequence of acute
    pain, 10–11
  definition of, 61–62
  in elderly people, 302–3
  evaluation of, 74–79
  headaches, 94–108, 109–116
  lack of education in management
    of, 63–64
  low-back pain, 108, 117–25
  meaning to patients of, 66–67
  Pain Diaries of, 88–90
  patient-physician conflicts
    over, 65–66

psychological aspects of, 241–42
resources on, 133–35
Survey of Pain Attitudes
  on, 79–83
treatment of, 90–94
types of, 62–63
unrelieved, effects of, 209–10
West Haven-Yale
  Multidimensional Pain
  Inventory on, 83–88
  see also cancer pain
Chronic Pain Diaries, 88–90
circumcision, 141–42
Cleeland, Charles, 204, 212, 228
cluster headaches, 102–3
corticosteroids, 235
codeine, 48, 155
Cohen, Felissa, 31
cold therapy, 93, 240–41
color therapy, 359
combined ("mixed")
    headaches, 104
communications
  about pain, 211
  with AIDS patients, 287
  physician-patient conflicts
    and, 65–66
community resources, for
    cancer, 276–79
Compazine (phenothiazine), 236
confusion (as side effect), 239
constipation, 238
controlled drugs, 4–5
coping strategies, 71–72
  in adolescents, 190–91
  in cancer patients, 244–46
  in children, 146, 159–60
costs
  of chronic pain, 61
  of home care, 294
  of hospice care, 337
  of low-back pain, 117
  of nursing homes, 314–15
  of poor pain management, 21

counterirritants, 241
Cousins, Norman, 292
Coyle, Nessa, 296, 331, 334
Croker, Nancy, 331–32
Cruzan, Nancy, 323
cryoanalgesia, 241
cryotherapy, 359
crystal healing, 359
CT (computerized tomography), 78
cutaneous examinations, 77

Dahl, June, 201
Dalessio, Donald J., 94
Dalton, Jo Anne, 41–44, 218
Daut, Randall, 204
deaths, 321–22
    from anesthetics, 29–30
    from cancer, 199
    impact on family of, 335
deconditioning, 68–70
    of arthritis pain, 126
Demerol, 49
dental problems, myofascial pain
        and, 106
dental surgery, 50–51
dependence, on opioids, 49, 235,
        239
depression, 243, 334
    in AIDS patients, 286
Desoxyn (amphetamine), 237
Dexedrine (amphetamine), 237
diagnoses
    assessment tools for, 78–79
    of cancer, 199
    of headaches, 95–96
    of osteoarthritis, 126
    pain histories in, 23–25
    patient evaluations in, 76–78
    of rheumatoid arthritis, 128
    see also evaluation of pain
diagnostic procedures, 25
diaries
    Chronic Pain Diaries, 88–90
    headache diaries and logs, 97, 98

Pain Diaries, for
    children, 155–56
    in self-management of
        arthritis, 132
Dilaudid, 49
Dillon, Paula, 201
disabilities, from low-back
        pain, 108–17
distraction, 155, 197, 360
doctors, see physicians
Donaldson, Gary, 9, 206–7
Donovan, Marilee, 34, 201
dorsal column stimulation, 93, 240
dosages, 31, 33–34
    ceiling effects in, 233
    for dying patients, 334
    of opioids, 32–33
    of opioids for cancer
        pain, 207–8, 234–35
    patient-controlled analgesia (PCA)
        for, 35–36, 151–54, 287, 334
    in WHO three-step analgesic
        ladder, 233
drowsiness, 239
drug abuse, 70–71
drug abusers, with AIDS and HIV
        infections, 288–89
Drug Enforcement Administration
        (DEA, U.S.), 4
drugs, see medications
Dubner, Ronald, 10
durable power of attorney, 330
Duragesic (Fentynal), 334
dying patients, 321–22

early adolescence, 187–88
Eastern Cooperative Oncology
        Group (ECOG), 202
education
    of nurses, pain in, 200–201
    in pain control, 55
    in pain management, lack
        of, 63–64, 203
Edwards, Lindsey, 71

Eiler, John, 302–3
Elavil (antidepressant), 236
elderly people, 6
  assessment of pain in, 304–7
  in nursing homes, 310
  pain care for, 302–4
  treatment of pain in, 307–8
electrodiagnostic studies, 78
emergency rooms, children in, 149
EMLA (topical anesthetic), 150
emotions, 357–58
enhancing (adjuvant)
    medications, 34, 233, 235–37
epidural administration of
    medications, 46–47, 238, 240
epidural anesthetics, 26–28
  for children, 142, 153–54
epidural endoscopy, 124–25
ergotamine products, 101
ethical issues, 2, 208–9
evaluation of pain, 74–78
  in adolescents, 191–94
  of arthritis, 128–30
  assessment tools for, 78–79
  in children, 144–47
  of headaches, 95–97
  of low-back pain, 120–23
  pain diaries for, 88–90
  Survey of Pain Attitudes
    for, 79–81
  West Haven–Yale
    Multidimensional Pain
    Inventory for, 82–88
  see also assessment of pain
Evans, Wayne O., 2, 68
examinations, in patient
    evaluations, 77
exercise
  for low-back pain, 124
  in treatment of chronic
    pain, 91–92

faith healing, 359
families
  as caregivers, 247, 335

of chronic pain patients, 72–73
  descriptions of pain by, 248–50
  experiences of pain of, 250–51
  see also parents
Family Member/Significant Other
    Pain Diaries, 88–90
family therapy, 92–93
Fear-Avoidance Beliefs
    Questionnaire, 122–23
federal government, 4
  children's cancer resources
    from, 260–62
  guidelines on pain management
    issued by, 9
  on rights of dying
    patients, 323–24
Federal Patient Self-Determination
    Act (1990), 324
femoral nerve blocks, 26
Fentanyl, 49
Fentanyl (Duragesic), 334
Ferrell, Betty, 322
  on assessment of pain among
    elderly people, 304
  on costs of uncontrolled cancer
    pain, 21
  on home care for pain
    management, 296–97
  on impact of cancer pain on
    family caregivers, 247–51
  on impact of deaths on
    family, 335
  on ineffective pain
    treatments, 225–26
  on nurses' fears of
    addiction, 31–32
  on nursing and pain
    management, 3
  on pain in nursing
    education, 200–201
  on pain in nursing home
    patients, 303, 310–11, 315
  Quality of Life Measuring Tool
    by, 227–31
  on undertreatment of pain, 20

Ferrell, Bruce
  on assessment of pain among
    cancer pain, 304
  on home care for pain
    management, 296–97
  on pain in nursing home
    patients, 303, 310–11, 315
field blocks, 26
Fishman, Baruch, 245
Foley, Kathleen, 199
  on opioids for cancer pain, 239
  on physical dependence, 235
  types of cancer pain distinguised
    by, 204–6
  on use of morphine for cancer
    pain, 234
foods, as cause of migraine
    headaches, 99–100
Friedman, Mark, 102
Fries, James F., 125, 132
Frymoyer, John, 108, 117, 124

general anesthetics, 28–29
girls, *see* women
glucocorticoids, 131
Graff-Radford, Steven B., 106, 108
Grossman, Stuart, 203
group therapy, 92
guided imagery, 55, 197, 359

Haldol (phenothiazine), 236
Harkins, Stephen, 66–67, 202,
    303
headache diaries and logs, 97, 98
headache histories, 95–96
headaches, 94–95
  chart on, 109–16
  cluster, 102–3
  combined, 104–6
  evaluation of, 95–97
  migraine, 97–102
  myofascial pain and, 106–8
  tension or
    muscle-contraction, 104
head pain, myofascial pain, 106–8

head surgery, 51
health, World Health Organization's
    definition of, 225
heat therapy, 359
heat treatments, 240
Henretig, F., 149
herbal healing, 359
Hester, Nancy
  on lack of research on pain in
    children, 142
  Pain Experience History used
    by, 145
  Pain Interviews used by, 156–57
  on Pain Plans for children, 147
  on withdrawal by children, 141
Hill, Stratton, 4
HIV infection, 284–85
  assessment of pain with, 286–87
  drug-abusing patients
    with, 288–89
  nondrug pain management
    for, 289
  prevalence of pain with, 285–86
  resources for, 290
  treatments for pain with, 287–88
Hofmann, A., 190
holistic medicine, 359
Holland, Jimmie, 241
home care, 54, 292–93
  for chronically ill children, 160
  cost-effectiveness of, 294
  evaluating quality of, 295–96
  locating agencies for, 294–95
  for pain management, 296–97
  resources for, 298–300
homeopathy, 359
Hospice Association of
    America, 337
Hospice Patients' Bill of
    Rights, 337–39
hospices, 335–37
  resources for, 340
hospitals, 292
  for children, 167–83
  children in, 148–49

hospitals (*continued*)
discussing pain management
plans with, 30–33
lack of education for pain
management in, 64
lack of pain policies in, 3–4
medical directives for, 325–27
pain in AIDS patients in, 285–86
pain centers, 342–56
patient-controlled analgesia used
in, 35–36, 151–54, 194
patients' rights in, 324
Houde, Raymond, 33, 234
humor, 246
Hurtz, R., 289
hypnosis, 360
hypnotherapy, 90, 360
hypnotics (medications), 50

ibuprofens, 47–48, 100, 155
imagery, 55, 90, 197, 244–45,
359
immune system
cancer pain and, 207
emotions and, 357–58
see also AIDS
individual therapy, 92
infants, 6, 140–42
Children's Pain Bill of Rights
for, 161
insufficient pain medication given
to, 142–43
Pain Plans for, 147–56
resources for, 162–83
undertreated postoperative pain
in, 143–44
see also children
Informed Consent, 21
instruction, in pain control, 55
intercostal nerve blocks, 26
International Association for the
Study of Pain Task Force, 342
intramuscular administration of
medications, 46, 238

intrathecal administration of
medications, 240
intravenous administration of
medications, 46, 238
intravenous diazepam
(Valium), 103
intravenous pentobarbital
(Nembutal), 103
Inturrisi, C., 239

Jacob, M. C., 82–83
Jacox, Ada, 14
Jensen, Mark, 217
Joranson, David, 4

Kane, R., 302, 307
Katz Activities of Daily Living
(ADL) assessment, 306–7
Kerns, Robert, 82–83
Kinney, Wesley, 74, 75, 76–78
Koo, Peter, 48
on dosages of opioids, 235
on lack of medical education in
pharmacology, 33–34
on multidisciplinary teams for
pain management, 286
on phantom limb pain, 27
on physician-patient
communications, 31
on treatment of AIDS pain, 288
on treatment of chronic cancer
pain, 231
Kübler-Ross, Elisabeth, 322
Kwentus, J., 303

Lamer, William M., Jr., 327–31
late adolescence, 188–89
legal issues, 2, 209
durable power of attorney, 330
medical directives, 326–29
on rights of dying
patients, 323–24
state laws and regulations, 4–5
LeShan, 241

Levoprome (phenothiazine), 236
Levorphanol, 50
Lidocaine (local anesthetic), 150
Liebeskind, John, 10–11, 207
liquid administration of
    medications, 46, 237
lithium carbonate, 103
living wills, 323
local anesthetics, 150
local nerve blocks, 26
Loeser, John D.
    on depression and pain, 75
    on incorrect medication, 70
    on low-back pain, 117, 118
    on nervous system
        injuries, 62–63
    on pain centers, 13
Lorig, Kate, 125, 132
Loscalzo, Matthew, 245
low-back pain, 108–20
    evaluation of, 120–23
    treatment of, 123–25

McAnarney, E., 194
McCaffery, Margo
    on attitudes communicated by
        nurses, 45
    on children in emergency
        rooms, 149
    on children in health care
        settings, 148
    on depression and pain, 12
    on descriptions of chronic pain
        patients, 65
    on misidentification of "drug
        abuse," 70–71
    on pain in infants, 140–41
    on pain in nursing
        education, 200–201
    on parental responsibility for
        children, as patients, 144
    on parents with children in
        recovery rooms, 147
    patients characterized by, 208

McGill Pain Questionnaire, 41–44,
    78
    Short-Form, 304, 305, 332, 333
McGuire, Deborah, 3, 218
Mackie, J., 143–44
macrobiotics, 360
Marcaine (local anesthetic), 150
Marks, Richard, 34
Mason, James, 200
massage, 55, 93
Massie, Mary Jane, 241
Mather, L., 143–44
Matthews-Simonton, Stephanie, 245
Max, Mitchell, 35, 203
Mayer, Tom, 118
medical charts
    "drug abuse" indicated
        on, 70–71
    pain recorded on, 38
medical directives, 325–29
medical education, 2
    in pain management, lack
        of, 63–64, 203
medical histories, 76, 96
    headache histories, 95–96
    pain histories, 23–25
medications
    administration of, 46–47
    administration of, to dying
        patients, 321
    for adolescents, 196–97
    for arthritis, 130–31
    availability in nursing homes
        of, 315
    for cancer pain, 233–39
    for children, dosages of, 153
    for cluster headaches, 103
    for combined headaches, 104
    dosages of, 31
    guide to, 365–81
    inadequately given to infants and
        children, 142–43
    for low-back pain, 123
    for migraine headaches, 100–102

medications (*continued*)
nondrug alternatives to, 54–56
no standard dosages for, 33–34
patient-controlled analgesia (PCA)
for, 35–36, 151–54, 194, 287,
334
pharmaceutical companies
for, 363–64
polypharmacy, 70–71, 76–77
regulation of, 4–5
side effects of, 36–37
for tension headaches, 104
in treatment of pain among
elderly people, 307
types of, 47–50
WHO three-step analgesic ladder
for, 231–33
meditation, 245, 360
Mehta, M., 207
Melzack, Ronald
on classes of pain, 40–41
on descriptions of pain, 191
on evaluation of pain, 74
gate control theory of, 69
on measurement of pain, 211
on pain and quality of life, 5
on unfounded fears of
addiction, 11
Memorial Pain Assessment
Card, 222, 223
memory, in infants, 141
men
early adolescence in, 187–88
puberty in, 187
mental imagery, 244–45
Methadone, 49
Miaskowski, Christine, 284
midadolescence, 188
migraine headaches, 97–99
Minnesota Multiphasic Personality
Inventory, 79
"mixed" (combined)
headaches, 104
mobilization treatments, 241

modality-oriented clinics, 343
Modig, J., 28
Moinpour, Carol, 199–200, 225
moral issues, 2
morphine, 48–49, 234, 235
availability in nursing homes
of, 315
for children, 155
for dying patients, 321, 334
fear of addiction to, 11
oral administration of, 332–33
Mount, Balfour, 241–42, 244
Moyers, Bill, 358
MRI (magnetic resonance
imaging), 78
MS Contin (morphine), 235, 333
mucosal administration of
medications, 46, 237
multidisciplinary pain centers, 342
multidisciplinary pain
clinics, 342–43
multidisciplinary teams, 246
muscle-contraction (tension)
headaches, 104
music, 55, 90, 245–46, 360
myelography, 78
myofascial pain, 106–8

Nash, Justin, 67, 68
National Association of Children's
Hospitals and Related
Institutions, Inc., 167–83
National Association for Home
Care, 294
National Chronic Pain Outreach
Association, 133–34
National Citizens' Coalition for
Nursing Home Reform, 311,
319
National Headache Foundation, 95
naturopathy, 360
nausea, 238
neck pain, myofascial pain, 106–8
neck surgery, 51

Nembutal (intravenous pentobarbital), 103
nerve blocks, 78, 240
  for children, 154
neurological examinations, 77
neurostimulation, 93, 240
neurosurgery, 51
Newshan, Gayle, 289
Ngeow, Jeffrey, 27–28
Nicassio, Perry, 71–72
nitrous oxide, 150
nondrug alternative treatments, 54–56
  for AIDS and HIV infection, 289
  for cancer pain, 240–41
  for pain among elderly people, 307–8
nonprescription drugs, *see* medications
nonsteroidal anti-inflammatory drugs (NSAIDs), 47–48, 101, 123, 155, 233
nose sprays, 46, 237
Numeric Pain Intensity Scale, 37–38, 297, 332, 361
Nuprin Pain Report, 12, 94
nurses
  attitudes communicated by, 45
  care for dying patients by, 324–25
  dosages cut by, 31, 208
  medication withheld by, 8–9
  pain management in education of, 3, 200–201
  patients' communications about pain to, 211–12
nursing homes, 310–12
  checklist for, 316–18
  evaluating care in, 314
  pain complaints among patients in, 303–4
  pain management in, 315–16
  resources on, 319
  staffing of, 313–14
  visiting, 312–13

occupational therapists, 246
occupational therapy, 92, 131
Oden, Rollin, 37
opioids, 70
  administration of, 10
  for AIDS patients, 285
  for arthritis, 131
  for cancer pain, 207–8, 233–35
  doses of, 32–33
  "enhancing drugs" given with, 34
  fears of addiction to, 11, 201
  given to infants and children, 142–43
  not stocked by some pharmacies, 202
  restrictions on, 4
  side effects of, 36–37, 238–39
  types of, 48–50
  used with adolescents, 194–96
  weak, for migraine headaches, 102
  in WHO three-step analgesic ladder, 233
oral administration of medications, 46, 194, 232, 234, 237
  of morphine, 332–33
orthopedic surgery, 53
Osler, Sir William, 119–20
osteoarthritis, 125–27
osteopathy, 360
Osterweil, Dan, 310–11
Ouslander, J., 302
Oxymorphone, 50

Page, Gayle, 10
Paice, Judith, 239
pain
  acute, 7–11
  in adolescents, study of, 190–91

pain (*continued*)
  assessment of, 37–45
  children's coping strategies
    for, 146
  children's words for, 145
  chronic, 11–13
  chronic cancer, 13–15
  definition of, 6
  from diagnostic procedures, 25
  among elderly people, 303–4
  families' descriptions of, 248–50
  families' experiences of, 250–51
  felt by infants, 140–42
  individual responses to, 206–7
  meaning to patients of, 66–67
  in nursing homes, 310–11
  physician-patient conflicts
    over, 65–66
  undertreated, 200–203
  unrelieved, effects of, 209–10
  see also cancer pain; chronic
    pain
pain behavior, 75
  subjective, 77–78
pain centers, 342–43
  list of, 343–53
pain clinics, 343
Pain Diaries, 88–90
  for cancer pain, 222, 224
  for children, 155–56
Pain Experience Histories, 145–46
pain histories, 23–25
Pain Interviews, 156–57
pain management
  in adolescents, 194–97
  anesthetics in, 26–30
  assessment of pain in, 210
  benefits of, 1
  of cancer pain, 202, 231–41
  discussing with hospitals,
    30–33
  ethical, moral, and legal issues
    in, 2
  federal guidelines on, 9
  for home care, 54
  home care for, 296–97
  lack of education in, 63–64
  lack of hospital policies on, 3–4
  laws and regulations on, 4–5
  medical education in, 2–3
  nondrug, 289
  in nursing homes, 311, 315–16
  Pain Patient's Bill of Rights
    for, 57
  participation of adolescents
    in, 190
  patient participation in, 5–6
  planning with physicians, 19–22
  to prevent acute pain from
    becoming chronic pain, 10–11
pain patches, 333–34
Pain Patient's Bill of Rights, 57
  Children's, 161
Pain Plans, 30–33
  for infants and children, 147–56
  see also pain management;
    treatments
pain treatment facilities, 342
parents
  children's pain plans developed
    by, 147–48
  as guardians of rights of
    children, 144
  Pain Experience Histories
    for, 145
  Pain Interviews for, 157
Parent's Daily Pain Chart for Young
    Children, 151, 152
patch administration of
    medications, 46, 237, 333–34
patient-controlled analgesia
    (PCA), 35–36
  in adolescents, 194
  for AIDS patients, 287
  in children, 151–54
  for dying patients, 334
patient records
  "drug abuse" indicated
    on, 70–71
  pain recorded on, 38

patients
    advance planning by, 322–27
    of alternative therapies, 357
    cancer, coping strategies
        of, 244–46
    cancer, undertreatment of pain
        of, 201
    children as, 144
    communications about pain
        by, 211–12
    conflicts between physicians
        and, 65–66
    cycle of poor pain control
        in, 207–8
    with drug-abuse
        histories, 288–89
    dying, 321–22
    evaluations of, 76–78
    health-care decisions by, 21
    in hospices, rights of, 337–39
    individual responses to pain
        in, 206–7
    meaning of pain to, 66–67
    in nursing homes, 310–11
    Pain Patient's Bill of Rights
        for, 57
    participation in pain management
        by, 5–6
    rights of, 323–24
    self-reporting of pain by, 8
    undertreatment of pain in, 34–35
Patient's Personal Daily Pain
    Chart, 38–39
Payne, Richard, 284–85
pediatric oncology units, 262–76
perineal surgery, 52–54
peripheral nerve stimulation, 93
phantom limb pain, 27
pharmaceutical companies, 363–64
pharmacies
    controlled drugs stocked by, 4–5
    opioids not stocked by, 202
phenothiazines, 236
Philips, Clare, 69
physical dependence, 234–35, 239

physical examinations, 77
physical relief techniques, 56
physical therapists, 91, 246
physical therapy, 93, 126–27
physicians
    anesthesiologists, 29–30
    care for dying patients
        by, 324–25, 331–32
    children's pain plans developed
        by, 147
    children's pain
        professionals, 163–67
    conflicts between patients
        and, 65–66
    lack of education in pain
        management of, 63–64
    low dosages prescribed by, 35
    medical directives for, 325–27
    monitoring of prescribing
        practices of, 4
    pain histories taken by, 23–25
    pain management in education
        of, 2–3, 203
    pain underestimated by, 8
    patients' communications about
        pain to, 211–12
    planning pain management
        with, 19–22
    rheumatologists, 132
Pizzo, Philip A., 143
Poker Chip Tool (of pain
    assessment), 157, 158
Polatin, Peter, 118
Poletti, Rosette, 334
polypharmacy, 70–71, 76–77
Portenoy, Russell, 71
    on fears of cancer pain, 13
    on lack of medical education on
        pain, 3
    on prevalence and characteristics
        of symptoms of
        cancer, 226–27
    on relief of cancer pain, 228
    on undertreatment of cancer
        pain, 203

postoperative pain
  federal guidelines on pain
    management for, 9
  in infants, 142
  undertreated in infants and
    children, 143–44
power of attorney, durable, 330
prayer, 55
prescription drugs, *see* medications
prevention
  of migraine headaches, 100
  of myofascial pain, 107–8
Price, Donald, 66–67, 202, 303
privacy
  for adolescents, 189
  of hospice patients, 338
procedure-related pain, in
  children, 150–51
Prolixin (phenothiazine), 236
proxy decision makers, 325
psychological dependence, 234, 239
psychological factors
  in acute cancer pain, 204–6
  in cancer pain, 241–46
  in causes of migraine
    headaches, 100
  in chronic pain, 71–72
  in patient evaluations, 76
  in treatment of chronic pain, 90
puberty, 187

quality of life, 5
  cancer pain and, 225–27
  of dying patients, 327
  in evaluation of headaches, 97
  of hospice patients, 339
  measurement of, 227–31
  near end of life, 331
Quality of Life Measuring
  Tool, 227–31
Quinlan, Karen Ann, 323

radical head and neck surgery, 51
recovery rooms, parents with
  children in, 147–48

rectal administration of
  medications, 46, 238
Reeves, John, 78, 108
reflexology, 360
regional analgesia, 153–54, 240
regional blocks, 26, 142
regulations, 4–5, 202
  on nursing homes, 311, 315–16
relaxation techniques, 197, 244–45
religious healing, 359
resources
  for AIDS and HIV infection, 290
  for cancer pain, 252–56
  for chronic pain, 133–35
  for elderly people, 308
  for home care, 298–300
  on hospices, 340
  on nursing homes, 319
  pain centers, 343–53
respiratory depression, 239
rheumatoid arthritis, 127–28
rheumatologists, 132
rights
  Children's Pain Bill of
    Rights, 161
  of hospice patients, 337–39
  of nursing home patients, 313
  Pain Patient's Bill of Rights,
    57
  of patients, 323–24
Roland and Morris Disability
  Questionnaire, 120–22
rolfing, 360
Roy, Ranjan, 72
Rudy, R., 82
Rustad, Lynne, 72–73

Saberski, Lloyd, 124–25
Sachar, Edward, 34
Sarno, John, 118–19
Saunders, Dame Cicely, 334
Savedra, Marilyn, 188, 190, 196
Schechter, Neil
  on cancer pain in children, 160,
    162

on children's understanding of
pain, 146
on opioids given to children,
142
on undertreatment of pain in
children, 6, 140, 154
Schienle, Donald, 302–3
Schwartz, S. I., 29, 30
sedation, 239
of adolescents, 194
of children, 149
sedatives, 50
Selbst, Steven, 149
self-hypnosis, 197, 244–45
self-management of
arthritis, 131–32
Shapiro, Barbara, 303
Sharrock, Nigel, 28
Shawyer, Martha, 242
shiatsu, 360
Short-Form McGill Pain
Questionnaire, 304, 305, 332,
333
side effects of medications, 36–37,
238–39
in children, 153
Silverman, Howard, 331–32
Sinatra, Raymond, 9–10
Sinequan (antidepressant), 236
sleep, 33
side effects of medications
and, 37
Smith, Robert, 2, 208–9
social workers, 246
soft tissue surgery, 53–54
Solomon, Mildred Z., 324
Solomon, Seymour, 100, 103
spinal administration of
medications, 47, 238
spinal anesthetics, 28
Spross, Judith, 202–3
staffing, of nursing homes, 313–14
state laws, 4–5
on rights of dying
patients, 323–24

states, home care agencies licensed
by, 295
Stehlin, John, 199
steroid therapy, 103
stress
in infants, 140
in myofascial pain, 106, 107
subcutaneous administration of
medications, 46, 238
subcutaneous anesthetics, 26
subjective pain behavior, 77–78
substance abusers, with AIDS and
HIV infections, 288–89
Sullivan, Louis, 61
support groups, for cancer, 276–79
surgery
abdominal and perineal, 52–54
anesthetics for, 26–30
chest and chest-wall, 51–52
on children, pain plans
for, 147–48
on children, pain related
to, 150–51
dental, 50–51
discussing pain management
plans for, 30–33
federal guidelines for pain
management following, 9
on infants, 142
neurosurgery, 51
preparing children for, 148–49
radical head and neck, 51
see also postoperative pain
Survey of Pain Attitudes, 79–81
swimming, 92
symptoms
aura symptoms, 97–99
of cancer, pain as, 204
of cancer, prevalence and
characteristics of, 226–27
headaches as, 94
Syrjala, Karen L., 75, 78, 212

tablets, 46, 237
TAC (topical anesthetic), 150

tactile strategies, 360
teenagers, *see* adolescents
Tegretol (anticonvulsant), 236
tension (muscle-contraction)
    headaches, 104
tension myositis syndrome
    (TMS), 119
therapeutic heat, 92
therapeutic touch, 289
therapies
    alternative, 357–60
    for osteoarthritis, 126–27
    see also treatments
thermography, 78
Thorazine (phenothiazine), 236
Tofranil (antidepressant), 236
tolerance (to opioids), 239
topical analgesic cream, 131
topical anesthetics, 26
    for children, 150
topical capsaicin (Zostrix), 103,
    131
Torgerson, W.S., 40–41
tranquilizers, 50, 334
Transcutaneous Electrical Nerve
    Stimulation (TENS), 93, 240,
    360
transdermal administration of
    medications, 46
transdermal patches, 333–34
Tranxene (anxiolytic), 236
treatments
    for acute pain, 8–10
    in adolescents, 194–97
    for arthritis, 130–32
    for cancer pain, 233–41
    for chronic pain, 90–94
    for cluster headaches, 103
    for low-back pain, 118–19,
        123–25
    medical directives on, 325–27
    for migraine headaches, 100–102
    for myofascial pain, 107
    nondrug, 54–56

for pain in AIDS
    patients, 287–88
for pain among elderly
    people, 307–8
physical relief techniques, 56
for tension headaches, 104
undertreatment of cancer
    pain, 200–203
tricyclic antidepressants, 50, 287
trigger point injections, 240
trigger points, 77
    for myofascial pain, 106
Turk, Dennis, 67–70, 73, 74, 82
Twycross, Robert G., 322
Tylenol (acetaminophen), 47–48,
    100, 123, 233
    for children, 154

ultrasonography, 78
Uniform Controlled Substance Act
    (model state law), 5

Valium (anxiolytic), 236
Valium (intravenous
    diazepam), 103
vascular surgery, 53
Ventafridda, V., 233
videos, for pain control, 55
Vistaril (anxiolytic), 236
visualization of pain, 245
vomiting, 238
Von Roenn, Jamie, 14

Wall, Patrick D., 66, 69
Warfield, Carol, 144
Weisman, Steven, 160, 162
Weissman, David, 4, 201
West Haven-Yale Multidimensional
    Pain Inventory (MPI), 82–88
Wilensky, Jamie, 91–92
Wilkie, Diana, 8, 14
Williams, Anna, 296
Wisconsin Cancer Pain
    Initiative, 202

women
  early adolescence in, 187–88
  epidural anesthetics during
    childbirth by, 28
  puberty in, 187
Wong-Baker Faces Pain Rating
    Scale, 157, 159
Woolf, Clifford, 140
World Health Organization
    (WHO), 20, 225, 234, 334
  "analgesic ladder" by, 231–33

Xanax (anxiolytic), 236

Yaksh, Tony, 9
Yaster, Myron, 23, 211
  on children in pain, 141–42,
    146, 147
  on patient-controlled
    analgesia, 36, 153, 194
  on sedation of children, 149
Young Child's Pain Assessment
    Scale, 156

Zayas, Victor, 142
Zerwekh, Joyce, 3
Zostrix (topical capsaicin), 103, 131

About the Author

Jane Cowles authored the landmark 1976 book *Informed Consent.* Women facing a breast cancer crisis learned they had a right to a second opinion and a fair explanation of options before any medical or surgical treatment. Today second opinions are standard medical practice. Her "Breast Cancer Patient's Bill of Rights" has been translated into three languages.

As a medical journalist and cancer therapist specializing in second opinions, Cowles has written on a wide variety of patient advocate topics in national magazines. She has been featured on national television and in print.

Cowles is on the Board of Directors of the American-Italian Foundation for Cancer Research in New York, where she resides with her husband.

Additional copies of *Pain Relief! How to Say "No" to Acute, Chronic, and Cancer Pain* may be ordered by sending a check for $22.95 (please add the following for postage and handling: $2.00 for the first copy, $1.00 for each added copy) to:

MasterMedia Limited
17 East 89th Street
New York, NY 10128
(212) 260-5600
(800) 334-8232
(212) 546-7638 (fax)

Jane Cowles, Ph.D., is available for speeches and workshops. Please contact MasterMedia's Speakers' Bureau for availability and fee arrangements. Call Tony Colao at (800) 4-LECTUR

Other MasterMedia Books

To order MasterMedia Books, either visit your local bookstore or call (800) 334-8232.

AGING PARENTS AND YOU: A Complete Handbook to Help You Help Your Elders Maintain a Healthy, Productive and Independent Life, by Eugenia Anderson-Ellis, is a complete guide to providing care to aging relatives. It gives practical advice and resources to the adults who are helping their elders lead productive and independent lives. Revised and updated. ($9.95 paper)

YOUR HEALTHY BODY, YOUR HEALTHY LIFE: How to Take Control of Your Medical Destiny, by Donald B. Louria, M.D., provides precise advice and strategies that will help you to live a long and healthy life. Learn also about nutrition, exercise, vitamins, and medication, as well as how to control risk factors for major diseases. Revised and updated. ($12.95 paper)

DARE TO CONFRONT! How to Intervene When Someone You Care About Has an Alcohol or Drug Problem, by Bob Wright and Deborah George Wright, shows the reader how to use the step-by-step methods of professional interventionists to motivate drug-dependent people to accept the help they need. ($17.95 cloth)

THE LIVING HEART BRAND NAME SHOPPER'S GUIDE (Revised and Updated), by Michael E. DeBakey, M.D., Antonio M. Gotto, Jr., M.D., D.Phil., Lynne W. Scott, M.A., R.D./L.D., and John P. Foreyt, Ph.D., lists brand-name supermarket products that are low in fat, saturated fatty acids, and cholesterol. ($14.95 paper)

THE PREGNANCY AND MOTHERHOOD DIARY: Planning the First Year of Your Second Career, by Susan Schiffer Stautberg, is the first and only undated appointment diary that shows how to manage pregnancy and career. ($12.95 spiral-bound)

CITIES OF OPPORTUNITY: Finding the Best Place to Work, Live and Prosper in the 1990's and Beyond, by Dr. John Tepper Marlin, explores the job and living options for the next decade and into the next century. This consumer guide and handbook, written by one of the world's experts on cities, selects and features forty-six American cities and metropolitan areas. ($13.95 paper, $24.95 cloth)

THE DOLLARS AND SENSE OF DIVORCE, by Dr. Judith Briles, is the first book to combine practical tips on overcoming the legal hurdles by planning finances before, during, and after divorce. ($10.95 paper)

OUT THE ORGANIZATION: New Career Opportunities for the 1990s, by Robert and Madeleine Swain, is written for the millions of Americans whose jobs are no longer safe, whose companies are not loyal, and who face futures of uncertainty. It gives advice on finding a new job or starting your own business. ($12.95 paper)

CRITICISM IN YOUR LIFE: How to Give It, How to Take It, How to Make It Work for You, by Dr. Deborah Bright, offers practical advice, in an upbeat, readable, and realistic fashion, for turning criticism into control. Charts and diagrams guide the reader into managing criticism from bosses, spouses, children, friends, neighbors, in-laws, and business relations. ($17.95 cloth)

BEYOND SUCCESS: How Volunteer Service Can Help You Begin Making a Life Instead of Just a Living, by John F. Raynolds III and Eleanor Raynolds, C.B.E., is a unique how-to book targeted at business and professional people considering volunteer work, senior citizens who wish to fill leisure time meaningfully, and students trying out various career options. The book is filled with interviews with celebrities, CEOs, and average citizens who talk about the benefits of service work. ($19.95 cloth)

MANAGING IT ALL: Time-Saving Ideas for Career, Family, Relationships, and Self, by Beverly Benz Treuille and Susan Schiffer Stautberg, is written for women who are juggling careers and families. Over two hundred career women (ranging from a TV anchorwoman to an investment banker) were interviewed. The book contains many humorous anecdotes on saving time and improving the quality of life for self and family. ($9.95 paper)

THE CONFIDENCE FACTOR: How Self-Esteem Can Change Your Life, by Dr. Judith Briles, is based on a nationwide survey of six thousand men and women. Briles explores why women so often feel a lack of self-confidence and have a poor opinion of themselves. She offers step-by-step advice on becoming the person you want to be. ($9.95 paper, $18.95 cloth)

THE SOLUTION TO POLLUTION: 101 Things You Can Do to Clean Up Your Environment, by Laurence Sombke, offers step-by-step techniques on how to conserve more energy, start a recycling center, choose biodegradable products, and even proceed with individual environmental cleanup projects. ($7.95 paper)

TAKING CONTROL OF YOUR LIFE: The Secrets of Successful Enterprising Women, by Gail Blanke and Kathleen Walas, is based on the authors' professional experience with Avon Products' Women of Enterprise Awards, given each year to outstanding women entrepreneurs. The authors offer a specific plan to help you gain control over your life, and include business tips and quizzes as well as beauty and lifestyle information. ($17.95 cloth)

SIDE-BY-SIDE STRATEGIES: How Two-Career Couples Can Thrive in the Nineties, by Jane Hershey Cuozzo and S. Diane Graham, describes how two-career couples can learn the difference between competing with a spouse and becoming a supportive power partner. Published in hardcover as *Power Partners.* ($10.95 paper, $19.95 cloth)

WORK WITH ME! How to Make the Most of Office Support Staff, by Betsy Lazary, shows you how to find, train, and nurture the "perfect" assistant and how to best utilize your support staff professionals. ($9.95 paper)

MANN FOR ALL SEASONS: Wit and Wisdom from The Washington Post*'s Judy Mann,* by Judy Mann, shows the columnist at her best as she writes about women, families, and the impact and politics of the women's revolution. ($9.95 paper, $19.95 cloth)

THE SOLUTION TO POLLUTION IN THE WORKPLACE, by Laurence Sombke, Terry M. Robertson and Elliot M. Kaplan, supplies employees with everything they need to know about cleaning up their workspace, including recycling, using energy efficiently, conserving water and buying recycled products and nontoxic supplies. ($9.95 paper)

THE ENVIRONMENTAL GARDENER: The Solution to Pollution for Lawns and Gardens, by Laurence Sombke, focuses on what each of us can do to protect our endangered plant life. A practical sourcebook and shopping guide. ($8.95 paper)

THE LOYALTY FACTOR: Building Trust in Today's Workplace, by Carol Kinsey Goman, Ph.D., offers techniques for restoring commitment and loyalty in the workplace. ($9.95 paper)

DARE TO CHANGE YOUR JOB—AND YOUR LIFE, by Carole Kanchier, Ph.D., provides a look at career growth and development throughout the life cycle. ($9.95 paper)

MISS AMERICA: In Pursuit of the Crown, by Ann-Marie Bivans, is an authorized guidebook to the Pageant, containing eyewitness accounts, complete historical data, and a realistic look at the trials and triumphs of the potential Miss Americas. ($19.95 paper, $27.50 cloth)

POSITIVELY OUTRAGEOUS SERVICE: New and Easy Ways to Win Customers for Life, by T. Scott Gross, identifies what the consumers of the nineties really want and how businesses can develop effective marketing strategies to answer those needs. ($14.95 paper)

BREATHING SPACE: Living and Working at a Comfortable Pace in a Sped-Up Society, by Jeff Davidson, helps readers to handle information and activity overload, and gain greater control over their lives. ($10.95 paper)

TWENTYSOMETHING: Managing and Motivating Today's New Work Force, by Lawrence J. Bradford, Ph.D., and Claire Raines, M.A., examines the work orientation of the younger generation, offering managers in businesses of all kinds a practical guide to better understand and supervise their young employees. ($22.95 cloth)

REAL LIFE 101: The Graduate's Guide to Survival, by Susan Kleinman, supplies welcome advice to those facing "real life" for the first time, focusing on work, money, health, and how to deal with freedom and responsibility. ($9.95 paper)

BALANCING ACTS! Juggling Love, Work, Family, and Recreation, by Susan Schiffer Stautberg and Marcia L. Worthing, provides strategies to achieve a balanced life by reordering priorities and setting realistic goals. ($12.95 paper)

REAL BEAUTY . . . REAL WOMEN: A Handbook for Making the Best of Your Own Good Looks, by Kathleen Walas, International Beauty and Fashion Director of Avon Products, offers expert advice on beauty and fashion to women of all ages and ethnic backgrounds. ($19.50 paper)

MANAGING YOUR CHILD'S DIABETES, by Robert Wood Johnson IV, Sale Johnson, Casey Johnson, and Susan Kleinman, brings help to families trying to understand diabetes and control its effects. ($10.95 paper)

STEP FORWARD: Sexual Harassment in the Workplace, What You Need to Know, by Susan L. Webb, presents the facts for dealing with sexual harassment on the job. ($9.95 paper)

A TEEN'S GUIDE TO BUSINESS: The Secrets to a Successful Enterprise, by Linda Menzies, Oren S. Jenkins, and Rickell R. Fisher, provides solid information about starting your own business or working for one. ($7.95 paper)

GLORIOUS ROOTS: Recipes for Healthy, Tasty Vegetables, by Laurence Sombke, celebrates the taste, texture, and versatility of root vegetables. Contains recipes for appetizers, soups, stews, and baked, broiled, and stir-fried dishes—even desserts. ($12.95 paper)

THE OUTDOOR WOMAN: A Handbook to Adventure, by Patricia Hubbard and Stan Wass, details the lives of adventurous outdoor women and offers their ideas on how you can incorporate exciting outdoor experiences into your life. ($14.95 paper)

FLIGHT PLAN FOR LIVING: The Art of Self-Encouragement, by Patrick O'Dooley, is a life guide organized like a pilot's flight checklist, which ensures you'll be flying "clear on top" throughout your life. ($17.95 cloth)

HOW TO GET WHAT YOU WANT FROM ALMOST ANYBODY, by T. Scott Gross, shows how to get great service, negotiate better prices, and always get what you pay for. ($9.95 paper)

FINANCIAL SAVVY FOR WOMEN: A Money Book for Women of All Ages, by Dr. Judith Briles, divides a woman's monetary lifespan into six phases, discusses the specific areas to be addressed at each stage, and demonstrates how to create a sound lifelong money game plan. ($14.95 paper)

TEAMBUILT: Making Teamwork Work, by Mark Sanborn, teaches business how to improve productivity, without increasing resources or expenses, by building teamwork among employers. ($19.95 cloth)

THE BIG APPLE BUSINESS AND PLEASURE GUIDE: 501 Ways to Work Smarter, Play Harder, and Live Better in New York City, by Muriel Siebert and Susan Kleinman, offers visitors and New Yorkers alike advice on how to do business in the city as well as how to enjoy its attractions. ($9.95 paper)

MIND YOUR OWN BUSINESS: And Keep It in the Family, by Marcy Syms, COO of Syms Corporation, is an effective guide for any organization, small or large, facing what is documented to be the toughest step in managing a family business—making the transition to the new generation. ($18.95 cloth)

KIDS WHO MAKE A DIFFERENCE, by Joyce M. Roché and Marie Rodriguez, with Phyllis Schneider, is a surprising and inspiring document of some of today's toughest challenges being met—by teenagers and kids! Their courage and creativity allowed them to find practical solutions. ($8.95 paper; with photos)

ROSEY GRIER'S ALL-AMERICAN HEROS: Multicultural Success Stories, by Roosevelt "Rosey" Grier, is a wonderful collection of personal histories, told in their own words by prominent African-Americans, Latins, Asians, and native Americans; each tells of the people in their lives and choices made to achieve public acclaim and personal success. ($9.95 paper; with photos)

OFFICE BIOLOGY: Why Tuesday Is the Most Productive Day and Other Relevant Facts for Survival in the Workplace, by Edith Weiner and Arnold Brown, teaches how in the '90s and beyond we will be expected to work smarter, take better control of our health, adapt to advancing technology, and improve our lives in ways that are not too costly or resource-intensive. ($21.95 cloth)

ON TARGET: Enhance Your Life and Ensure Your Success, by Jeri Sedlar and Rick Miners, is a neatly woven tapestry of insights on career and life issues gathered from audiences across the country. This feedback has been crystalized into a highly readable guidebook for exploring who you are and how to go about getting what you want from your career and your life. ($11.95 paper)

SOMEONE ELSE'S SON, by Alan A. Winter, explores the parent-child bond in a contemporary story of lost identities, family secrets, and relationships gone awry. Eighteen years after bringing their first son home from the hospital, Trish and Brad Hunter discover they are not his natural parents. Torn between their love for their son, Phillip, and the question of whether they should help him search for his biological parents, the couple must also struggle with the issue of their own biological son. Who is he—and do his parents know their baby was switched at birth? ($18.95 cloth)

STRAIGHT TALK ON WOMEN'S HEALTH: How to Get the Health Care You Deserve, by Janice Teal, Ph.D., and Phyllis Schneider, is destined to become a health-care "bible" for women concerned about their bodies and their future health. Well-researched, but devoid of confusing medical jargon, this handbook offers access to a wealth of resources, with a bibliography of health-related books and contact lists of organizations, healthlines, and women's medical centers. ($14.95 paper)

THE STEPPARENT CHALLENGE: A Primer for Making It Work, by Stephen J. Williams, Sc.D., shares firsthand experience and insights into the many aspects of dealing with step relationships—from financial issues to lifestyle changes to differences in race or religion that affect the whole family. Peppered with personal accounts and useful tips, this volume is must reading for anyone who is a stepparent, about to become one, or planning to bring children to a second or subsequent marriage. ($13.95 paper)

MAKING YOUR DREAMS COME TRUE: A Plan for Easily Discovering and Achieving the Life You Want, by Marcia Wieder, introduces an easy, unique, and practical technique for defining, pursuing, and realizing your career and life interests. Filled with stories of real people and helpful exercises, plus a personal workbook, this clever volume will teach you how to make your dreams come true—any time you choose. ($9.95 paper)

WHAT KIDS LIKE TO DO, by Edward Stautberg, Gail Wubbenhorst, Atiya Easterling, and Phyllis Schneider, is a handy guidebook for parents, grandparents, and babysitters who are searching for activities that kids *really* enjoy. Written by kids for kids, this easy-to-read, generously illustrated primer can teach families how to make every day more fun. ($7.95 paper)